W9-CDD-832

Men's Health

TODAY 2009

SYMPTOMS AND SOLUTIONS

**Mark A. Goldstein, MD, Myrna Chandler Goldstein, MA,
and Larry P. Credit, OMD**

RODALE

Notice

This book is intended as a reference volume only, not as a medical manual. The information given here is designed to help you make informed decisions about your health. It is not intended as a substitute for any treatment that may have been prescribed by your doctor. If you suspect that you have a medical problem, we urge you to seek competent medical help.

Mention of specific companies, organizations, or authorities in this book does not imply endorsement by the author or publisher, nor does mention of specific companies, organizations, or authorities imply that they endorse this book, its author, or the publisher.

Internet addresses and telephone numbers given in this book were accurate at the time it went to press.

© 2009 by Mark A. Goldstein, MD, Myrna Chandler Goldstein, and Larry P. Credit, OMD

All rights reserved. No part of this publication may be reproduced or transmitted in any form or by any means, electronic or mechanical, including photocopying, recording, or any other information storage and retrieval system, without the written permission of the publisher.

Men's Health is a registered trademark of Rodale Inc.

Portions of this book were previously published © 2008 by Rodale Inc. as *Your Best Medicine*.

Printed in the United States of America
Rodale Inc. makes every effort to use acid-free ∞, recycled paper ♻.

Book design by Christopher Rhoads

ISBN-13 978–1–60529–807–8 hardcover

ISBN-10 1–60529–807–7 hardcover

2   4   6   8   10   9   7   5   3   1   hardcover

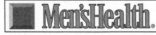 If you want to build muscle, improve your sex life, and do nearly everything better, visit our Web site at menshealth.com

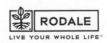
LIVE YOUR WHOLE LIFE™

We inspire and enable people to improve their lives and the world around them

For more of our products visit **rodalestore.com** or call 800-848-4735

Contents

Integrative Medicine:
The Best of All Worlds 1

Angina 10

Atherosclerosis 17

Back Pain 23

Cataracts 35

Celiac Disease 40

Colon Polyps 45

Coronary Artery Disease 48

Depression...55

Diabetes 64

Diverticulosis/Diverticulitis...................74

Emphysema 80

Erectile Dysfunction 85

Essential Tremor 92

Gastroesophageal Reflux
Disease (GERD) 96

Glaucoma 102

Gout...109

Gum Disease.....................................115

Hearing Loss 123

Heart Palpitations 130

Hemorrhoids 134

High Blood Pressure...........................138

High Cholesterol 149

Indigestion 156

Influenza...161

Insomnia...166

Kidney Stones 173

Macular Degeneration........................179

Male Menopause 186

Memory Loss 190

Metabolic Syndrome..........................195

Muscle Cramps..................................199

Nail Fungus......................................203

Obesity 206

Osteoarthritis...................................214

Parkinson's Disease...........................222

Peripheral Neuropathy.......................229

Peripheral Vascular Disease 234

Prostate Enlargement 240

Prostatitis 245

Rosacea..250

Shingles..255

Sleep Apnea 261

Source Notes....................................266

Index...271

Integrative Medicine:
The Best of All Worlds

In this book, you're going to find treatments from both conventional medicine and complementary disciplines. Combining the two in a treatment plan has come to be known as an integrative approach to care.

For many years, conventional and complementary medicine operated in separate universes, with little common ground except their mutual objective of helping patients to heal from illness or—in the case of chronic conditions—to minimize symptoms. Why are they coming together now? Mostly because health care consumers like you have demanded it. They recognized that conventional and complementary therapies alike have benefits as well as risks—and that combining the two can optimize healing while, in many cases, reducing costs.

In this chapter, we'll provide brief overviews of conventional and complementary medicine in turn. This information will provide a foundation for the condition-specific "prescriptions."

What Is Conventional Medicine?

Until relatively recently, the words "complementary medicine" seldom were spoken in a medical setting. For the most part, the care and treatment provided by doctors fell within the conventional realm.

Conventional medicine—sometimes called allopathic medicine or mainstream medicine—has been practiced by generations of traditionally trained physicians. Those who wish to pursue a career in medicine must complete 4 years of study (beyond a bachelor's degree), followed by an internship, a residency, and possibly a fellowship. Generally, students who attend one of the nation's 125 medical schools are taught to use medications, surgery, and other conventional modalities to treat medical conditions. They may not learn about complementary disciplines, unless they choose to do so. (Many schools are offering training on the relationship between body and mind, so doctors-to-be can recognize when treatment may need to involve a mental health practitioner.)

Among the key differences between conventional and complementary medicine is that conventional modalities must undergo a certain level of scientific scrutiny before they become available to the general public. Every day, medical researchers in laboratories throughout the United States are conducting thousands of studies in a continual effort to develop new diagnostic procedures, medications, and surgical techniques. To a certain extent, these endeavors are overseen and regulated by the federal government.

In recent years, many medical doctors have embraced evidence-based medicine—that is, the use of the best evidence from research studies to guide their clinical decisions. Thanks to the Internet, they now have quick and easy access to these findings, which allows them to provide their patients with the most up-to-date medical care possible.

Conventional medicine also places an emphasis on prevention. From a very young age, children are given vaccines to help protect against a host of different illnesses. Likewise, adults are encouraged to get certain shots—such as the one that prevents influenza—and to undergo regular screenings designed to detect various illnesses in their earliest and most treatable forms.

But conventional medicine isn't without challenges, particularly with regard to cost and access to care. There's a serious shortage of medical doctors—especially those who specialize in certain areas of medicine—in rural communities. Further, more than 46 million Americans have no health insurance, while another 40 million have inadequate coverage. These people all too often neglect preventive care, and they may put off treatment for their health problems until they require emergency intervention.

Perhaps not surprisingly, those with greater financial resources tend to receive better medical care in the conventional medical system. The recent emergence of "boutique practices" promises to widen the gap even more, with some doctors limiting their practices to a preset number of patients. Patients, in turn, pay thousands of dollars above their normal health insurance premiums for improved access to their doctors.

Despite the problems within a conventional medical system, it is a good idea to have a traditionally trained physician as your primary care provider. To some degree, whom you choose may be determined by your health plan, as some plans require their members to utilize certain physicians or practices. Beyond that, you want a doctor who's board-certified, meaning that he or she has met the training requirements and passed the certification exam of a medical organization such as the American Board of Internal Medicine. These exams are designed to assess competency in various medical specialties.

Also be sure to ask whether a doctor has hospital admitting privileges. This means that if you ever require hospitalization, your doctor can admit you to the appropriate facility.

These days, it's relatively easy to check out a doctor's training and credentials online through the Web sites of organizations such as the American Medical Association (www. ama-assn.org). Still, many people find their primary care providers by word of mouth— through family members, friends, and colleagues who are happy with the quality of care that a particular doctor provides. At the end of the day, perhaps what matters most is finding someone with whom you feel comfortable and in whom you have the confidence to entrust your care.

What Is Complementary Medicine?

Complementary medicine—also known as alternative or holistic medicine—is an umbrella term for a number of healing disciplines, some of which date back thousands of years. A typical complementary treatment plan takes into account all of the elements that influence a person's health—including the physical, mental, emotional, spiritual, and social, and sometimes the environmental. Complementary therapies also tend to be quite sensitive to the mind-body connection—that is, how a person's mental and emotional state can influence physical health and vice versa. A complementary practitioner will actively involve a patient in his or her own care by teaching the person to use remedies and techniques that not only support healing but also prevent future illness.

Where conventional medicine tends to focus on alleviating the symptoms of a disease, complementary therapies attempt to identify and treat the root cause. These perspectives may seem at odds, but as practitioners and patients are coming to realize, combining conventional and complementary modalities—that is, an integrative approach to care—often can be more effective than using either alone.

One of the enduring criticisms of complementary medicine is that very few of the treatments have been subject to the same rigorous scientific scrutiny as conventional medicine. Indeed, though certain complementary disciplines have thousands of years

of anecdotal evidence to support their therapeutic powers, the scientific literature remains rather scant. Gradually that is changing, due in large part to the creation of the National Center for Complementary and Alternative Medicine in 1999. This government-funded institution—under the auspices of the National Institutes of Health—is training researchers, financing clinical trials, and disseminating authoritative information about various complementary therapies to physicians and laypeople alike.

Within complementary medicine, the philosophies and practices of the disciplines can vary greatly. If you're thinking about adding one of these therapies to your health care regimen, it's important for you to consider your personal preferences and comfort level when weighing your options. For example, acupuncture, massage, and therapeutic touch are all effective treatments for headaches, but they're very different in what they entail. Choosing the one that's best for you requires some research, and perhaps a bit of trial and error.

More and more insurance companies are expanding their coverage to include complementary therapies, so before you make a decision, you may want to check the provisions of your own health plan. Other factors that you should take into account: how far you'll be traveling to a qualified practitioner, how often you'll require in-office visits and treatments, and whether you can use the treatments at home, on your own.

Depending on the discipline, finding a

qualified practitioner can take some legwork. Often the Web sites for these organizations have tools that allow you to search for practitioners by location.

What follows are brief descriptions of the complementary disciplines that you're most likely to encounter in this book. You'll find more detailed remedies in the condition entries.

Acupressure

Based on the principles of acupuncture and traditional Chinese medicine, acupressure is the application of pressure to specific points on the body via deep circular movements of the thumbs, fingers, elbows, or palms. This pressure is said to release *chi*, or healing energy, which circulates throughout the body along specific pathways called meridians. By clearing blockages in the energy flow, acupressure improves the body's ability to heal itself.

Acupuncture

The main difference between acupuncture and acupressure is that the former uses hair-thin, sterile, disposable needles rather than firm pressure to release *chi*. Studies have shown that acupuncture treatment is able to stimulate various physical reactions, including changes in brain activity, blood pressure, blood chemistry, heart rate, endocrine function, and immune system response.

Alexander Technique

Developed by the Australian actor Frederick Matthias Alexander, who suffered from chronic hoarseness when performing, the Alexander Technique (AT) identifies poor postural habits and replaces them with improved body mechanics. An AT instructor teaches basic exercises that improve balance, posture, and coordination and help relieve posture-related problems such as back pain.

Aquatic Therapy

Also known as water therapy, aquatic therapy involves performing gentle, rhythmic movements and exercises in a warm (92° to 99°F), shallow pool. Participants may be seated or standing during their therapy sessions, and they may walk or float in the water. Since many aquatic therapy facilities have an additional pool that's set to a cooler temperature, a therapy session may include time in both pools.

Ayurveda

Developed in India more than 5,000 years ago, Ayurveda is a holistic (whole-body) discipline that tailors treatment to a person's body type (*prakriti*) and energy type (*dosha*). Each of the three energy types—*vata*, *pitta*, and *kapha*—corresponds to particular body types. Although everyone has a combination of the three *doshas*, one (sometimes two) tends to be most prevalent.

Once an Ayurvedic practitioner has determined your dominant *dosha*, he will make recommendations that collectively will bring the three energy types into balance. A typical Ayurvedic treatment plan will combine a number of approaches, including nutritional therapy, herbal remedies, physical exercise, massage, and meditation.

Biofeedback

In biofeedback, an electric monitoring device is placed on the surface of the skin to record data on vital functions such as heart rate, blood pressure, muscle tension, brain wave activity, and skin temperature. These data are transmitted to a biofeedback machine, which "translates" them into sounds (beeps), visual images (flashes), or dial readings. By paying attention to these signals, you become more aware of stress-related physical changes and better able to control them—usually through relaxation techniques such as deep breathing, meditation, and/or visualization. The goal of biofeedback training is to learn how to achieve and maintain a relaxed state even when you are not using a biofeedback machine.

Bodywork

Bodywork is a general term for a number of therapeutic approaches that use hands-on techniques to manipulate and balance the musculoskeletal system. These approaches relieve pain, facilitate healing, increase energy, and promote relaxation and well-being. Examples of bodywork techniques include acupressure, craniosacral therapy, reflexology, Rolfing, shiatsu, therapeutic touch, and trigger point therapy.

Chiropractic

Based on the premise that good health requires a strong, agile, and aligned spine, chiropractic medicine involves spinal manipulation and adjustment. This moves the backbone into its proper position, thereby facilitating the correct functioning of the nervous system and the well-being of the entire body. A chiropractic session also may include nutritional counseling.

Craniosacral Therapy

Craniosacral therapy is the gentle manipulation of the craniosacral system, which includes the brain, spinal cord, cerebrospinal fluid, dural membrane, cranial bones, and sacrum. The pressure applied to these parts is no more than the weight of a nickel. By reducing stress and correcting systemic imbalances, craniosacral therapy may stimulate the body's innate healing powers.

Diet

Proper nutrition is vital to the healing process, and to optimal health. In general, we advocate a well-balanced diet that's high in fiber and low in unhealthy fats, with an abundance of whole grains, fresh fruits and vegetables, and lean proteins. Try to avoid hydrogenated fats, fried foods, and processed foods containing artificial colors and other chemicals. For certain medical conditions, we recommend eating some foods that help heal the body while avoiding other foods that can contribute to or aggravate the problem.

Feldenkrais Method

Similar to the Alexander Technique, the Feldenkrais Method teaches you to become more aware of your movement patterns and to correct unhealthy habits by relearning proper body mechanics. Sessions may be one-on-one or group instruction. In a private session, the instructor manually guides you through the various movements, a technique called Functional Integration. Group sessions involve a technique called Awareness Through Movement, in which the instructor provides verbal cues to the movement sequences. The goal of the Feldenkrais Method is to reduce pain, increase mobility, and enhance well-being.

Herbal Medicine

Herbal remedies are among the most popular and accessible of the complementary therapies. Each herb has its own set of therapeutic properties, and often it's necessary to use a particular part of the plant—perhaps the roots, stems, leaves, or flowers—to obtain an optimal dose of the medicinal constituent(s). Herbal remedies are available as pills, teas, tinctures, creams, and ointments. Herbalists may recommend multiple herbs to treat a particular condition.

Although herbs are available over-the-counter, they are potent substances that can interact with medications and cause side effects. For this reason, we strongly advise talking with your doctor or a qualified herbalist before adding any herbal remedy to your self-care regimen.

Homeopathy

Homeopathy is a healing system based on the principle that substances capable of producing symptoms of sickness in healthy people can have a healing effect when given in very minute quantities to sick people who exhibit the same symptoms. Homeopathic remedies—which are derived from plants, animals, and minerals—work in part by encouraging symptoms to run an accelerated course through the body, thereby speeding the healing process.

Although high-dose homeopathic remedies are available from homeopaths and other trained practitioners, you can find lower-dose products in health food stores, some drugstores, and online. Most remedies are tiny pills that dissolve when placed under the tongue.

Hydrotherapy

Hydrotherapy is the use of water in any of its various forms—liquid, solid, or vapor—to relieve discomfort and promote healing. As a therapeutic discipline, hydrotherapy dates all the way back to ancient Greece and Rome. Today, it's most likely to entail steam baths, saunas, hot tubs, whirlpools, and/or applications of hot and cold packs or ice. All of these treatments have different physiological effects, which makes hydrotherapy a versatile remedy capable of soothing sore or inflamed muscles, reducing fever, rehabilitating injured limbs, relieving headache, and promoting relaxation.

Hypnotherapy

In a hypnotherapy session, the therapist guides the patient into a trancelike state, characterized by extreme suggestibility, heightened imagination, and relaxation. The therapist then uses posthypnotic suggestion to alter the patient's perceptions and behaviors. Hypnotherapy may be beneficial for improving a person's emotional state or helping to overcome addictive behaviors such as smoking and overeating.

Naturopathy

Naturopathy is a holistic healing system that utilizes an array of natural therapies, such as nutritional therapy, herbal medicine, exercise, acupuncture, massage, and hydrotherapy. Together, these therapies strengthen and support the body's innate ability to heal itself.

Nutritional Supplements

Even if you're eating a relatively healthy diet, you may not be getting sufficient amounts of all the vitamins, minerals, and other nutrients that your body needs to carry out its most basic functions. One reason is that nutrient-depleted soils tend to produce nutrient-deficient foods. Storing, cooking, and otherwise processing foods can further deplete their nutrient supplies. Add to this the nutrient-robbing properties of certain medical conditions as well as certain medications (both prescription and over-the-counter), and your body may be at risk for nutritional shortfalls.

Supplements can help cover your nutritional bases when, for whatever reason, your diet may be coming up short. In this book, we recommend supplements both for general nutritional support and for targeted treatment of conditions that may cause or result from a vitamin or mineral deficiency. In nearly every condition entry, you will find recommendations for specific supplements.

Just as for herbal remedies, we do strongly advise talking with your doctor before adding nutritional supplements to your self-care regimen. Though they are natural and generally safe, they can cause harm—especially when taken in too-large amounts or when used in combination with certain herbs or medications.

Qigong

Much like acupressure and acupuncture, qigong facilitates the flow of *chi*, or energy, along specific pathways throughout the body. It does this through a series of gentle movements, postures, meditations, and breathing patterns. By encouraging the flow of *chi*, qigong supports healing while increasing stamina, flexibility, and relaxation.

Reflexology

In reflexology, certain points on the feet, hands, and ears correlate to specific parts of the body. As a reflexologist stimulates these points (using pressure and massage techniques), he or she can direct blood, energy, nutrients, and nerve impulses to the corresponding parts, thereby stimulating the healing process.

Reiki

Reiki—a 2,500-year-old Tibetan Buddhist practice—is based on the belief that a universal life force flows around us and connects us to one another. This force can be channeled through the hands of a trained practitioner to help restore the flow of a person's innate healing energy. The practitioner may use a light touch, or he may simply place his hands over the affected area. This releases old energy while directing new energy to cells, stimulating the body's systems and normalizing its functions.

Relaxation/Meditation

In this book, we often recommend meditation and/or other relaxation techniques to counteract the harmful effects of stress and to support healing. In some cases, we have provided specific exercises that you can try on your own. In general, though, whenever you see a reference to "relaxation/meditation," feel free to use any technique that helps calm you and helps reduce your heart rate and blood pressure. Among your choices: biofeedback, deep breathing, hypnosis, meditation, tai chi, and yoga.

Rolfing

Developed by Ida Rolf, PhD, Rolfing involves deep manipulation and massage of the connective tissues in order to relieve physical and emotional tension. Practitioners, called Rolfers, may use their fingers, thumbs, forearms, and elbows to physically alter the body's posture and structure. This fosters proper postural alignment, increases mobility, and reduces pain throughout the body.

Shiatsu

Shiatsu, a Japanese term meaning "finger pressure," is a hands-on therapy in which practitioners use their fingers, palms, and thumbs to identify irregularities within the body and to correct those irregularities by applying pressure to specific points—the same points used in acupressure and acupuncture. (In fact, you may hear shiatsu described as "needle-free acupuncture.") In this way, shiatsu unblocks and facilitates energy flow, which in turn relieves muscular tension, improves lymph circulation, and fosters the body's natural healing powers.

Tai Chi

Similar to qigong, tai chi—also a traditional Chinese discipline—consists of a series of slow, gentle movements that require a significant amount of concentration as well as synchronized breathing. The movements help unite body and mind, build inner strength, and stimulate energy flow throughout the body.

Therapeutic Massage

Therapeutic massage involves kneading or otherwise manipulating muscles and soft tissues to alleviate pain, muscle spasms, and stress and to promote relaxation. Swedish massage is the most common technique; others include deep-tissue massage, neuromuscular massage, and sports massage.

Therapeutic Touch

A practitioner trained in therapeutic touch is able to redirect energy flow simply by moving his or her hands over a client's body, without actually touching the person. In this way, therapeutic touch has much in common with Reiki. By properly channeling energy, or *chi*, therapeutic touch can relieve pain, promote relaxation, and restore balance to the body.

Traditional Chinese Medicine

Traditional Chinese medicine (TCM) embraces a range of therapeutic disciplines, all developed in China over thousands of years. Acupressure, acupuncture, herbal medicine, qigong, and tai chi are components of TCM.

Trager Approach

Developed by Milton Trager, MD, the Trager Approach uses a series of gentle, rhythmic movements and touch to create deep relaxation and increased mobility. There are no rigid procedures in this discipline; rather, the practitioner tailors the movements to each individual, helping to relax tight muscles without pain.

Trigger Point Therapy

Also known as myotherapy and neuromuscular therapy, trigger point therapy targets so-called trigger points—tender spots on the muscle tissue that radiate pain to other areas of the body. Applying pressure to these areas helps to relieve tension, relax muscle spasms, improve circulation, and break the cycle of pain.

Angina

The characteristic chest pain of angina is caused by ischemia—a lack of bloodflow and, hence, a lack of oxygen supply to the heart muscle, or myocardium. Angina may manifest simply as chest pain, or as heaviness, tightness, squeezing, pressure, or a burning sensation in the chest, back, arms, neck, throat, or jaw.

Angina (sometimes referred to as angina pectoris) is a common problem in midlife and beyond. An estimated 6.4 million Americans have the condition, with about 400,000 new cases being diagnosed each year.

Of the four main types of angina, the two most common are stable and unstable angina. Stable angina, also known as common angina, is predictable chest pain. It is caused by factors that increase the heart's demand for oxygen, such as exercise, cold weather, emotional turmoil, and large meals. A high proportion of stable angina attacks take place between 6:00 a.m. and noon. An attack generally lasts no more than 2 to 5 minutes. This type of angina tends to respond well to rest and medication, and it causes no permanent damage to the heart.

Unstable angina, on the other hand, is not predictable. The pain may occur while you are resting, sleeping, or participating in less than strenuous activities. It may increase in intensity and persist for more than 20 minutes at a time. Unstable angina may be a warning sign of an impending heart attack, which is why it must be handled as a medical emergency. The good news is that when unstable angina is treated with aggressive medical therapy, up to 80 percent of patients will stabilize within 48 hours.

The less common types of angina are variant angina, also known as Prinzmetal's angina, and microvascular angina. Variant angina is triggered by a spasm of a coronary artery. It's most likely to occur while you are resting, between the hours of midnight and 8:00 a.m. The majority of people who experience this type of angina have narrowed arteries from plaque deposits. Treatment provides immediate pain relief.

Microvascular angina also causes chest pain, but without any evidence of coronary artery blockage. Instead, the pain—which can occur during exercise or rest—is caused by poorly functioning blood vessels.

A Quick Guide to Symptoms

- ☐ Mild to moderate to severe chest pain
- ☐ A feeling of something heavy pressing on the chest
- ☐ Intense chest pain or a burning sensation
- ☐ Pain radiating to the neck, jaw, shoulder, arm, or back
- ☐ Palpitations
- ☐ Fatigue
- ☐ Shortness of breath

Causes and Risk Factors

The lack of sufficient oxygen flow to the heart may be associated with a number of medical problems. The most widespread cause is coronary artery disease, a condition in which the walls of the arteries that carry blood to the heart are narrowed by fatty deposits, and thus have a reduced capacity to carry blood. Other, less common causes of angina include abnormal heart valves, abnormal heart rhythm, coronary artery spasm (temporary narrowing of the artery), anemia, polycythemia (too many red blood cells, resulting in thickening of the blood), and hyperthyroidism.

Signs and Symptoms

The symptoms of angina may vary in intensity from mild to moderate to severe. Severe symptoms do not necessarily mean that you are about to have a heart attack, and mild symptoms do not always mean that your problem is insignificant. People with angina often describe feeling as though there were something heavy pressing on their chests. Sometimes the pain is intense; sometimes it's more of a burning sensation. The pain may extend to the neck, jaw, shoulder, arm, or back. Some people experience palpitations, fatigue, or shortness of breath. The skin may be more sensitive to heat.

Conventional Treatments

To manage angina effectively, conventional medicine tends to focus on lifestyle changes and medication. In severe cases, surgery may be necessary.

Lifestyle Changes

For angina associated with coronary artery disease, treatment often begins with lifestyle changes. Your doctor may recommend improving your diet, starting an exercise program, losing weight, quitting smoking, reducing your alcohol consumption, and keeping stress in check.

Medications

Anticoagulants. If you have angina, you may be advised to take low-dose aspirin or another anticlotting medication. Aspirin inhibits the action of blood platelets, which is how it helps keep blood from clotting. It's important to note that the prolonged use of aspirin may increase your risk of gastrointestinal ulcers and bleeding. Other medications that inhibit blood platelets include clopidogrel (Plavix) and ticlopidine (Ticlid).

Beta-blockers. Beta-blockers are drugs that reduce heart rate and lower blood pressure. Although they do not stop angina attacks, they may reduce the frequency of attacks and the need for nitrate medications (see below). Examples of beta-blockers are propranolol (Inderal), atenolol (Tenormin), and carvedilol (Coreg). Possible side effects of beta-blockers include a moderate decline in HDL ("good") cholesterol, along with fatigue and lethargy. Among those who use these medicines, there have been reports of vivid dreams, nightmares, memory loss, cold

If you are experiencing chest pain, you must get to an emergency room without delay. Call 911 or your local emergency medical services number, or ask someone to call for you.

extremities, and depression. Some people have a diminished capacity for exercise, decreased heart function, sexual dysfunction, and gastrointestinal upset.

Calcium-channel blockers. These medications reduce heart rate and dilate blood vessels, thereby increasing the supply of oxygen while decreasing the demand for it. Examples of calcium-channel blockers are verapamil (Calan, Isoptin), nifedipine (Adalat, Procardia), nicardipine (Cardene), diltiazem (Cardizem, Tiazac), and amlodipine (Norvasc). Withdrawal from calcium-channel blockers should be gradual. If you are taking a calcium-channel blocker, do not mix it with grapefruit juice, as this may intensify its effects.

Nitrates. These are the most frequently prescribed drugs for angina. They relax the blood vessels, allowing more blood to flow and reducing the workload of the heart. The most popular of the nitrates is nitroglycerin. It is administered as a pill that you place under your tongue, or between your upper lip and gum, and allow to dissolve. It also is available in a metered-dose spray.

The basic dosage regimen for nitroglycerin is as follows.

- One dose at the first signs of an angina attack

- A second dose 5 minutes after the onset of pain, if pain persists

- A third dose 10 minutes after the onset of pain, if pain persists

If pain doesn't subside within 15 minutes of onset, then you must seek emergency medical assistance.

Since nitroglycerin is very volatile, it can easily lose its potency. Do not purchase more than 100 tablets at one time. Store them in a cool, dry place in their original container, but discard the cotton filler and close the cap tightly. Always carry nitroglycerin tablets with you. Ask your pharmacist to suggest a suitable container.

In addition to prescribing nitroglycerin for acute episodes of angina, your doctor may recommend a long-acting nitrate medication. This drug is available as a topical ointment, patches, and oral tablets. The ointment should be placed, not rubbed, on the chest, stomach, or thigh. Before it's reapplied, the previous application must be removed. The patch should be affixed each morning to a hairless, injury-free area on the back, chest, upper arm, stomach, or thigh. To avoid skin irritation, change the application site each time. Be sure to wash your hands after handling a patch or the ointment.

Since the long-acting forms of nitrate medication may lose their effectiveness over time, many health care providers suggest nitrate-free periods. However, abruptly stopping a nitrate medication may trigger an angina attack, so withdrawal always should be gradual.

Potential short-term side effects of nitrate medications include dizziness, headache, flushing, blurred vision, nausea, rapid heartbeat, and sweating. There are no known long-term side effects. If you experience low blood pressure or dizziness, it may help to lie down and elevate your legs.

Ranolazine (Ranexa). Approved for the treatment of chronic angina, ranolazine (Ranexa) may be given to patients who have not responded to other medications.

Other medications. If your blood cholesterol is too high, your doctor may prescribe a cholesterol-lowering medication. Likewise, for elevated blood pressure, a blood pressure medication may be recommended.

Surgery

If lifestyle changes and medication do not relieve your angina symptoms, your doctor may recommend surgery. There are a number of procedures available.

Angioplasty. In a balloon angioplasty, the physician inserts a catheter with a tiny balloon at the end into an artery in the arm or groin. Where the artery is narrowed, the balloon is inflated, flattening deposits against the arterial wall. To keep the area open, a stent—a small metal tube—may be placed in the artery.

Coronary bypass surgery. In this procedure, the surgeon removes pieces of veins and arteries from the legs (and possibly the chest), and sews them into the arteries of the heart. This allows the blood to "bypass" the blocked arteries and flow through the replacement vessels. Although these surgeries tend to be very successful, they are major medical procedures, requiring at least a week of hospitalization and several weeks of recovery time.

Complementary Treatments

Complementary approaches to angina include lifestyle changes that reduce stress, strengthen the heart muscle, and increase arterial circulation. These treatments are most effective when used in conjunction with conventional medicine.

Acupuncture

Several studies of acupuncture have shown that it can be effective in reducing angina pain, while also promoting relaxation and reducing stress. To locate an acupuncturist in your area, visit the Web site of the National Certification Commission for Acupuncture and Oriental Medicine (NCCAOM) at www. nccaom.org.

Ayurveda

Originating in India more than 5,000 years ago, Ayurveda is a healing system that combines nutrition, herbal remedies, exercise, massage, and meditation. Ayurveda views the heart as the most important organ and the seat of human consciousness. Further, problems such as angina occur because the heart is not receiving proper attention—characterized not just by poor diet and a lack of physical activity, but also by a lack of emotional attachment and spirituality. In Ayurveda, the emotions play a major role in heart health and always factor into treatment.

Ayurveda has been successful in treating the frequency and severity of angina attacks. One helpful remedy is Abana, a combination of herbs and minerals based on your *prakriti*, or body type. Other recommendations may include diet and lifestyle changes, yoga, and meditation.

An Ayurvedic practitioner will make dietary and lifestyle recommendations based on your *dosha*, which is the cornerstone of Ayurvedic diagnosis and treatment. The objective is to restore balance to your dosha, so you can achieve better health. To find a qualified practitioner in your area, begin by visiting the Web site for the Ayurvedic Institute at www.ayurveda.com.

Bodywork

Two forms of bodywork—acupressure and shiatsu—may help alleviate the symptoms of angina. In these techniques, a practitioner applies controlled pressure to selected points along the heart and pericardium meridians—pathways through which the healing energy of the body flows. By strengthening and toning the meridians, these techniques may reduce the frequency and severity of angina attacks.

A practitioner of acupressure or shiatsu can show you how to use these techniques on your own, so when necessary, you can help relieve mild angina pain. To find a qualified practitioner in your area, visit either of the following Web sites: www.aobta.org (American Organization for Bodywork Therapies of Asia) or www.ncbtmb.org (National Certifi-cation Board for Therapeutic Massage and Bodywork).

Diet

A healthy diet rich in nutrients and fiber allows blood to flow more freely, reducing pressure on the heart muscle. Foods high in saturated fat and cholesterol, such as red meat and butter, as well as processed and refined foods—especially fried and sugary foods, and anything containing hydroge-nated fats—should be avoided. Steer clear of salty foods, too; sodium causes the body to retain fluids, creating more work for your heart. If you do consume meat products, choose only those that are low in fat, such as skinless poultry.

Be sure to include in your diet foods that contain essential fatty acids, as they help reduce inflammation and blood clots, and regulate heart rhythm. Pink salmon and other cold-water fish, olive oil, and raw nuts are all good choices. Vitamin C—found in abundance in raw fruits and vegetables such as grapefruit, kiwifruit, oranges, peaches, bell peppers, and tomatoes—is vital for heart health. So, too, is magnesium, found in green, leafy vegetables such as spinach, parsley, kale, and mustard and turnip greens as well as raw almonds.

Because caffeine increases production of stress hormones, putting you at greater risk for heart problems, limit your con-sumption of coffee to 1 cup a day. Cut back on other caffeine-containing beverages and foods as well.

Herbal Medicine

Ginkgo biloba. Ginkgo is an antioxidant herb that supports circulation. It is sold both raw and in capsule form. The recommended daily dose is 120 milligrams, twice a day, of an extract standardized to 24 percent flavone glycosides and 6 percent terpene lactones. The flavone glycosides give ginkgo its antioxidant benefits, while terpene lactones increase circulation and have a protective effect on nerve cells. *Note:* If you're taking any blood-thinning medication, be sure to check with your doctor before trying ginkgo supplements.

Green tea. Green tea contains high levels of substances called polyphenols, which have powerful antioxidant properties. It also helps to lower cholesterol and blood pressure, and to keep arteries from clogging. Green tea may be taken as a tea or in capsules. By drinking 3 cups of green tea per day, you'd get 240 to 320 milligrams of polyphenols. In capsule form, a standardized extract of EGCG (a polyphenol) may provide 97 percent polyphenol content, which is the equivalent of drinking 4 cups of tea per day.

Hawthorn. Like green tea, hawthorn works to lower cholesterol and blood pressure. In addition, hawthorn helps to strengthen the heart muscle, improve circulation, and rid the body of unnecessary fluid and salt. Hawthorn is available in capsule or tincture form, standardized to 2.2 percent total bioflavonoid content. The recommended daily dose of hawthorn capsules varies widely, ranging from 100 to 300 milligrams, two or three times per day. Be aware that higher doses may significantly lower blood pressure, which may cause you to feel faint. For the tincture, the recommended dose is 4 to 5 milliliters, three times per day. It can take up to 2 months for hawthorn to have any noticeable effect on your health.

Nutritional Supplements

A number of nutritional supplements are very helpful for maintaining a healthy heart and reducing angina symptoms. These supplements can be taken together.

- Vitamin B_6: 50 milligrams daily, in divided doses of 25 milligrams. Improves the absorption of calcium, L-carnitine, and magnesium.

- Vitamin C: 1,000 milligrams daily, in divided doses of 500 milligrams. Converts cholesterol into bile, lowering LDL cholesterol; strengthens arterial walls; and stops the buildup of cholesterol.

- Vitamin E: 400 IU daily. Increases the oxygen supply to heart tissue and reduces excessive blood clotting.

- Calcium: 1,500 milligrams daily, in divided doses of 750 milligrams. Lowers total cholesterol while increasing HDL cholesterol.

- Coenzyme Q_{10}: 200 milligrams daily, in divided doses of 100 milligrams. Increases the oxygen supply to heart tissue.

- L-carnitine: 1,000 milligrams daily, in divided doses of 500 milligrams. Lowers total cholesterol while increasing HDL cholesterol.

- Magnesium: 800 milligrams daily, in divided doses of 400 milligrams. Regulates heartbeat, helps lower total cholesterol, and helps increase HDL cholesterol.

Relaxation/Meditation

Many complementary health care practitioners recommend various relaxation techniques to help reduce stress, control emotions, and lower blood pressure. In clinical trials, a combination of biofeedback, yoga, and meditation has been the most successful in reducing blood pressure.

Lying still and focusing on your breath can quiet the mind and relieve tension, too. Try this exercise for yourself: Lie flat on your back on the floor or your bed and place both hands on your abdomen. Slowly inhale through your nose, pushing your abdomen upward as if inflating a balloon. Then slowly exhale through your mouth, feeling your abdomen deflate as you do. Continue for 8 to 10 full cycles of inhalation and exhalation. Repeat as often as you're able throughout the day.

Lifestyle Recommendations

Stay active. If you have angina, you may be tempted to stop exercising, but don't give in. Instead, work with your doctor to develop an appropriate exercise plan. If you have not been getting regular exercise, you might start with something as brief as a 5-minute walk. Then gradually increase the duration of your walks as your fitness level improves.

By lowering your blood pressure and slowing your heart rate, exercise will improve bloodflow in your arteries. It also alleviates stress and supports weight loss. So over time, a sound exercise routine will help reduce angina symptoms.

Raise the head of your bed. To decrease the likelihood and/or frequency of angina attacks at bedtime, raise the head of your bed up to 4 inches by putting wooden blocks under the bed frame. This will lower the pressure on your arteries, reducing angina pain.

Stop smoking. Because it decreases the amount of oxygen in the blood, forcing the heart to work harder, the carbon monoxide produced by cigarette smoking only aggravates angina. Smoking also causes blood platelets to stick together, which may lead to an arterial blockage. And smoking interferes with certain prescription medications, making them less effective.

Preventive Measures

Maintain a desirable weight. If you are overweight, lose the extra pounds. Excess weight places additional strain on the cardiovascular system, increasing the risk of angina. Ask your doctor to refer you to a dietitian or a supervised weight-loss program.

Atherosclerosis

Also known as "hardening of the arteries," atherosclerosis is the buildup of plaque—a substance made of cholesterol, cellular waste products, and other materials—in the walls of the arteries. Over time, plaque makes the arteries stiffer than normal and either partially or completely blocks the flow of blood and oxygen. A narrowing of the artery is called a stenosis; a total blockage is an occlusion. The reduction in bloodflow is known as ischemia.

Atherosclerosis is the leading cause of death and disability in the United States. More than 5 million Americans have been diagnosed with it, while at least 5 million more are thought to have it but not know about it.

Atherosclerosis tends to occur near the branching points of the arteries. Most often, it affects medium-size arteries, such as those that feed the heart (coronary arteries), the brain (cerebral arteries), and the neck (carotid arteries), as well as those in the kidneys. It also can affect the aorta—the largest artery, which carries blood from the heart to the rest of the body.

Causes and Risk Factors

Atherosclerosis is thought to begin with an injury to the inner lining of an artery—perhaps caused by high blood pressure, a virus, nicotine, drugs, or an allergic reaction. In an attempt to repair the injury, white blood cells release a chemical that promotes plaque for-mation and acts as a soothing coating for the arterial wall. As the plaque continues to grow, it reduces bloodflow. If the surface of the plaque breaks off, it can cause a clot, impeding or stopping bloodflow and leading to a heart attack, stroke, or kidney failure.

The risk for atherosclerosis increases with age. Those who have high blood pressure, high cholesterol, diabetes, and/or a family history of atherosclerosis are more vulnerable to the disease, as are those who smoke. In a 3-year study of 10,914 middle-age adults, both active smoking and exposure to environmental tobacco were associated with the progression of atherosclerosis. The effect was most significant for those with diabetes and high blood pressure.

Signs and Symptoms

Particularly in its early stages, atherosclerosis produces no symptoms. However, as the level of blockage increases, it can lead to a number of symptoms, which tend to vary according to the affected artery. They include chest pain (angina), dizziness, calf pain during exercise, and transient ischemic attacks (TIAs, or "mini-strokes"). In men, atherosclerosis also may cause erectile dysfunction.

Conventional Treatments

The development of atherosclerosis is a life-long, additive process. With early intervention,

A Quick Guide to Symptoms

- ☐ Chest pain (angina)
- ☐ Dizziness
- ☐ Calf pain during exercise
- ☐ Transient ischemic attacks (TIAs or "mini-strokes")
- ☐ Erectile dysfunction

it's possible to slow and even stop the course of the disease.

Lifestyle Changes

In conventional medicine, the treatment of atherosclerosis often begins with lifestyle changes. Your doctor will review your habits and behaviors, with an eye toward possible modifications. Among the strategies that your doctor may suggest are eating a healthier diet, starting an exercise program, losing weight, quitting smoking, cutting back on your alcohol consumption, and reducing the amount of stress in your life.

Medications

To reduce the possibility of a blood clot, your doctor may recommend taking a daily low-dose aspirin. If you have chest pain (angina), you may need nitroglycerin, which helps open your arteries.

Other medications for treating atherosclerosis include beta-blockers, which slow the heart rate and decrease blood pressure. They also appear to lower the risk of fatal heart attacks. (To learn more about beta-blockers, see Angina on page 18.) Your physician also may prescribe an angiotensin-converting enzyme (ACE) inhibitor to facilitate bloodflow from the heart, thus reducing the heart's workload. Examples of ACE inhibitors are lisinopril (Prinivil and Zestril) and captopril.

Many people with atherosclerosis have elevated cholesterol. If you do, your doctor may advise you to take a cholesterol-lowering medication. These drugs include statins, niacin, fibrates, and bile acid sequestrants. (These are described in detail in High Cholesterol, beginning on page 149.) Similarly, if you have high blood pressure, you may require medication to bring it under control. (To explore your options, see High Blood Pressure on page 138.)

Surgery

If lifestyle changes and medication do not improve your atherosclerosis, your doctor may recommend surgery. One option is a procedure known as balloon angioplasty, which involves inserting a catheter with a tiny balloon at the end into an artery in the arm or groin. The catheter is threaded through the artery until the balloon can be inflated in the areas that are narrowed by plaque. As the balloon inflates, it pushes the plaque against the artery wall, which opens up the artery. To keep it open, a stent—a small metal tube—may be put in place.

For some patients who are unable to undergo balloon angioplasty, an atherectomy may be necessary. As in angioplasty, a tube is inserted into the narrowed coronary artery. Then a high-speed drill at the end of the tube shaves the plaque from the artery wall. The shaved plaque is removed via the catheter.

Complementary Treatments

The best complementary approach to slowing or stopping the progression of atherosclerosis involves dietary modification, nutritional supplementation, herbal therapies, and stress reduction techniques.

Ayurveda

Ayurveda is an ancient healing discipline that originated in India more than 5,000 years ago. Ayurvedic practitioners consider the heart to be the most important organ and the seat of human consciousness. Any problems with the heart occur because it's not being given proper care and attention—not just through diet and exercise, but also through emotional attachment and spirituality. In Ayurveda, the emotions play a key role in heart health and are a factor in treatment. A typical Ayurvedic "prescription" may include diet, herbs, yoga, meditation, and lifestyle changes.

Because Ayurvedic practitioners tailor their recommendations to each person's *dosha*, or mind/body type, it's best to see a practitioner for a consultation. The Ayurvedic Institute may be able to direct you to the names of qualified professionals in your area. Visit the organization's Web site at www.ayurveda.com.

Diet

A healthy diet is critical to a healthy cardiovascular system. It should include lots of vegetables, fruits, whole grains, and nuts and seeds (walnuts, almonds, and sesame seeds). Avoid fried foods, sugar, and processed foods, all of which can compromise cardiovascular health. Also avoid foods rich in saturated fats and cholesterol, such as fatty meats, egg yolks, milk fat, and margarine. Replace whole-fat dairy products with their low-fat and nonfat counterparts.

By building your diet around fresh, whole plant foods, you naturally increase your intake of water-soluble fiber. This is the fiber that helps lower cholesterol and high blood pressure not only by reducing the absorption of fat but also by escorting fat from the intestines. Good sources of water-soluble fiber include fruits, legumes, and whole grains, especially oat and wheat bran.

Remember, too, to drink more water to help water-soluble fiber do its job. The minimum recommendation is eight 8-ounce glasses of water daily.

Any foods rich in essential fatty acids, beta-carotene, the B vitamins, vitamins C and E, magnesium, and the trace mineral selenium are beneficial for cardiovascular health. Essential fatty acids come from salmon and other cold-water fish, as well as flaxseed oil. Almost all fruits and vegetables contain beta-carotene, though in varying amounts. You can get your B vitamins from dark green, leafy vegetables, whole grains, avocados, beets, bananas, potatoes, low-fat or nonfat dairy products, nuts, beans, fish, and chicken. Good sources of vitamin C include almost all fruits and green vegetables, especially strawberries, cranberries, melons, oranges, mangoes, papayas, peppers, spinach, kale, broccoli, tomatoes, and potatoes. Vitamin E is available in vegetable oils, nuts, seeds, and wheat germ; green, leafy vegetables and whole grains provide smaller amounts. Magnesium is found in green, leafy vegetables such as spinach, parsley, broccoli, chard, kale, and mustard and turnip greens, as well as in raw almonds, wheat germ, potatoes, and tofu. As for selenium, good food sources include seafood, chicken, whole grain cereals, and garlic.

Antioxidant compounds known as anthocyanosides improve capillary circulation. The European species of blueberry, the bilberry, contains the most anthocyanosides of any food. Other excellent sources include blueberries, cherries, raspberries, red or purple grapes, and plums. An Israeli study, published in the August 2006 issue of *Atherosclerosis*, found that participants were able to reduce their risk of developing atherosclerosis by drinking 6 ounces of pomegranate juice every day for 3 months. Interestingly, the sugars in pomegranate juice did not elevate blood sugar levels in those participants who were diabetic. Instead, the sugars attached to certain antioxidants that help protect against atherosclerosis.

Herbal Medicine

Garlic. Beyond its antioxidant properties, garlic fights atherosclerosis not only by lowering cholesterol and blood pressure but also by improving the elasticity of blood vessel walls.

The recommended daily dose is two to three cloves of fresh garlic, or 500 milligrams in supplement form. If you have a choice, select fresh garlic over supplements; the supplements contain concentrated extracts, which may raise the risk of excessive bleeding.

Ginkgo biloba. Ginkgo is an antioxidant herb that supports healthy circulation. It is available both raw and in capsule form. The recommended daily dose is 120 milligrams, twice a day, of an extract standardized to 24 percent flavone glycosides and 6 percent terpene lactones. The flavone glycosides give ginkgo its antioxidant benefits, while terpene lactones improve circulation and have a protective effect on nerve cells. *Note:* If you're taking a prescription blood-thinning medication, be sure to check with your doctor before trying ginkgo supplements.

Green tea. Green tea contains high levels of substances called polyphenols, which have powerful antioxidant properties. It also helps to lower cholesterol and blood pressure and to keep arteries from clogging. Drinking 3 cups of green tea per day provides 240 to 320 milligrams of polyphenols. In capsule form, a standardized extract of EGCG (a polyphenol) may provide 97 percent polyphenol content, which is the equivalent of drinking 4 cups of tea per day.

Hawthorn. Like green tea, hawthorn helps to lower cholesterol and blood pressure. It also plays a role in strengthening the heart muscle, improving circulation, and ridding the body of unnecessary fluid and salt. Hawthorn is available in capsule or tincture form, standardized to 2.2 percent total bioflavonoid content. For the capsules, the recommended daily dose varies widely, from 100 to 300 milligrams, two or three times per day. Be aware that higher doses may significantly lower blood pressure, which may cause you to feel faint. For the tincture, the recommended dose is 4 to 5 milliliters, three times per day. Hawthorn does work slowly; it may take up to 2 months before you notice any effects.

Nutritional Supplements

The following nutritional supplements are very beneficial to maintaining a healthy heart.

- B-complex vitamins: Take as directed on the label. The B vitamins work best when they're taken together. B_6, B_{12}, and folic acid help reduce homocysteine, an amino acid that contributes to the artery-clogging process. In addition, B_6 improves the absorption of calcium, L-carnitine, and magnesium.

- Vitamin C: 1,000 milligrams daily, in divided doses of 500 milligrams. Converts cholesterol into bile, which lowers "bad" LDL cholesterol; strengthens the arterial walls; and stops cholesterol buildup in the arteries.

- Vitamin E: 400 IU daily. Prevents the oxidation of LDL cholesterol, protects and supports arterial walls and the heart muscle, improves circulation, and fortifies immune function. For the best absorption, pair your vitamin E capsules with selenium (see below). *Note:* Because vitamin E may thin the blood, consult your doctor before taking vitamin E if you already are using a blood-thinning medication.

- Calcium: 1,500 milligrams daily, in divided doses of 750 milligrams. Lowers total cholesterol while increasing "good" HDL cholesterol.

- Chromium: 200 micrograms daily. Helps prevent cholesterol buildup in the arteries.

- Coenzyme Q_{10}: 200 milligrams daily, in divided doses of 100 milligrams. Increases the oxygen supply to the heart tissues.

- L-carnitine: 1,000 milligrams daily, in divided doses of 500 milligrams. Lowers total cholesterol while increasing HDL cholesterol.

- Magnesium: 800 milligrams daily, in divided doses of 400 milligrams. May reduce angina symptoms. Also helps lower total cholesterol while increasing HDL cholesterol.

- Selenium: 400 micrograms daily, in divided doses of 200 micrograms. Thins the blood, helping to prevent heart disease and future heart attacks. *Note:* Consult your doctor before taking selenium if you already are on blood-thinning medication. For best absorption, do not take selenium at the same time as vitamin C.

Relaxation/Meditation

Conventional physicians and complementary health practitioners alike recommend relaxation techniques to help alleviate stress, defuse negative emotions, and lower blood pressure. Clinical trials have demonstrated that by combining biofeedback, yoga, and meditation, you can improve your ability to lower your blood pressure. Other effective relaxation techniques include qigong, tai chi, and visualization.

One 2006 study found that practicing mental relaxation or deep breathing can reduce both blood pressure and heart rate. To try deep breathing, first lie flat on your back either on a bed or on the floor. Place both hands on your abdomen. Slowly inhale through your nose, pushing your abdomen up as if inflating a balloon. Then slowly exhale through your mouth, feeling your abdomen deflate as you do. Continue deep breathing for 8 to 10 complete cycles of inhalation and exhalation. Repeat as often as needed throughout the day to keep stress in check.

Lifestyle Recommendations

Be active. By lowering blood pressure and slowing heart rate, exercise improves arterial bloodflow. It also may reduce plaque deposits, thereby reversing the atherosclerotic disease process. Of course, exercise is important for losing weight and managing stress, both cardiovascular risk factors.

If you have atherosclerosis, you may be tempted to avoid exercise. Instead, work with your doctor to develop an appropriate fitness program. If you have been relatively inactive, you should start with something as brief as a 5-minute walk, then gradually increase your duration over time. Aim for at least 20 minutes, three or four times a week.

Preventive Measures

Relax. Take steps to reduce the amount of stress in your life. As mentioned earlier, meditation, yoga, and other relaxation techniques can help offset the cardiovascular effects of stress.

Cut back on coffee consumption. Drinking coffee increases the body's production of stress hormones, which may place coffee drinkers at greater risk for cardiovascular problems. So far, studies have failed to establish a direct link between atherosclerosis and caffeine intake. Still, if you have other cardiovascular risk factors, you may want to limit your coffee intake to 2 cups a day.

Reduce your alcohol intake. Research into the effects of alcohol consumption on the heart has been mixed. Some studies have shown that red wine may be beneficial for the cardiovascular system, as the flavonoids in the wine help keep fatty deposits from forming in the arteries. On the other hand, alcohol can raise blood pressure and overtax the liver, causing cholesterol to build up in the arteries. While the jury is out, your best bet is to consume alcohol only in moderation. This means no more than two 5-ounce glasses daily.

Stop smoking. Beyond the fact that smoking elevates blood pressure, the carbon monoxide produced by cigarette smoke lowers the amount of oxygen in the blood, forcing the heart to pump harder. Smoking also causes blood platelets to stick together, which can lead to arterial blockages. In some instances, smoking can interfere with prescription medications.

Back Pain

Back pain may affect the upper or lower back, and often the neck and legs as well. The pain may be accompanied by other symptoms, such as weakness, numbness, and tingling.

Generally, back pain is classified as either acute or chronic. Acute back pain tends to occur suddenly, and it lasts anywhere from a few days to as long as 3 months. It may subside for a while, only to return later on. When pain persists for more than 3 months, it is considered chronic back pain.

Back pain is extremely common, affecting more than 65 million Americans every year. Four in five of us adults will experience a bout of back pain at some point in our lives. Acute low back pain is the fifth most common reason for physician visits.

Causes and Risk Factors

Back pain has a number of potential causes, including injuries and accidents, muscle strains and spasms, infection, and disorders such as Paget's disease, Parkinson's disease, ankylosing spondylitis (an inflammatory disease of the spine), and osteoarthritis. In cases of acute back pain, however, the cause often remains unknown.

It's not unusual for back trouble to begin in the vertebrae—the 33 bone segments that make up the spinal column. If greater than normal pressure is exerted on one of the cushioning disks that separate the vertebrae, the disk may become herniated (ruptured), causing great pain. For someone with osteoporosis, a vertebral compression fracture could occur even with mild pressure, as in the case of a sneeze. In rare instances, a tumor may be responsible for compressing the spinal column.

Pain also may occur when the bony protrusions on the back of each vertebra deteriorate or become misaligned. Sometimes the spine undergoes painful arthritic changes, a condition known as spinal stenosis.

Degenerative disk disease (DDD), also known as internal disk disruption and intervertebral disk disease, is the erosion of the disks in the spinal column. As we age, the normally soft, cushioning disks, which serve as shock absorbers between the vertebrae and prevent the vertebrae from hitting one another, become less flexible and less able to function effectively. Since they have diminishing amounts of blood and water, they lose some of their height. The disks become more vulnerable to tears, particularly in the outer layer, which has nerve cells. When this occurs, the gelatinous material inside the disk may bulge outward. The resulting herniated disk may put pressure on nerves. Adjacent vertebrae may rub against each other, which may pinch nerves and/or produce bone spurs (enlargements of normal bony structures).

Degenerative disk disease occurs most often in the cervical (upper) or lumbar (lower) spine and less often in the thoracic (middle) spine. If it affects the cervical spine, it may be

A Quick Guide to Symptoms

- ☐ Persistent pain in your back
- ☐ Pain may be dull and throbbing or sharp and piercing
- ☐ Pain may occur only when you're performing certain tasks, or when you're standing or sitting in a certain position
- ☐ Pain may radiate from your back into your legs, hips, buttocks, or pelvis
- ☐ Pain may trigger tingling or numbness in the calf or foot
- ☐ Pain that worsens when bending or lifting heavy objects

called cervical disk disease.

DDD is extremely common. Though the statistics vary widely, there is a reasonable chance that you may have some evidence of disk degeneration by the time you reach midlife. While the very process of aging may cause degenerative disk disease, the condition also may result from trauma, infection, or injury to the disk. Working at a job that requires repeated heavy lifting or that involves vehicle vibration (being a truck driver, for example) can raise risk. Even lei-

There are no self-tests for back pain, but if you have it, you know it. You may wish to keep a diary of your pain: When are your symptoms the worst? When do they seem better? This can help you and your doctor pinpoint the source of the problem.

sure activities that place repetitive strain on the back may play a role in DDD.

Pain in the lower back most often occurs because of a problem with the sciatic nerve, the major nerve that carries sensations between the lower back and legs. As many as 40 percent of Americans experience this type of pain, known as sciatica, during their lifetimes. Frequently the culprit is a herniated disk that pinches the nerve, producing pain that radiates into one or both legs. But sciatica can also be the result of an inflamed piriformis muscle (located in the buttocks), lumbosacral strain (muscle strain in the lower back), spinal stenosis, a ruptured disk, strained ligaments, endometriosis, uterine masses, prostatitis, arthritis, and weak abdominal and back muscles.

In some people, back pain may be an indicator of a problem with a nearby organ. For example, both kidney disease and pancreatitis can produce profound back pain. Likewise, conditions such as rheumatoid arthritis can cause painful inflammation of the spine.

Even certain medications may have back pain as a side effect. For example, anticoagulants (blood thinners) are known to trigger bleeding and internal bruising that may trigger back pain.

A number of factors raise the risk of back pain—among them obesity, smoking, and a sedentary lifestyle. People who participate in strenuous sports or who do a good deal of heavy lifting arc at cvcn higher risk, as are those who have poor posture, who sit or stand in one position for long periods of time, or who improperly lift heavy items. Many people seem to have a genetic tendency for back pain; that is, they are born with spinal abnormalities that make them more vulnerable to problems. The risk of back pain also increases with age.

Signs and Symptoms

If you have back pain, you already know it. It may be dull and throbbing or sharp and piercing, as though someone just stabbed you with a knife. Back pain may occur only when you perform certain tasks or stand or sit in certain positions, or it may be relatively constant. Because the pain may radiate from the back into the legs, it can cause stiffness and restrict movement. It also may trigger tingling or numbness in the calf or foot. In some instances, back pain may interfere with bladder or bowel control.

Conventional Treatments

When acute back pain is not associated with an underlying medical problem, it tends to improve with minimal treatment, often within a few months. Bed rest, once the standard prescription, no longer is recommended. Now doctors advise patients to resume normal activity as soon as possible.

Immediate Pain Relief Measures

Unless acute back pain is the result of an obvious serious medical problem, your best first step may be one or a combination of the following treatments.

- Take an over-the-counter pain reliever such as acetaminophen, aspirin, or another non-steroidal anti-inflammatory drug (NSAID).

- Apply cold, then heat. For the cold treatments, you can use a gel pack or a bag of frozen vegetables, wrapped in a towel. Leave it in place for 20 minutes, and repeat every hour for the first 24 hours. Then switch to heat treatments, such as a heating pad or a warm towel. Apply for 20 minutes of every hour, and continue for as long as needed, up to several days.

- Apply an over-the-counter pain patch.

- Wear a supportive back brace for a short period of time.

- Get a good night's sleep. It might help to avoid caffeine from the afternoon on; to take a warm bath before bedtime; or to practice a relaxation technique such as deep breathing.

Electrical Nerve Stimulation

Transcutaneous electrical nerve stimulation (TENS) uses low-level electrical pulses to reduce back pain. In a typical course of treatment, the TENS unit administers 80 to 100 pulses per second for 45 minutes, three times per day. The sensations are barely felt.

In a similar procedure known as percutaneous electrical nerve stimulation (PENS), small needles deliver the pulses directly to acupuncture points. While this approach appears to provide some relief for many people with chronic back pain, it is not thought to be effective for sciatica.

Exercise

When dealing with acute back pain, it is important to find a balance between inactivity and overexertion. While you should avoid exercises that trigger pain, you do want to incorporate some level of activity into your daily schedule. Within 2 weeks of the onset of pain, most people should be able to begin walking, cycling on a stationary bike, swimming, or light jogging. It's best to steer clear of any exercise that places too much pressure on your back—for example, if it involves twisting or bending—as well as sports that are high-impact.

Exercise also is beneficial for people who are dealing with chronic back pain. In fact, those who engage in exercise tend to return to their normal routines faster than those who are sedentary. A review of randomized trials of various activities, including strengthening and stretching programs as well as physical therapy, found them to be reasonably equal in their effectiveness.

If you have chronic back pain, you may find the following to be particularly useful.

- **Aerobic activities that are low-impact.** These strengthen muscles in the back and abdomen, without straining the back. Examples include bicycling, swimming, and walking.

- **Exercises to strengthen the lower back.** Both partial situps and pelvic tilts can improve lower back strength. To perform partial situps, lie on your back with your knees slightly bent. Raise your head and shoulders off the floor for 2 seconds, then return to the starting position. Repeat 5 to 10 times. For a pelvic tilt, lie on your back with your arms stretched out to your sides. Your knees should be bent, with your feet shoulder-width apart and your heels on the floor. With your shoulders back, squeeze your buttocks and raise your pelvis, keeping your lower back on the floor. Hold for 1 second, then return to the starting position. Repeat 25 to 30 times.

Medications

COX-2 inhibitors. One group of medications found to be effective for relieving back pain is the COX-2 inhibitors, which include celecoxib (Celebrex) and meloxicam (Mobic). These drugs suppress the enzyme cyclooxygenase-2 (COX-2), which causes joint inflammation and pain, while preserving the COX-1 enzyme, which protects the stomach lining. Patients taking COX-2 inhibitors tend to have fewer gastrointestinal side effects than those taking NSAIDs. Nevertheless, many who use COX-2 inhibitors do experience gastrointestinal problems. Some report other side effects as well, such as headache, dizziness, and kidney problems.

People who are using anticoagulant drugs may be at greater risk for bleeding with COX-2s. In a small number of cases, higher doses of celecoxib have been associated with hallucinations, fluid buildup in the legs, high blood pressure, and excess potassium in the blood.

Because of safety concerns, one COX-2 inhibitor, rofecoxib (Vioxx), was taken off the market in 2004. Some researchers question the safety of all COX-2 medications.

Nonsteroidal anti-inflammatory drugs (NSAIDs). Doctors commonly advise their patients with back pain, especially those with chronic back pain, to take nonsteroidal anti-inflammatory drugs. These include aspirin, ibuprofen (Motrin, Advil), and naproxen (Aleve, Naprosyn). NSAIDs may be quite effective, though they may require a week or two to produce significant pain relief.

NSAIDs are known to cause gastrointestinal problems such as ulcers, stomach upset, and internal bleeding. These symptoms may occur even with intravenous administration of the medications. NSAIDs also may increase blood pressure, especially among those who already have high blood pressure. Other possible side effects include headaches, skin rash, ringing in the ears, dizziness, and depression. There is some evidence that NSAIDs may damage cartilage and/or cause kidney damage. The longer you take NSAIDs, the more likely they are to cause side effects, which is why you should use them with caution.

If your doctor determines that you are at risk for developing an ulcer from an NSAID, a number of medications may help prevent one. Among these are the proton-pump inhibitors, which include omeprazole (Prilosec), lansoprazole (Prevacid), rabeprazole (Aciphex), and pantoprazole (Protonix). In comparisons of people who took these medications with those who did not, the proton-pump inhibitors produced an 80 percent reduction in ulcer occurrence.

The drug misoprostol may be helpful in preventing (but not treating) NSAID-induced ulcers. The medication Arthrotec is a combination of misoprostol and the NSAID diclofenac. In one study, patients who took Arthrotec developed between 65 and 80 percent fewer ulcers than those who took NSAIDs alone.

Sometimes NSAIDs are combined with muscle relaxants such as cyclobenzaprine (Flexeril), diazepam (Valium), carisoprodol (Soma), or methocarbamol (Robaxin). Similarly, antidepressants known as tricyclics may be prescribed along with NSAIDs, even to people who are not depressed. This class of drugs includes amitriptyline (Elavil, Endep), desipramine (Norpramin), doxepin (Sinequan), imipramine (Tofranil), amoxapine (Asendin), nortriptyline (Pamelor, Aventyl), and maprotiline (Ludiomil). Although the tricyclic antidepressants have been successful in relieving pain, they may cause significant side effects, such as weight gain, sexual dysfunction, mental disturbance, sleep disturbance, and a sudden reduction in blood pressure upon standing that may lead to dizziness or fainting.

Other medications. For some patients with severe back pain, narcotics are an option. Narcotics fall into two categories: opiates and opioids. Opiates, such as morphine and codeine, are derived from natural opium; opioids—methadone is one example—are synthetic. Since these medications are potentially addictive, people who use them require close medical supervision. With this caveat, narcotics can be very successful in controlling chronic pain. Methadone, for instance, tends to lessen the intensity of pain, enabling people to participate in strength-building exercises, which are an important component of managing back pain.

Another choice for severe pain associated with nerve impingement, such as sciatica, is the injection of substances directly into the affected area. Perhaps the best known of these is the one-time injection of corticosteroid into the area around the spinal column. Other options include injections of local anesthetics, hypertonic saline (saltwater solution), hyaluronidase (an enzyme from mammalian testes), and botulinum toxin (Botox). Better known for reducing wrinkles, Botox temporarily paralyzes muscle tissues, and in doing so may relieve back pain for several months. But none of the injectable options offers a cure.

To relieve pain caused by degenerative disk disease, your doctor may recommend chymopapain and other injections. After the administration of a general or local anesthetic, the enzyme chymopapain is injected directly into the herniated disk. It dissolves the portion of the disk that is pressing against a nerve. Common side effects are back pain, stiffness, soreness, and muscle spasms in the lower back. Less common are dizziness, a burning sensation in the lower back, nausea, leg cramps, pain or mild weakness, reduced sensitivity to pain, and numbness or tingling in the legs or toes. There is a long list of rare side effects, the most serious of which are leg paralysis, severe allergic reaction, and death.

Some side effects of chymopapain may not appear until days or even weeks after treatment. If you believe that you may be having a reaction to the medication, consult your doctor. You should be especially vigilant if you have sudden, intense back pain or weakness or if you develop a skin rash, hives, or itching.

Surgery

The vast majority of back pain does not require surgery. Even severe pain caused by a herniated disk or spinal stenosis usually responds to more conservative treatments. Nevertheless, in those cases in which more conservative options fail to bring adequate relief and the pain becomes debilitating, surgery may be necessary. It also may be recommended when there is progressive weakening of the legs or evidence of a physical abnormality, such as a bone spur.

Be aware that all of the surgical procedures described below may cause complications, such as nerve and muscle damage, infection, and scarring. Also note that like any surgery, back surgery requires a period of recuperation afterward.

Discectomy. This procedure involves surgically removing the fragment of a spinal disk that is causing pressure and pain. One of the most common complications of a discectomy is the formation of scar tissue, which may lead to persistent pain.

Electrothermal surgery. In this procedure—formally known as an intradiskal electrothermal treatment (IDET)—the surgeon inserts a needle into the compromised disk, using x-rays for guidance. Electricity then heats and shrinks the injured disk tissue. Once healed, the disk is stronger, and often the pain is significantly reduced.

Laminectomy or laminotomy. Both of these procedures target the lamina, which is the back section of the vertebra. In a laminectomy, the entire lamina is removed; in a laminotomy, only a portion is removed. While these procedures tend to bring immediate pain relief, they are not always successful. Moreover, in more than half of all cases, the pain recurs to some degree.

Spinal fusion. Sometimes, when two or more vertebrae are positioned in such a way that they cause pain when they move, the surgeon may recommend fusing them together to eliminate the painful motion. A number of surgical methods are used for spinal fusion.

Total disk replacement. In this relatively new procedure, an individual disk is replaced with an artificial one. Complete pain relief occurs for about 20 percent of patients, while 65 percent of patients report improvement in back pain.

Complementary Treatments

Complementary medicine offers a number of approaches that have been successful in treating various types of back pain. Since complementary therapies can improve posture, relax tight muscles, address poor body mechanics, and alleviate pain, they should always be tried before scheduling surgery.

Acupuncture

An article published in *Annals of Internal Medicine* analyzed 33 acupuncture studies and concluded that acupuncture is a viable treatment for the relief of chronic back pain. To locate an acupuncturist in your area, visit the Web site of the National Certification Commission for Acupuncture and Oriental Medicine (NCCAOM) at www.nccaom.org.

Aquatic Therapy

Aquatic therapy is effective for relaxing tired, aching back muscles. People who cannot tolerate traditional exercise programs find the water to be the perfect medium for promoting pain relief, because it's buoyant. Health clubs, resorts, and gyms have back pain programs that are available to the general public. There are also physical therapy clinics that offer individual and group aquatic therapy classes specifically for low back pain. Treatments are generally provided by physical therapists, athletic trainers, and licensed aquatic therapists.

Bodywork

Various bodywork approaches have been shown to effectively relieve back pain, while also helping to address the underlying cause of the pain.

Acupressure. Acupressure—the application of pressure at specific points—can eliminate obstructions in the flow of healing energy. This helps your back muscles and ligaments to relax, and your body to return to a healthier structure.

Craniosacral therapy. Through gentle manipulation of the craniosacral system, this therapy can reduce stress and correct systemic imbalances, allowing the body to heal itself and restore normal function.

Reflexology. Through application of pressure to specific areas of the hands and feet, reflexology can restore the natural flow of energy in the zones of the body. For the spine, the reflex area is located along the edge of each foot, from the big toe down to the heel, representing the area of the neck down to the base of the spine. Tenderness in this area means that circulation to the spine or back is blocked. You may even feel what seem to be tiny crystals when working on this area of the foot. If so, continue to apply gentle pressure, moving along the area until it feels smooth.

Rolfing. Rolfing involves deep manipulation of the connective tissue to restore the body's natural alignment.

Shiatsu. The deep finger pressure of shiatsu massage can help release obstructions in the muscles and vital energy system. Shiatsu can both stimulate and relax, bringing about relief from pain.

Therapeutic massage. Therapeutic massage helps relieve muscular tension and pain. It has an overall calming effect on the body and mind.

Trigger point therapy. Also known as myotherapy, trigger point therapy focuses on trigger points—tender, congested spots on muscle tissue that radiate pain to other areas of the body. Applying pressure to these areas helps alleviate tension, relax muscle spasms, improve circulation, and reduce pain.

Chiropractic

In chiropractic treatment, the chiropractor manipulates and adjusts the spine, placing the backbone in its proper position and thereby diminishing pain. The chiropractor may also integrate various massage therapy techniques to alleviate tension and spasm.

Diet

Maintain a healthy weight by eating lots of whole grains, fruits, and vegetables. This not only helps alleviate the pressure exerted by excess weight but also supports healing by properly nourishing the body. Aim for a minimum of six servings of whole grains, five servings of vegetables, and four servings of fruit each day.

Eliminate foods high in fat and sugar. Beyond their adverse effect on your weight, they rob your body of essential nutrients and interfere with their absorption.

But don't skip meals, particularly breakfast, in your quest to maintain a healthy weight. Strong muscles need food; weakened muscles create injured muscles. In the morning, 95 percent of your energy reserve is depleted. So be sure to eat breakfast to start your day off right.

Also, many people who are trying to lose weight eat the right kinds of food, but don't eat enough. Be sure to take in enough calories to fuel your muscles, so they're able to support your spine.

Energy Balancing

Stress and negative emotions can cause back muscles to tighten, resulting in muscle pain and tension. Energy balancing techniques can help to restore the flow of the body's natural healing energy, removing blockages and reducing pain and stress.

Reiki. Through the hand movements of a trained practitioner, Reiki releases old energy and allows new energy to flow into the body—revitalizing and strengthening each cell, stimulating the body's systems, and normalizing function.

Therapeutic touch. Therapeutic touch moves the body's energy, preventing it from stagnating and causing pain.

Herbal Medicine

Capsaicin. Extracted from the seeds of hot chili peppers, capsaicin reduces substance P, a naturally occurring compound that fosters inflammation and the delivery of pain impulses from the central nervous system. The over-the-counter creams Zostrix and Capzasin-P contain capsaicin in an easy-to-use form. Simply rub a small amount of cream on the affected area four times a day.

During the first few days of use, you may experience a localized sensation of warmth and stinging. This will pass, and pain relief will begin within 1 to 2 weeks.

Ginger. Ginger has a long-standing reputation for reducing the pain associated with inflammation. It is sold in tincture or powder form. Recommended doses are 2 milligrams of tincture, three times a day, or 3 grams of the dried powder, three times a day. Fresh ginger can be grated onto food or added when cooking. Use up to 3 tablespoons of raw ginger or 6 to 8 tablespoons of cooked ginger per day.

Note: If you are taking aspirin or using warfarin (Coumadin), consult your doctor before using therapeutic doses of ginger, since it can increase the potency of these medications and cause unexpected bleeding.

Movement Reeducation Therapies

Relearning proper body movements. can result in decreased pain, greater mobility, and improved posture.

Alexander Technique. You may benefit from a series of sessions with an Alexander Technique instructor, who will teach you how to avoid poor postural habits and replace them with healthy body mechanics.

Feldenkrais Method. Practitioners of the Feldenkrais Method train their clients to become more aware of movement patterns and practice proper body mechanics. This can relieve stiffness, inflammation, and pain.

Qigong and tai chi. These "moving meditations"—which date back to ancient times—use gentle, rhythmic postures and movements to facilitate the flow of energy throughout the body.

Many hospitals offer qigong and tai chi classes, as do YM/YWCAs, community colleges, and some churches. Check your local newspaper, or watch the bulletin board of your local library or community fitness center.

Trager Approach. The Trager Approach uses movement reeducation to release tight muscles. As it is a passive treatment, it is especially useful for people with limited mobility. Over time, the body's nervous system is reeducated to respond in the proper manner to relieve pain and discomfort.

Nutritional Supplements

It is important to maintain proper levels of nutrients to support back health.

- Multivitamin/mineral: Take as directed on the label. Look for a supplement that contains vitamins A, B-complex, C, and E, as well as beta-carotene, calcium, copper, magnesium, selenium, and zinc. Such a supplement has anti-inflammatory properties and, more generally, ensures proper nutrient levels.

- Bromelain: 500 milligrams daily. An enzyme derived from pineapple, bromelain has anti-inflammatory properties.

- Essential fatty acids—omega-3 (flaxseed and fish oil) and omega-6 (borage, evening primrose, and black currant seed oils): Available in oil and capsule form; take as directed on the label. They increase the levels of anti-inflammatory agents in the body.

Personal Fitness Training

When a study published in *Annals of Internal Medicine* reviewed 61 trials involving more than 6,390 adults, it came to the conclusion that physical activity reduced acute and chronic back pain. Other studies have shown that exercises performed with the supervision of a knowledgeable professional, such as a personal trainer, yield better long-term results than exercises performed without professional supervision.

The best exercises for a painful back are those that strengthen and stabilize the core muscles—the muscles of the abdomen, pelvis, buttocks, and hips. These are the muscles that support the back. Appropriate exercises include strength training and Pilates.

To locate a certified personal trainer in your area, visit the Web site of the American College of Sports Medicine at www.acsm.org. Click on "General Public" on the left side of the homepage, then on the link to "ProFinder."

Relaxation/Meditation

Since emotional stress often is a factor in low back pain, it can be helpful to reduce stress and increase relaxation. Therapies such as deep breathing, visualization, guided imagery, and meditation are useful for reducing stress.

John E. Sarno, MD, a physician and professor of rehabilitation medicine, has successfully worked with patients suffering from chronic back pain. He feels that chronic back pain is not a mechanical dysfunction, but rather is emotional in origin. To help reinforce the "pain as emotion" idea, Dr. Sarno discontinues all physical interventions during treatment, and instead instructs patients to practice positive affirmations to interrupt and eventually reverse the pain cycle.

Though it is not necessary to cease physical therapy when treating back pain, for best results, it is helpful to accept the mind-body connection and to work on healing the mind as well as the back.

Therapeutic Massage

Studies have found therapeutic massage to be effective in reducing the pain of DDD by relaxing muscles and improving circulation. It also supports flexibility and allows for greater mobility, while offsetting the effects of stress. Therapeutic massage can be especially helpful when combined with movement reeducation therapies and exercise.

For help in locating a qualified massage therapist, visit the Web site of the National Certification Board of Therapeutic Massage and Bodywork at www.ncbtmb.com.

Lifestyle Recommendations

Brace your back when sneezing. To avoid aggravating a back injury when sneezing, bend your knees and brace your back by holding on to a nearby support.

Maintain correct posture. To maintain healthy posture, keep your ears, shoulders, and hips in a straight line with your head and your stomach pulled in. Also, avoid excessive standing; standing for long periods of time places extra stress on your back.

For tasks such as washing your face or brushing your teeth, it is necessary to lean forward over the sink. If you have back pain, this position can be extremely difficult. To reduce the strain on your lower back, place one foot on a stool or box. If this is not possible, keep your feet shoulder-width apart, bend your knees slightly, and lean forward at the hips. Throughout this process, try to keep your back straight.

Take breaks on road trips. During longer drives, it is best to stop every hour and get out for a brief walk. Avoid lifting any heavy objects immediately after the drive, as your muscles and joints will be stiff and more vulnerable to injury. Depending on your personal preferences, you might consider using a contoured back pillow in your car.

Apply ice as needed. Ice reduces swelling and can alleviate the pain from back muscle strain. Fill a paper cup with water and freeze it. Then peel back the paper, and you're ready for an ice massage. Move the ice continuously over the painful area for 4 to 5 minutes. As an alternative, use a bag of frozen peas, which will conform to the shape of the painful area. After icing, you might switch to heat.

Relax before bedtime. If back pain compromises your ability to fall asleep, try some of these pampering strategies.

• Take a warm bath right before climbing into bed.

• Fill your room with the aroma of lavender. You can use the essential oil as a room spritzer or apply a few drops to a lamp ring and heat on a lightbulb.

• Listen to quiet music and release the tension of the day with deep abdominal breaths, slowly inhaling and exhaling.

Stretch carefully. When stretching, make sure that you feel the stretch in your muscles rather than in your joints. If you feel it in your joints, you are probably pulling the ligaments that connect the muscles to the joints. Ligaments are more likely to tear than stretch.

Push, don't pull. If at all possible, move a heavy object by pushing rather than pulling.

When you push an object, you can use your legs and body weight, which takes the pressure off your lower back.

Take care in lifting heavy objects. If you *must* lift a heavy object, try to heed the following suggestions.

- To give a wider base of support, spread your feet apart.
- Stand close to the object you plan to lift.
- Do not arch your back.
- Bend at your knees.
- Lift with your leg muscles instead of your back muscles.
- While bending or lifting, do not twist from your waist.

Choose appropriate chairs. It is best to sit in chairs with straight backs or low-back support. Look for a chair that swivels and has arm rests. An adjustable chair back is preferable. When you are sitting, your knees should be higher than your hips; you might wish to place your feet on a low stool, if necessary.

Join a support group. If you have chronic back pain, you might consider joining a support group. You'll learn new ways to manage your pain in a more effective manner, and the psychological support of your fellow members may facilitate healing. To find a group in your area, ask your doctor or local hospital for a referral.

Preventive Measures

Get regular exercise. While regular exercise is an important component of any treatment plan for back pain, it also is a means of preventing back problems. By participating in regular exercise that incorporates stretching to increase flexibility, abdominal exercises to support your back, and cardiovascular activity such as walking, you will stretch and strengthen your back muscles as well as lubricate your joints, making them less vulnerable to injury. People who are active also are less likely to be obese, another risk factor for back pain. Aim for at least 40 minutes of physical activity per day.

Stop smoking. Probably because smoking impairs blood circulation, smokers are at higher risk for back problems. Further, smoking disrupts the delivery of vital nutrients to the spinal disks, leaving them more vulnerable to damage when under stress.

Cataracts

Cataracts form when protein in the lens of the eye clumps together. The once-transparent lens becomes cloudy and no longer allows light to pass through and focus on the retina. This leads to a gradual loss of clarity of vision, which over time may seriously interfere with sight and the activities of everyday living.

Approximately 40 percent of Americans between ages 55 and 64 have some degree of opaqueness in the lenses of their eyes. In fact, after age 65, at least half of all Americans have some clouding of the lens, though there may be no noticeable impairment of vision.

Causes and Risk Factors

The most significant risk factor for cataracts is the aging process—the risk of cataracts increases with age. But other factors play a role as well. For example, women are at greater risk than men, and African Americans are at greater risk than whites. Family history also is important.

The presence of any of the following medical conditions may increase the likelihood of developing cataracts: diabetes, glaucoma (and glaucoma treatments), high blood pressure, and connective tissue diseases such as rheumatoid arthritis. Prolonged sun exposure, long-term corticosteroid use, excess abdominal fat, smoking, excess alcohol use, and radiation exposure also have been associated with an increased risk of cataracts. People who have had an eye injury or eye surgery are more vulnerable, too.

Signs and Symptoms

Cataracts tend to develop very slowly and are rarely noticeable in their early stages. There is no pain. Instead, symptoms center around diminished vision. People may experience blurred vision, double vision, or even ghost images. Their night vision may decline, and their perception of colors tends to fade.

People with cataracts may become more sensitive to light or perceive light from the sun or a lamp as too bright. Yet in order to see, they may require ever-increasing amounts of lighting. They also may need frequent changes in their eyeglass prescriptions and/or contact lenses. Those who were farsighted may notice a shift toward nearsightedness.

Conventional Treatments

During the early stages of cataracts, the easiest and best treatments entail modest lifestyle changes. Visit your eye-care professional annually, and obtain eyeglass prescriptions or contact lenses that adequately address your changing needs. When you read, make sure that you have proper lighting. In fact, it might be a good idea to improve the lighting throughout your home. Halogen lights and 100- to 150-watt incandescent bulbs are particularly good. If necessary, buy and use a magnifying glass. Wear sunglasses outside. Reduce or discontinue night driving. For many people, these changes are sufficient to help them live with mild to moderate cataracts.

A Quick Guide to Symptoms

- ☐ Blurred vision
- ☐ Double vision
- ☐ Ghost images
- ☐ Increased sensitivity to light
- ☐ Diminished perception of colors
- ☐ Difficulty seeing at night
- ☐ Frequent changes in eyeglass prescriptions

Surgery

At some point, a cataract may so impede vision that surgery becomes necessary. In cataract surgery, the clouded lens is removed and replaced with an artificial lens. In most cases, this is an outpatient procedure that's performed under local anesthesia and completed in less than an hour. You will probably be given medication to help you relax.

The most common procedure is called phacoemulsification, in which the surgeon breaks up the clouded lens by emulsifying it with ultrasound waves. The remaining fragments are removed with suction. The lens capsule, or outer layer of the lens, remains intact.

If the cataract is quite large, the surgeon may recommend an extracapsular cataract extraction. In this procedure, a slightly larger incision is made, and the hard center of the lens is removed. The softer outer layer is removed by suctioning, and the capsule shell is left intact.

Once the cataract is gone, an artificial lens is implanted in the empty lens capsule. This implant, which is called an intraocular lens (IOL), may be made from silicone, acrylic, or plastic. It becomes a permanent part of the eye and requires no care.

Shortly after the surgical procedure, you will be able to return home (though you won't be able to drive for a while). You may feel drowsy, so you should rest and relax for the next 24 hours. Don't lift any heavy objects, either. Your physician will probably want to check your eye the next day and again in a month to six weeks. Your vision will likely remain blurred for several weeks.

Expect some pain for a few days; you can treat it with an over-the-counter medication. If you experience vision loss, severe pain, light flashes, numerous floaters (tiny spots that appear to float in your field of vision), marked eye redness, or nausea, coughing, or vomiting, contact your doctor immediately.

While complications from cataract surgery are rare, they do occur. Two of the primary risks are infection and retinal detachment. (The retina is the "screen" at the back of the eye on which images focus.) During your surgical follow-up visits, your doctor will be looking for these problems. Generally, when complications are treated early, the eye heals well.

Cataract surgery has been known to cause glaucoma, a condition in which the pressure inside the eye rises. To reduce the possibility of this occurring, you should minimize physical activity—especially exercise—during the postoperative period. If you must retrieve something for which you'd normally bend over, kneel down to the level of the object instead. Sit down when you put on your shoes. Sleep on your back or on the side that hasn't been operated on. You may resume reading, walking, eating, and watching television the evening after you've had surgery.

Complementary Treatments

When dealing with cataracts, complementary health care practitioners focus on stimulating bloodflow and strengthening the eyes. This is achieved primarily through improved nutrition and dietary supplements.

Diet

Studies show that antioxidant-rich foods, along with a healthy lifestyle, can reduce the risk of developing cataracts. Among the most beneficial antioxidants for eye health are lutein and zeaxanthin. Good sources of lutein and zeaxanthin include corn, egg yolks, and green vegetables, particularly broccoli, kale, and spinach. They also are found in cabbage, collard greens, green beans, green peas, and lettuce. Aim for at least four or five servings of these foods each week; one serving a day is even better. Research suggests that people who eat lots of spinach are at lower risk for developing cataracts.

Also be sure to get plenty of vitamin C in your diet. The lens of the eye actually absorbs vitamin C, so the more you consume, the more the lens will contain. Good food sources of vitamin C include oranges, melons, tomatoes, strawberries, red and green peppers, and sweet potatoes.

Beyond these specifics, it's a good idea to adhere to the basic principles of healthy

Cataract surgery is very common. It is the most frequently performed surgery among Americans age 65 and older. In the United States, there are about 1.5 million cataract surgeries every year.

eating—building meals around whole grains, vegetables, and fruits while avoiding foods high in hydrogenated fats, such as solid shortening, margarine, and anything deep-fried. A good benchmark is four servings of fruit, five servings of vegetables, and six servings of whole grains per day.

Foot Reflexology

In foot reflexology, the eye points are located at the base of the second and third toes. By applying finger pressure to this area, you help to improve circulation to the eyes. Tenderness

A Second Cataract

In about 15 to 20 percent of cases, the back of the lens capsule—the supporting part of the lens capsule, which is not removed during cataract surgery—becomes cloudy. This can occur months or years after the procedure. There is a quick treatment for this medical condition. It's called the neodymium: yttrium-aluminum-garnet (YAG) laser capsulotomy.

In a 5-minute procedure, the surgeon uses a laser beam to create a small opening in the clouded capsule, thereby allowing light to pass through. To ensure that the surgery has not raised eye pressure, you will probably be asked to remain at your doctor's office for an hour after the procedure.

here means that circulation to the eyes is blocked.

When working this area, you may feel what seem to be tiny crystals underneath the skin. If so, continue to apply gentle pressure, moving along the area until it feels smooth.

Herbal Medicine

Ginkgo biloba and bilberry extract are two herbal remedies that aid in improving the delivery of oxygen to the eyes. And because they're antioxidants, scavenging for free radicals, they help to slow the progression of cataracts.

The recommended dose of ginkgo is 120 milligrams, twice a day, of an extract standardized to 24 percent of flavone glycosides and 6 percent terpene lactones. The flavone glycosides give ginkgo its antioxidant benefits; the terpene lactones increase circulation and have a protective effect on nerve cells. *Note:* If you are taking a blood-thinning medication such as aspirin, consult your doctor before using ginkgo.

The recommended dose of bilberry is one 100-milligram capsule, standardized to 25 percent anthocyanosides, three times a day.

Homeopathy

Homeopathy is a healing system in which substances that produce symptoms of illness in healthy people are believed to have a healing effect when given in very minute quantities to sick people who exhibit the same symptoms. For cataracts, one commonly recommended homeopathic remedy is *Cineraria*. A derivative of the plant known as dusty miller, it is applied as drops to the eyes—1 drop per eye,

four or five times a day. This remedy has been used to treat corneal cloudiness. For optimal effectiveness, treatment must continue for several months.

Although high-dose homeopathic remedies are available from homeopaths and other trained practitioners, lower doses can be purchased in retail stores and online.

Nutritional Supplements

The best way to get the antioxidants that support eye health is through diet. If this is not possible, however, you may want to consider vitamin and mineral supplements. The nutrients below are helpful for maintaining eye health and, when taken in combination, may reduce your risk of developing cataracts.

- Vitamin A: 10,000 IU daily. Necessary for eye health; protects eyes from free radicals.

- B-complex vitamins: One capsule twice daily, with meals. The B vitamins help maintain eye health. They work best when taken together.

- Vitamin C: 1,000 milligrams daily, in divided doses (500 milligrams at breakfast and 500 milligrams before bed). Reduces the risk of developing cataracts. Because vitamin C and selenium interfere with each other's absorption, it's best to take these supplements separately.

- Vitamin E: 400 IU daily, taken at lunch or dinner. An antioxidant, vitamin E helps neutralize the free radicals that damage cell membranes.

- Copper: 2 milligrams daily. Plays a role in eye health.

- Lutein: 10 milligrams daily. An antioxidant that's present in the eye.

- Magnesium: 500 milligrams daily. Supports the absorption of vitamin C.

- Selenium: 200 micrograms daily, taken at lunch or dinner. Like vitamin E, selenium is an antioxidant. The two are better absorbed when taken together.

- Zinc: 30 milligrams daily. Zinc is another antioxidant, present in the retina of the eye. *Note:* Long-term use of zinc may impair the absorption of copper, potentially causing copper-induced anemia.

Lifestyle Recommendations

Certain prescription and over-the-counter medications may increase your risk of developing cataracts. They are photosensitizing— that is, they absorb light energy, which makes you more sensitive to sunlight. Moreover, the tissue of the eyes is chemically modified due to the photochemical reaction produced by the absorption of light. Among the drugs that have this effect are antihistamines, nonsteroidal anti-inflammatory drugs (including aspirin, ibuprofen, and drugs that contain them), antidepressants, oral diabetes medications, and sulfa drugs.

Even if it is medically necessary for you to use one or more of these medications on an ongoing basis, you may be able to limit your use. Ask your doctor. You should never stop or alter the dosage of any medication without your doctor's knowledge and approval.

Preventive Measures

Move your body for healthy eyes. Because it improves circulation, exercise enhances the delivery of nutrients to the eyes and facilitates the removal of waste products. The best form of exercise for the eyes is aerobic. Consider walking on a regular basis, gradually working up to daily 30-minute constitutionals.

Maintain proper weight. A high body mass index is a risk factor for cataract development. Excess abdominal weight, in particular, has a strong association with cataracts.

Stop smoking. The direct correlation between cataracts and smoking is well documented. In fact, it is believed that about 20 percent of cataract cases are related to smoking. Both men and women who smoke have significantly higher rates of cataracts than nonsmokers. Smoking is associated with high levels of the heavy metal cadmium in the lens. It also produces cyanide, a retinal toxin. If you smoke, quit. And do your best to avoid secondhand smoke.

Protect yourself from the sun. Most eye-care professionals agree that ongoing exposure to sunlight increases the risk of cataracts. When you head outdoors, it is a good idea to wear a protective hat and sunglasses that block out 100 percent of ultraviolet-A (UVA) and ultraviolet-B (UVB) rays and filter out at least 85 percent of blue-violet rays.

Be aware that certain medications, such as tetracycline, sulfa drugs, corticosteroids, and hydrocortisone, make the skin and the eyes more sensitive to light. Ask your doctor if any of your medications have this effect. If so, you need to be extra vigilant about protecting yourself from the sun.

Celiac Disease

Also known as celiac sprue, gluten-sensitive enteropathy, and nontropical sprue, celiac disease is a genetically transmitted autoimmune disorder. When someone with celiac disease eats foods containing the protein gluten (found in wheat, barley, and rye, and in oats from cross-contamination), an immune reaction occurs in the small intestine. Over time, the surface of the small intestine—with its hairlike projections known as villi—sustains damage. As a result, food cannot be absorbed properly (a problem known as malabsorption), and the nutrients vital to your body are eliminated in stool instead. This may lead to nutrient deficiencies in the nervous system, bones, brain, liver, and other organs, and may serve as a trigger for other illnesses. In addition, because of the damage to the villi, which contain the enzyme that helps to digest dairy products, many people with celiac disease are lactose intolerant.

Celiac disease is far more common than most of us may realize, affecting about one in 133 people by at least one estimate. Close relatives of those with celiac disease are at significantly higher risk themselves, with a one-in-22 chance of developing the condition. That said, only about 3 percent of cases of celiac disease have been diagnosed. This means that in the United States, more than 2.1 million Americans could have celiac disease and not know it.

People with celiac disease are at increased risk for other autoimmune disorders such as insulin-dependent (type 1) diabetes, thyroid disease, Sjögren's syndrome, and Addison's disease. Because of malabsorption, they are at higher risk for osteoporosis. Celiac disease has been linked to nervous system disorders such as seizures (epilepsy) and nerve damage. People who have celiac disease but continue to consume gluten are more likely to develop intestinal lymphoma and bowel cancer.

In Italy, researchers attempted to determine the prevalence of celiac disease in adults diagnosed with non-Hodgkin's lymphoma. Of 650 patients with lymphoma, six had antibody tests consistent with celiac disease. The researchers concluded that celiac disease is associated with an elevated risk of non-Hodgkin's lymphoma.

Causes and Risk Factors

Celiac disease has a strong genetic component. Though you may be born with the potential to develop the condition, experts believe that its onset requires some sort of environmental, physical, or emotional trigger, such as a particularly stressful situation or a bacterial or viral infection to which the immune system responds inappropriately. And you must be eating a diet that contains wheat, barley, rye, or oats.

Celiac disease may have some connection to breastfeeding. Those who were breastfed for longer periods tend to develop celiac disease later in life, and their symptoms may be atypical. Moreover, when and how celiac disease manifests may have something to do with how old a person is when he or she starts eating gluten-containing foods and how much gluten the person is consuming.

Although anyone may develop celiac disease, people of European descent are at increased risk. Women are diagnosed more often than men.

Signs and Symptoms

The symptoms of celiac disease can vary widely from one person to the next. Most people experience some form of gastrointestinal distress such as abdominal pain and bloating, constipation, and/or diarrhea. Their symptoms may be similar to other conditions such as irritable bowel syndrome and Crohn's disease. They may notice weight loss and general weakness, and they may pass foul-smelling stools that float.

Other symptoms of celiac disease include stomach upset, joint pain, skin rashes, depression, irritability, gas, behavioral changes, pale sores inside the mouth (aphthous ulcers), chronic fatigue, migraines, rheumatoid conditions, muscle cramps, dental and bone disorders, and tingling in the legs and feet (neuropathy). In some cases, there are no obvious symptoms, even though there is damage to the small intestine.

If you suspect that you are experiencing symptoms of celiac disease, you should see your doctor. But until you receive an official diagnosis, do not eliminate gluten from your diet. If you do, there is no way to ensure the accuracy of your diagnostic tests.

Dermatitis Herpetiformis

Though sometimes confused with celiac disease, dermatitis herpetiformis is a separate illness. Just like celiac disease, dermatitis herpetiformis is an autoimmune disorder that is caused by gluten intolerance—only it affects the skin, producing severe, itchy blisters that tend to appear on the elbows, knees, and buttocks. While people with this disorder do not experience the digestive symptoms of celiac disease, they may still show signs of intestinal damage.

Conventional Treatments

The most important treatment for celiac disease is to strictly avoid foods that contain gluten.

Dietary Modifications

Treatment for celiac disease involves the complete elimination of all gluten from the diet. This can be difficult, as gluten not only is found in obvious sources such as bread and pasta, it also may be hidden in sauces, soups, salad dressings, medications, supplements, and other products such as lipstick and postage stamps. There also is the consideration of possible cross-contamination: In kitchens where there are gluten-containing ingredients, it is very easy for gluten to find its way into "gluten-free" foods.

You will need to read product labels very carefully. Frequently it may take a phone call to a manufacturer to find out if a specific product contains gluten. When in doubt about a product, avoid it.

A Quick Guide to Symptoms

- ☐ Gastrointestinal problems such as abdominal pain and bloating, constipation, and/or diarrhea
- ☐ Weight loss
- ☐ General weakness or chronic fatigue
- ☐ Foul-smelling stools that float
- ☐ Joint pain or rheumatoid conditions
- ☐ Skin rashes
- ☐ Pale sores inside the mouth (aphthous ulcers)
- ☐ Depression, irritability, or behavior changes
- ☐ Gas
- ☐ Migraines
- ☐ Muscle cramps
- ☐ Dental and bone disorders
- ☐ Tingling in the legs and feet (neuropathy)

It is very important that you adhere to a gluten-free diet. If you accidentally ingest gluten, there is a good chance that you will develop symptoms such as abdominal pain and/or diarrhea. Even if you don't have symptoms, the gluten will do damage to the lining of your small intestine.

On occasion, people following a gluten-free diet will not get better, because the damage to the small intestine is so severe. Their doctors may recommend another course of treatment, such as intravenous nutritional support.

Complementary Treatments

Complementary medicine strives to reduce or eliminate the symptoms associated with celiac disease, often with help from acupuncture, lifestyle modification, and dietary supplements.

Acupuncture

Acupuncture is very helpful for treating the pain associated with celiac disease. To locate a qualified acupuncturist in your area, visit the Web site of the National Certification Commission for Acupuncture and Oriental Medicine (NCCAOM) at www.nccaom.org.

Diet

A review of dietary studies, published in the *American Journal of Clinical Nutrition*, confirmed that the most effective treatment for celiac disease is a gluten-free diet. Among patients who strictly adhered to a gluten-free regimen, there was a rapid improvement in symptoms.

Of course, following a gluten-free diet means steering clear of the gluten-containing grains—barley, rye, and wheat—and any products made with them. Among the acceptable grains and flours are arrowroot, buckwheat, corn, flax, millet, quinoa, rice, soy, and tapioca.

On January 1, 2006, the Food Allergen Labeling and Consumer Protection Act (FALCPA) went into effect, requiring any food that contains one of the top eight food allergens (eggs, fish, milk, peanuts, shellfish, soy, tree nuts, and wheat) to declare this information on the food label. The new law also directs the FDA to develop and implement a policy for use of the term *gluten-free* on product labels by August 2008.

Naturopathy

Naturopathic medicine is very effective in the treatment of digestive disorders such as celiac disease. The first step in the naturopathic healing process is to determine the underlying cause of an illness. Once this is done, the naturopath assumes the role of educator, showing a client why and how to restructure his diet and lifestyle. In naturopathy, proper diet and nutritional supplements are fundamental to healing and strengthening the various systems of the body. In order for a naturopathic program to be most beneficial, a person must be willing to make a commitment to change, as it may be necessary to restructure lifelong habits.

To find a naturopathic practitioner in your area, visit the Web site for the American Association of Naturopathic Physicians at www.naturopathic.org.

Nutritional Supplements

Because of their impaired ability to absorb vitamins and minerals, people with celiac disease often run the risk of developing nutrient deficiencies. Taking a daily multivitamin/mineral supplement may help to maintain proper levels of vital nutrients within the body. A B-complex supplement also is recommended, as the B vitamins are not well absorbed in the presence of celiac disease. Beyond the B-complex, a sublingual (under the tongue) supplement of 1,000 micrograms of vitamin B_{12} each day is recommended to support proper digestion and nutrient absorption.

Lifestyle Recommendations

Be wary of beer. Beer, ale, and lagers contain gluten and so are off-limits for those with celiac disease. Because of the distillation process, spirits and wine are gluten-free.

Pay attention for cross-contamination. Cross-contamination can occur in many ways. Foods prepared on a common surface, shared utensils and toasters, flour sifters, foods cooked in the same oil, and shared condiments may easily be overlooked as potential gluten sources.

Take care when you eat out. A number of restaurants throughout the United States now offer gluten-free items on their menus. You might telephone or e-mail a particular restaurant in advance and ask if it's possible to accommodate your diet. Or list your food restrictions on an index card and ask your server to share the card with the chef. If you find a few restaurants that are particularly accommodating, be sure to patronize them often.

Take extra precautions. Remember that the following items may contain gluten: energy bars, communion wafers, prescription and over-the-counter medications, herbal and dietary supplements, and marinades.

Stay active. Regular exercise helps expedite the transit time of food through the digestive tract, reduces pressure inside the colon, and promotes normal functioning of the bowels. For improved bowel health, try to squeeze at least 30 minutes of exercise into every day, or at least as many days as possible. One of the best forms of exercise is walking. If you have been fairly sedentary, be sure to check with your doctor before beginning an exercise regimen.

Manage the stress in your life. When you are under stress, your digestive system can become a sort of "holding tank" for tension-causing emotions, contributing to digestive distress. Try to incorporate stress-reduction techniques into your daily routine. Among your options: biofeedback, deep breathing, hypnosis, massage, meditation, and yoga.

Join a support group. Following a gluten-free diet can be challenging. In a support group, you can learn about your illness, ask questions, share concerns, and see how others cope. If you aren't comfortable with a "live" group, you might try an online group instead.

Visit a registered dietitian. Many people with celiac disease benefit from one or two visits with a registered dietitian. You might ask your doctor or your local hospital to recommend someone who's particularly knowledgeable about your condition.

Preventive Measures

Right now, there is no way to prevent celiac disease. To reduce your chances of a symptom flare-up, it is very important to follow a gluten-free diet. Otherwise, the damage to your small intestine will not heal, and you will be much more likely to develop celiac-related health problems and complications.

Colon Polyps

Colon polyps are benign or precancerous growths that occur in the colon or rectum. They appear as bumps that vary greatly in size, from less than ¼ inch to several inches in diameter.

There are two main types of colon polyps. A biopsy is necessary to differentiate between them.

Hyperplastic polyps tend to be small and located in the rectum or left lower (sigmoid) section of the colon. They are benign and do not develop into cancer.

Adenomas—which account for about two-thirds of all colon polyps—are believed to be a precursor to almost all forms of colon cancer. Large adenomatous polyps are more likely to contain cancerous cells than smaller ones. A person who has an adenoma in his or her colon is about twice as likely to develop colon cancer as someone who doesn't.

Colon polyps are quite common. The average 50-year-old with no special risk factors for colon polyps has about a 25 percent chance of getting them.

Causes and Risk Factors

Though the cause of colon polyps remains unknown, it may have something to do with not getting enough dietary fiber. A lack of dietary calcium also seems to play a role. Other risk factors include eating lots of red meat and smoking cigarettes.

The odds of developing colon polyps increase with age, with the highest risk among those over age 50. There may be a genetic link as well; you're more likely to develop colon polyps if a first-degree relative has a history of colon polyps or colon cancer or if you've already had a polyp yourself. In rare instances, colon polyps/colon cancer syndromes run in families, and members of those families are more likely to develop polyps at a younger age.

Signs and Symptoms

In the vast majority of cases, colon polyps cause no symptoms. Sometimes there's painless bleeding from the rectum or blood in the stool. Other possible symptoms include anemia, rectal muscle spasms (which make you feel as though you're about to have a bowel movement), cramps, abdominal pain, and intestinal obstructions.

A Quick Guide to Symptoms

- ☐ Painless rectal bleeding
- ☐ Blood in the stool
- ☐ Anemia
- ☐ Rectal muscle spasms
- ☐ Cramps or abdominal pain
- ☐ Intestinal obstructions

Conventional Treatments

Most colon polyps can be removed during a colonoscopy in a procedure known as a polypectomy. Smaller polyps are removed with an instrument known as a biopsy forceps, which snips off small pieces of tissue. Larger polyps usually are separated from the colon lining with a wire loop and/or burned at the base with an electric current. Since the colon lining is not sensitive to cutting or burning, there is no pain from either procedure. On rare occasions, a polyp may be too large to be removed during a colonoscopy, in which case surgery will be necessary.

If a polyp is benign, no further treatment is required. If it is cancerous, your doctor likely will recommend surgery. Generally, the surgeon will remove the section of the colon affected by the cancer, then stitch together the healthy ends of the colon. More serious cases may call for a colectomy, in which the entire colon or a significant section of it is removed.

When caught early, cancerous polyps may require no further treatment beyond surgery. Your doctor must make this determination.

Complementary Treatments
Diet

As mentioned earlier, people who don't get enough dietary fiber or who eat large amounts of red meat, fatty foods, and processed foods are more likely to develop colon polyps. If you have polyps or are at risk for a recurrence, try cutting back on red meat and other animal products and eating more fiber-rich plant foods—whole grains, fruits, and vegetables—instead. Aim for at least five servings of vegetables, four servings of fruit, and six servings of whole grains each day. This should get you to the American Dietetic Association's recommendation of 20 to 35 grams of fiber daily.

One caveat: If you haven't been eating a lot of fiber and you add too much fibrous food too quickly, you may trigger uncomfortable symptoms such as diarrhea, gas, bloating, cramping, or constipation. Increase your intake gradually. Be sure to drink enough fluids, too—at least eight 8-ounce glasses of water or noncaffeinated, nonalcoholic beverages each day.

Herbal Medicine

A natural anti-inflammatory, aloe vera juice may have a soothing effect on colon polyps. When buying aloe vera juice, look for a product with the label designation "IASC Certified," which means that it has been processed according to the standards of the International Aloe Science Council. The juice should be derived from the gel, not the latex, and contain 98 percent aloe vera. (Check the label for aloin or aloe-emodin compounds, both of which are substances in aloe latex. Aloe latex has a laxative effect.) The recommended dose is 1 tablespoon after each meal.

Nutritional Supplements

Certain supplements may be helpful in treating adenomatous colon polyps.

- Calcium: 1,500 milligrams daily; 1,200 milligrams daily for men over age 50. May help protect against a recurrence of adenomatous polyps. The lower dosage for men over age 50 is because of a possible connection between high doses of calcium and an increased risk of prostate cancer.

- Magnesium: 750 milligrams daily. Supports calcium absorption.

Preventive Measures

One study identified several lifestyle factors that can help protect against colon polyps. They include taking aspirin (81 milligrams) or another nonsteroidal analgesic and getting

Anyone age 50 or older should be periodically screened for colon polyps.

Lifestyle Recommendations

Be vigilant about screenings. If you've already had an adenomatous polyp, you are at higher risk for getting another one. So don't put off your next colonoscopy. Catching a polyp early allows for its removal while it's still small.

Take an aspirin. Preliminary studies show that a daily aspirin reduces the incidence of colon polyps. Aspirin therapy also may help keep polyps from developing into colon cancer.

more dietary fiber and vitamin D. In particular, taking a supplement of vitamin D (400 IU) plus calcium (500 milligrams) on a daily basis is a good preventive strategy, as is consuming dairy products.

Don't smoke. If you smoke, you are more likely to develop colon polyps, among other medical conditions.

Stay active. In studies, moderate to vigorous exercise for 60 minutes a day was shown to reduce the cell growth that leads to polyp formation.

Coronary Artery Disease

Coronary artery disease, or CAD (sometimes called coronary heart disease), is caused by the gradual buildup of plaque deposits in the coronary arteries, a problem known as atherosclerosis. Over time, these deposits—which consist of fat, cholesterol, calcium, and other cellular sludge—narrow the coronary arteries. Less blood is able to flow to the heart, which may trigger chest pain, or angina. A sudden, complete blockage of an artery could lead to a heart attack.

CAD is the most common form of cardiovascular disease, affecting about 7 million Americans. It is also the leading cause of death in the United States. Every year, 500,000 Americans die from a heart attack caused by CAD.

Causes and Risk Factors

Recent studies suggest that inflammation plays an important role in coronary artery disease, as do other medical conditions such as high blood pressure (hypertension) and high blood levels of LDL cholesterol. Though people often are unaware that they have coronary artery disease—in its earliest stages, it may not produce symptoms—a number of factors are known to increase risk. These include a family history of heart disease, smoking, obesity, physical inactivity, diabetes, stress, and unexpressed anger.

Depression is a risk factor for the development of CAD in people who are otherwise healthy, as well as for adverse cardiovascular outcomes in those with known heart disease. In fact, depression is present in about 20 percent of outpatients and one-third of inpatients with CAD. What is not yet known is whether treating depression with medication will improve cardiovascular outcomes. Still, those with CAD should be considered at risk for depression.

While young people may develop coronary artery disease, it is much more common in those at midlife and older. Until then, men are more likely to have CAD than women.

The pain from a heart attack may be quite intense, and it lasts considerably longer than the pain of angina. But not all heart attacks cause chest pain. Other symptoms include pain in the jaw, neck, or back, as well as nausea, shortness of breath, weakness, or fatigue.

If you're experiencing these or any other symptoms of a heart attack, call 911 or your emergency medical number. It is vital to seek medical attention without delay.

Signs and Symptoms

As mentioned earlier, coronary artery disease doesn't always produce symptoms. Even though the narrowed arteries are impeding the flow of blood—and therefore the delivery of vital nutrients and oxygen to the heart (a condition called ischemia)—a person may not notice any difference in his or her health.

This is known as silent ischemia, and it is the most common manifestation of CAD.

When symptoms do occur, they may include shortness of breath, irregular heartbeat, and chest pain (angina). A heart attack caused by a blocked coronary artery is another symptom of CAD.

A Quick Guide to Symptoms

☐ **Shortness of breath**
☐ **Irregular heartbeat**
☐ **Chest pain (angina)**

Conventional Treatments
Lifestyle Changes

Treating coronary artery disease often begins with lifestyle changes. Your doctor probably will review various lifestyle factors with you to determine whether they require modification. He or she may recommend improving your diet, starting an exercise program, losing weight, giving up smoking, cutting back on alcohol, and reducing the stress in your life (or learning to cope with stressors that you can't avoid).

Medications

Aspirin. To reduce the likelihood of a blood clot developing and lodging in a narrowed coronary artery, your doctor may advise you to take a low-dose aspirin daily. Aspirin helps to prevent blood platelets from sticking together and forming clots.

Beta-blockers and calcium-channel blockers. Among the prescription medications that help treat CAD are beta-blockers and calcium-channel blockers.

Beta-blockers, such as atenolol (Tenormin) and metoprolol (Lopressor), slow heart rate and lower blood pressure, so the heart doesn't need as much oxygen. These drugs have been shown to reduce the risk of dying from a heart attack, to prevent recurrent heart attacks, and to improve the odds of survival among patients who've had heart attacks.

Calcium-channel blockers, such as verapamil (Calan) and nifedipine (Procardia), relax the muscles surrounding the coronary arteries, so the arteries can open up.

Cholesterol-lowering medications. Many people with coronary artery disease have elevated cholesterol levels. If this is true for you, your doctor may prescribe a cholesterol-lowering medication. There are several categories of these drugs (including statins, niacin, fibrates, and bile acid sequestrants), and they work in various ways. Besides lowering cholesterol, the statins have anti-inflammatory properties—and since CAD is an inflammatory process, it may respond particularly well to treatment with these drugs.

Nitrates. If you're experiencing chest pain (angina) from CAD, your doctor may recommend any of a class of medications called nitrates for use in emergencies. The best known of the nitrates is nitroglycerin, but these drugs are sold under a variety of generic and brand names. Some are meant to be swallowed; others dissolve under the tongue; and still others, in liquid form, are to be sprayed into the mouth. Nitrates work by opening the arteries and reducing the heart's need for oxygen.

Surgery

If lifestyle changes and medication do not relieve CAD symptoms, the next step may be surgery. Your doctor may recommend one of the following procedures.

Atherectomy. This procedure is an option for those patients who are not candidates for a balloon angioplasty (described next). In an atherectomy, a flexible hollow tube called a catheter is slowly threaded through a small incision underneath the arm or in the groin into the narrowed coronary artery. At the end of the tube is a tiny, high-speed drill, which shaves plaque from the arterial wall.

Balloon angioplasty and laser ablation. As in an atherectomy, a balloon angioplasty involves inserting a catheter into an artery and slowly threading it toward the heart. Once the catheter is in place in the narrowed area of the artery, a balloon at the tip of the tube is inflated. This compresses the plaque against the arterial wall, allowing blood to flow more freely.

In laser ablation, the cardiologist first uses a laser to burn away some of the arterial plaque. Then a balloon further opens the artery.

About 35 percent of people who undergo either of these procedures eventually develop more blockages in the treated area, a condition known as restenosis. To keep this from happening, the cardiologist may place a small metal rod, or stent, inside the artery to help keep it open. Among people who receive stents, the rate of restenosis is between 15 and 20 percent. The use of a polymer-based, paclitaxel-coated stent instead of a bare metal stent may lower the risk of restenosis even further.

Bypass surgery. In this procedure—the full name is coronary artery bypass graft surgery—the surgeon removes pieces of vein or artery from a patient's legs and/or chest and sews the pieces into the arteries of the heart. This allows blood to "bypass" the blocked arteries by flowing through the replacement vessels. Though these surgeries have an excellent success rate, they are major procedures, generally requiring at least 1 week of hospitalization and several weeks for recovery.

A newer procedure, called minimally invasive direct coronary artery bypass, may be performed on a beating heart without using a heart-lung machine. It also requires a smaller incision.

Transmyocardial laser revascularization. This procedure is particularly useful for patients who have angina that is not responsive to other treatment or who experience residual angina after bypass surgery. It may be performed by a cardiologist in a cardiac catheterization lab.

After numbing an area of the leg with anesthesia, the cardiologist inserts a catheter into a leg artery. Once the catheter reaches the heart, the laser makes 10 to 20 tiny channels in the heart muscle. Blood flows into these channels, giving the heart muscle the additional oxygen that it needs. The procedure may lead to the formation of additional vessels as well.

Complementary Treatments

The best complementary treatments for coronary artery disease are those that support a conventional treatment plan. A person with CAD always should be under a doctor's care.

Ayurveda

Ayurveda—a discipline with Indian roots dating back some 5,000 years—combines exercise, herbal remedies, massage, meditation, and nutrition in a holistic approach to healing. Ayurvedic practitioners view the heart as the most important organ and the seat of human consciousness. Health problems arise when we ignore the heart—not only through physical inactivity and poor diet but also through a lack of emotional attachment and spirituality. In Ayurveda, the emotions are key to the health of the heart and always are considered during treatment. An Ayurvedic treatment plan for coronary artery disease might include dietary and lifestyle changes, herbs, meditation, and yoga.

There is no professional organization that offers certification or membership to Ayurvedic practitioners. The Ayurvedic Institute may provide the names of practitioners in your area. Visit the institute's Web site at www.ayurveda.com.

Diet

Research shows that a diet heavy on fruits and vegetables—particularly leafy greens and vitamin C–rich produce—helps protect against coronary artery disease. According to an article in the March 2007 issue of the *American Journal of Clinical Nutrition*, some studies further suggest that these foods could reduce the risk of death from CAD. Try to eat at least four servings of fruits and five servings of vegetables, along with six servings of whole grains, each day.

Be sure to leave room in your diet for nuts and seeds such as walnuts, almonds, and sesame seeds, which help maintain a healthy heart. And don't forget the following foods and nutrients, all of which play roles in heart health.

- Fish oil from cold-water fish such as bluefish, herring, salmon, and tuna helps to lower blood pressure, cholesterol, and triglycerides. It also may prevent blood clots. Fish oil is rich in heart-friendly omega-3 fatty acids, which include EPA (eicosapentaenoic acid), DHA (docosahexaenoic acid), and ALA (alpha-linolenic acid). If you're not fond of fish or the aftertaste of fish oil supplements, you might try flaxseed oil instead. It's abundant in ALA, which the body converts to EPA and DHA.

- Beta-carotene is found in fruits and vegetables at the red-to-yellow end of the color spectrum. It's what gives these foods their vibrant hues.

- You can get a modest amount of vitamin C from virtually any fruit or vegetable. Among the very best sources are strawberries, cranberries, melons, oranges, mangoes, papayas, peppers, spinach, kale, broccoli, tomatoes, and potatoes.

• Vitamin E is found in vegetable oils, nuts, seeds, and wheat germ, with smaller amounts coming from leafy vegetables and whole grains.

• Food sources of the B vitamins include leafy dark green vegetables, whole grains, oranges, avocados, beets, bananas, potatoes, dairy products, nuts, beans, fish, and chicken.

• Magnesium—an important nutrient for heart health—comes from leafy green vegetables such as spinach, parsley, broccoli, chard, kale, and mustard and turnip greens, as well as raw almonds, wheat germ, potatoes, and tofu.

• Food sources of selenium include seafood, chicken, whole-grain cereals, and garlic.

• Anthocyanosides are compounds with antioxidant properties. They also help improve blood circulation in the capillaries. The European species of blueberry, called bilberry, contains the most anthocyanosides. Other good sources include blueberries, cherries, raspberries, red or purple grapes, and plums.

• Garlic, onions, cayenne pepper, ginger, turmeric, and alfalfa all reduce blood cholesterol, an important benefit for heart health. Garlic, onions, and cayenne pepper also help thin the blood, which keeps clots from forming.

• Foods derived from soybeans, such as tofu and soy milk, have been shown to help lower cholesterol as well.

Note: If you are taking a prescription medication—including any cholesterol-lowering drug—for a heart condition, talk with your doctor before making changes in your diet. This will reduce the likelihood of an interaction between the medication and any new foods or nutrients.

Herbal Medicine

Ginkgo biloba. Ginkgo is an antioxidant that supports circulation. It is sold raw or in capsule form. The recommended daily dose is 120 milligrams twice a day of extract standardized to 24 percent flavone glycosides and 6 percent terpene lactones. The flavone glycosides give ginkgo its antioxidant properties, while terpene lactones improve circulation. *Note:* If you are taking a prescription blood-thinning medication, be sure to consult your doctor before adding ginkgo supplements to your self-care regimen.

Green tea. Green tea contains high levels of substances called polyphenols, which have powerful antioxidant properties. It also helps to lower cholesterol and blood pressure, and to keep arteries from clogging.

Green tea may be taken as a tea or in capsules. Prepared tea bags are readily available in grocery and health food stores. To brew the tea from dried leaves, steep 1 teaspoon of the herb in 1 cup of boiling water for 2 to 3 minutes. (The tea can become bitter if it steeps too long.) Strain and allow to cool before drinking. Three cups of tea per day may provide 240 to 320 milligrams of polyphenols.

In capsule form, a standardized extract of EGCG (a polyphenol) provides 97 percent polyphenol content. This is the equivalent of drinking 4 cups of green tea per day.

Hawthorn. Hawthorn works to lower cholesterol and blood pressure. It also strengthens the heart muscle, improves circulation, and rids the body of unnecessary fluid and salt.

Hawthorn is available in capsule or tincture form, standardized to 2.2 percent total bioflavonoid content. The recommended daily dose of hawthorn capsules varies widely, ranging from 100 to 300 milligrams, two or three times per day. Be aware that higher doses may significantly lower blood pressure, which may cause you to faint. For the tincture, the recommended dose is 4 to 5 milliliters, three times per day.

It may take up to 2 months before you notice any effects from this herb.

Nutritional Supplements

All of the following nutritional supplements have proven benefits for heart health.

- B-complex vitamins: Take as directed on the label. Together the B vitamins help keep blood clots from forming and arteries from clogging.

- Vitamin B_6: 50 milligrams daily, in divided doses of 25 milligrams. Supports the absorption of calcium, magnesium, and vitamin C.

- Vitamin C: 1,000 milligrams daily, in divided doses of 500 milligrams. Essential for heart health. Vitamin C converts cholesterol into bile, strengthens the arterial walls, and stops cholesterol buildup.

- Calcium: 1,500 milligrams daily, in divided doses of 750 milligrams. Lowers total cholesterol while increasing HDL cholesterol.

- Chromium: 200 micrograms daily. Helps prevent cholesterol buildup; increases HDL cholesterol.

- Coenzyme Q_{10}: 200 milligrams daily, in divided doses of 100 milligrams. Supports the delivery of oxygen to the heart tissue. Also may help lower blood pressure and prevent oxidation of LDL cholesterol.

- Vitamin E: 400 IU daily; take with selenium (below) for optimal absorption. Stops the oxidation of LDL cholesterol, prevents damage to the arterial lining, improves circulation, and fortifies the immune system. *Note:* Because vitamin E may thin the blood, talk with your doctor before taking vitamin E if you are already on a blood-thinning medication.

- L-carnitine: 500 milligrams daily, in divided doses of 250 milligrams. Lowers total cholesterol while increasing HDL cholesterol.

- Magnesium: 800 milligrams daily, in divided doses of 400 milligrams. Helps to lower total cholesterol while increasing HDL cholesterol.

- Selenium: 400 micrograms daily, in divided doses of 200 micrograms. Helps prevent heart disease and future heart attacks by thinning the blood. For this reason, you should check with your doctor before taking selenium if you're already on a blood-thinning medication. Also, do not take selenium at the same time as vitamin C, as they interfere with each other's absorption.

Relaxation/Meditation

Many physicians recommend relaxation techniques to their patients with coronary artery disease to help alleviate stress as well as manage their blood pressure. In clinical trials, the combination of biofeedback, meditation, and yoga has proven effective in lowering blood pressure. For reducing stress, beneficial techniques include qigong, tai chi, visualization, and deep breathing exercises.

To try deep breathing, lie flat on your back on your bed or the floor. Place both hands on your abdomen. Slowly inhale through your nose, pushing your abdomen upward as though inflating a balloon. Then slowly exhale through your mouth, allowing your abdomen to "deflate" as you do. Repeat 8 to 10 times. Practice this exercise as often as necessary.

Lifestyle Recommendations

Exercise caution with coffee. To date, studies have not identified a definitive link between coffee consumption and heart disease risk. Still, there are points worth pondering. For example, caffeine can elevate stress hormones, which is not helpful if you're already under stress and dealing with high blood pressure. Caffeine also robs the body of essential nutrients, particularly calcium, magnesium, and the B vitamins, all of which are important for maintaining a healthy heart as you age. On the other hand, one study has shown that the caffeine in coffee may provide a beneficial boost for people with low blood pressure, or hypotension.

What does all of this mean? The current consensus is that moderate coffee consumption will not elevate your heart disease risk— "moderate" being the operative word. This means no more than 2 cups of coffee a day. Be sure that the rest of your lifestyle supports a healthy heart through proper diet, regular exercise, adequate sleep, and plenty of relaxation.

Stay active. If you have coronary artery disease, you may be tempted to stop exercising. Don't. And if you haven't been exercising regularly, now is the time to start. Your doctor can help you develop a program that's appropriate for your health status and fitness level. You can ease into your exercise program with something as simple as a 5-minute walk, then gradually increase the length of your workouts over time until you're putting in at least 40 minutes a day.

Regular exercise, particularly aerobic activity, lowers blood pressure and heart rate, which in turn improves bloodflow through the arteries. Further, exercise can help you lose weight and manage stress, which together help manage and reduce CAD symptoms.

Stop smoking. The carbon monoxide produced by cigarette smoking decreases oxygen in the blood, forcing the heart to work harder. Smoking also causes blood platelets to stick together, which raises the risk of blood clots and blocked arteries. In some instances, smoking may interfere with prescription medication as well.

Depression

We all have days when we feel unhappy and overwhelmed with problems. It would be abnormal to go through life in a perpetual state of gleefulness. But if negative feelings continue for at least 2 weeks and begin to interfere with work, family, and daily activities, you may be dealing with depression. Depression may impair your cognitive abilities as well as your mental and physical well-being. It may affect how you sleep and eat.

There are several forms of depression. The most common is major depression, in which you feel plagued with sorrow or grief and/or disinterested in everyday activities that you once enjoyed. You may be tired or have trouble sleeping, and you may gain or lose weight. Another form of depression is dysthymia, a low-intensity mood disorder that is not as intense as depression but can last for more than 2 years.

Some people cycle between periods of depression and periods of euphoria. This is called bipolar disorder (formerly manic depression), a condition that affects between 2 million and 3 million Americans. Others tend to experience depression in fall and winter but not in spring or summer. This condition, called seasonal affective disorder (SAD), affects about one in 20 adults—though only about 20 percent of them are men. Those who live in colder climates, where there is limited sun in the late fall and winter, are more likely to develop SAD.

At any point in time, about 19 million Americans suffer from depression. During the course of their lives, about one in five Americans will have at least one period of depression. Yet about one-third of those who are depressed are unaware of it, while two-thirds of those who do know they are depressed fail to obtain the treatment they need. Their doctors may not recognize the illness, or they may not seek help for fear of being stigmatized socially or penalized by their insurance companies. Of course, the very nature of the illness makes it less likely that someone with depression will seek help.

Causes and Risk Factors

Depression affects people of all ages and all walks of life. Often it's triggered by a major life event such as the death of a close family member or the collapse of a marriage. Childhood abuse or other past trauma, chemical dependency, and surviving a catastrophe also can bring about a depressive episode.

A number of other factors can increase a person's chances of developing depression. Family history is important; if you have family members who've dealt with depression, you may be at higher risk. People at midlife are vulnerable to depression, as they deal with various life adjustments and crises. Those who are highly creative are more likely than the general population to develop depression.

If you've already had one depressive

episode, you have a 50-50 chance of a recurrence. Your risk jumps to 70 percent with two depressive episodes.

Certain medications can cause depression with long-term use. The list includes the following:

- Diazepam (Valium) and chlordiazepoxide (Librium), which are anti-anxiety drugs

- Interferon (Avonex, Rebetron), an anti-inflammatory

- Prednisone (Deltasone, Orasone), a corticosteroid

- Propranolol (Inderal), a heart and blood pressure medication

- Tamoxifen (Nolvadex), an anticancer drug

A Quick Guide to Symptoms

- ☐ **Depressed mood**
- ☐ **A feeling of irritability, annoyance, or agitation**
- ☐ **Inability to find pleasure or joy in life**
- ☐ **Difficulty remembering and thinking clearly**
- ☐ **Disturbed sleep**
- ☐ **Neglect of appearance**
- ☐ **Disregard for basic responsibilities**
- ☐ **More conflicts with spouse or family members**
- ☐ **Diminished sex drive**
- ☐ **Reduced self-esteem**
- ☐ **A sense of hopelessness**
- ☐ **Weight gain or loss**
- ☐ **Thoughts of death or suicide**

People with certain medical conditions are at greater risk for depression. For example, about 30 percent of patients hospitalized for coronary artery disease have some form of depression, as do about half of all patients who've suffered heart attacks.

Depression also is common in people who've suffered strokes and in those with Alzheimer's or Parkinson's disease. And anyone who has ever dealt with chronic pain knows how easy it is to become profoundly depressed. Indeed, depression is routinely seen in people who are dealing with serious or chronic illness.

Signs and Symptoms

The most common symptom of depression is a depressed mood. You may be sad and tearful; you may feel that your situation is hopeless; you may have a sense of worthlessness. But not everyone with depression actually feels depressed. Instead, they may be irritable, annoyed, or agitated. Even if they don't feel sad, very little in life brings them pleasure or joy.

Depression may affect your memory and your ability to think clearly, making even the smallest decision seem too difficult. Depression also tends to interfere with sleep. You may awaken too early in the morning and be unable to fall back to sleep. Or you may spend a good deal of your day in bed; simply getting up requires a Herculean effort.

People who are depressed may neglect their appearance or disregard basic responsibilities, such as paying bills. On the job, they may be unable to keep up with their workload, and co-workers may notice changes in their behavior. It is not uncommon for people who are depressed to have more conflicts with spouses or family members.

Doctors will diagnose major depression in people who have at least five of the following symptoms: diminished energy, reduced self-esteem, a feeling of hopelessness, disturbed sleep, an inability to concentrate, impaired thinking, weight gain or loss, diminished sexual desire, restlessness or slowed movement, and thoughts of death or suicide. Major depression may occur along with another medical condition, such as anxiety disorder. Untreated, major depression may last for 6 to 18 months. Early treatment may prevent depression from becoming more severe, and continued treatment may prevent a recurrence.

Dysthymia has many of the same symptoms as major depression, but they tend to be less intense. They also last longer—at least 2 years. In fact, it is not unusual for dysthymia to persist for more than 5 years. In about three-quarters of cases, people with dysthymia have another medical condition.

As mentioned earlier, people with bipolar disorder experience manic symptoms in addition to depression. These include euphoria, irritability, grandiosity (a sense of importance out of proportion to reality), excessive talking, and disturbed sleep. Bipolar disorder may become much worse over time if it isn't treated properly.

Among people with seasonal affective disorder, the most common symptom is fatigue in the fall and winter. Their mood may change, with feelings of sadness. They also tend to eat more (especially carbohydrates) and sleep more than normal, which often leads to weight gain. A small number of those with SAD actually eat and sleep less.

Conventional Treatments

The best treatment for depression is a combination of medication and counseling. In recent years, however, insurers have begun limiting coverage for therapy and instead emphasize pharmacological treatment as a way to rein in costs. If a patient with depression seems in danger of harming himself or herself, the treating physician may recommend hospitalization.

Cognitive-Behavioral Therapy

The premise of cognitive-behavioral therapy is that you become what you think. Thus, if you continue to think negative, depressive thoughts, you're likely to remain depressed. Through sessions of CBT, you will learn to replace negative thoughts with positive ones. Your therapist may ask you to keep a journal of your thoughts and responses. Then, working together, the two of you will find alternatives to the negative thoughts.

CBT typically lasts for about 12 to 16 sessions. After these sessions, you will be able to practice the techniques by yourself. The combination of CBT and appropriate medication tends to be more effective than either treatment alone.

Electroconvulsive Therapy

Electroconvulsive therapy has improved dramatically since its earliest days, when it was known as shock therapy. Today, it's most often used as a treatment for severe depression, especially in cases that do not respond to medications. Generally, patients will receive 6 to 12 treatments over a period of about 4 weeks.

In a typical ECT session, a patient receives a muscle relaxant followed by a short-acting general anesthetic. Then a mild electric current is sent to the brain, causing a seizure that lasts for about 40 seconds. The entire treatment lasts only about 15 to 20 minutes, though recovering from the anesthesia adds time.

ECT does not require hospitalization. It does have a few potential side effects, including headache, nausea, muscle soreness, temporary confusion, memory lapses, and heart disturbances. ECT is successful in about 80 percent of cases.

Medications

In prescribing medications for depression, a physician has two main objectives: relieving symptoms and keeping depressive episodes from returning. Depending upon each unique set of circumstances, a patient may require treatment for only a brief period, for an extended period, or for the rest of his or her life.

Keep in mind that if you don't see improvement with one medication, it doesn't mean that none of the antidepressants will work for you. Research has shown that after initial treatment with an SSRI failed to provide relief from depression, about one in four patients experienced improvement in their symptoms once they switched to another antidepressant.

Antianxiety drugs. It is not unusual for depression and anxiety to occur together. Since antidepressants can take several weeks to begin working, your doctor may prescribe a short-term course of anti-anxiety medications. The most commonly prescribed of these medications, the benzodiazepines, work quickly—often in 30 to 90 minutes—to relieve anxiety. They have no effect on depression, however. Among the best known of the benzodiazepines are diazepam (Valium), alprazolam (Xanax), and chlordiazepoxide (Librium).

All of these drugs have potential side effects, such as sleepiness, dizziness, memory impairment, and reduced muscle coordination. It also is relatively easy to become addicted to them. When discontinuing these medications, do so gradually by slowly lowering the dosage. Then you're less likely to experience withdrawal symptoms such as insomnia, headache, trembling, nausea, irritability, and loss of appetite.

Anticonvulsants. Though generally used for seizure disorders, anticonvulsants such as valproate (Depakote) and carbamazepine (Tegretol) may be helpful for depression associated with bipolar disorder. Both have potential side effects. Valproate may cause digestive problems, sleepiness, increased appetite, and weight gain, while carbamazepine has been linked to headache, nausea, dizziness, sleepiness, skin rash, and confusion.

Anticonvulsants are known to cause liver problems in some people. For this reason, your doctor probably will want to do a blood test to check your liver function both before prescribing one of these drugs and during treatment.

Antipsychotic medications. Depression accompanied by hallucinations or delusions—a condition known as psychosis—may require treatment with an antipsychotic medication such as haloperidol (Haldol) or trifluoperazine (Stelazine). Though these medications generally are effective, they frequently cause side effects such as sleepiness, blurred vision, dry mouth, weight gain, constipation, and increased sun sensitivity.

Designer antidepressants. The so-called designer antidepressants relieve depression by elevating serotonin and inhibiting the uptake of norepinephrine, both of which are brain neurotransmitters. One of these drugs, venlafaxine (Effexor), may increase blood pressure. Another, mirtazapine (Remeron), may cause blurred vision, weight gain, and slight elevations of cholesterol and triglyceride levels. Because it may induce drowsiness, it may be helpful for those with insomnia.

Bupropion (Wellbutrin) has relatively few side effects, including a low incidence of sexual dysfunction. Still, in high doses, it has been linked to anorexia, bulimia, and an increased risk of seizures, usually in those with a history of seizures.

Lithium. Lithium, a well-known mood stabilizer, has been available in the United

If you think you may be depressed, you might want to complete a confidential diagnostic questionnaire. These forms are available online through a number of groups, such as the National Mental Health Association (www.depression-screening.org).

States since the 1970s. In 60 to 80 percent of people with bipolar disorder, it effectively controls mania and reduces sadness.

Some medications may raise blood levels of lithium by inhibiting its excretion by the kidneys. Among the medications known to have this effect are the nonsteroidal anti-inflammatory drugs such as ibuprofen (Advil, Motrin, and other over-the-counter products), naproxen (Aleve, Naprosyn), and ketoprofen (Orudis). Likewise, certain blood pressure medications may decrease blood levels of lithium. These medications include hydrochlorothiazide (Diuril, HydroDiuril) and angiotensin-converting enzyme inhibitors such as benazepril (Lotensin), captopril (Capoten), enalapril (Vasotec), fosinopril (Monopril), lisinopril (Prinivil, Zestril), moexipril (Univasc), perindopril (Aceon), quinapril (Accupril), ramipril (Altace), and trandolapril (Mavik). Your doctor likely will monitor your blood levels of lithium while you are taking the drug.

By itself, lithium can cause a number of unpleasant side effects, such as diarrhea, nausea, confusion, fatigue, hand tremors, thirst, and excessive urination.

Monoamine oxidase inhibitors. Monoamine oxidase inhibitors (MAOIs), such as phenelzine (Nardil) and tranylcypromine (Parnate), are effective antidepressants. They must be used with caution, however, since they can cause insomnia, drowsiness, weight gain, sexual dysfunction, and other side effects. Further, if someone who's taking an MAOI eats foods rich in the amino acid compound tyramine—such as red wine, vermouth, canned figs, fava beans, dried meat and fish, and cheese—the combination may trigger a sudden and dangerous rise in blood pressure.

MAOIs may interact with certain over-the-counter medications such as decongestants and cough medications. And if an MAOI is taken at the same time as an SSRI (see below), the combination can cause a fatal reaction. For this reason, MAOIs should never be used with other antidepressants. Still, this class of drugs may be helpful when other antidepressants have not been effective.

Mood stabilizers. Mood stabilizers are prescribed for people with bipolar disorder. They help control the swings between mania and depression by stimulating the release of the neurotransmitter glutamate.

Selective serotonin reuptake inhibitors. Commonly known as SSRIs, this class of drugs—which includes fluoxetine (Prozac), sertraline (Zoloft), paroxetine (Paxil), fluvoxamine (Luvox), escitalopram (Lexapro), and citalopram (Celexa)—works by raising the concentration of serotonin in the brain. These drugs need time to take effect—typically 2 to 4 weeks, longer in some people. Still, they've been very successful in treating depression.

SSRIs have some unpleasant side effects, including nausea, agitation, insomnia, restlessness, weight gain, and sexual dysfunction. Rarer, but potentially life-threatening, is a side effect known as serotonin syndrome. Usually it occurs when an SSRI interacts with another antidepressant, most commonly an MAOI, though it also can happen with a supplement that influences serotonin, such as the herb St. John's wort. Symptoms of serotonin syndrome include blood pressure and heart rhythm fluctuations, confusion, hallucinations, fever, seizures, and coma.

Tricyclic antidepressants. This class of drugs—which includes imipramine (Tofranil) and amitriptyline (Elavil, Endep)—has been in use since the 1950s. These drugs do have significant side effects, such as weight gain, sexual dysfunction, mental disturbances and sleep disturbances, and a sudden drop in blood pressure upon standing, which could lead to fainting. These drugs may be effective when other classes of antidepressants haven't produced the desired results.

Phototherapy

Phototherapy, or light therapy, is a common treatment for people with seasonal affective disorder. Since this type of depression is associated with a lack of sunlight, phototherapy involves exposure to very bright light from a specialized light box. The patient places the box on a table or desk and sits near it for 15 minutes to 2 hours every day. Some research suggests that phototherapy is most effective when done in the morning.

Talk Therapy

There are several forms of talk therapy, or psychotherapy. You might meet with a therapist on your own, or with a few family members present. There's also group therapy, in which several people—all unrelated—meet together for treatment.

Just as the forms of talk therapy vary, so do the training and credentials of the professionals who offer it. A psychiatrist is a trained therapist who also is a medical doctor, and so is able to prescribe medication. Psychologists usually have doctorate degrees; they may provide counseling, but in general, they can't write prescriptions. Some social workers and psychiatric nurses are qualified therapists, as are some members of the clergy.

Talk with your doctor about the various options in talk therapy. Together, the two of you can decide which option is best for you.

Complementary Treatments

To treat depression, the best complementary approaches are those that stimulate the release of brain chemicals to relieve symptoms, raise your energy level, and improve your sense of well-being.

Acupuncture

Studies have shown that electroacupuncture may be as effective in relieving depression as the prescription drug amitriptyline, a tricyclic antidepressant. Acupuncture treatment prompts the release of serotonin, enkephalins, and endorphins, neurotransmitters that help improve mood and reduce pain.

Acupuncture works best when combined with movement therapies such as exercise, tai chi, and yoga. Together they facilitate the flow of stagnant energy, or qi.

To find an acupuncturist in your area, visit the Web site of the National Certification Commission for Acupuncture and Oriental Medicine (NCCAOM) at www.nccaom.org.

Diet

Avoid refined foods and processed foods as much as possible. The same goes for trans-fatty acids, found in french fries, doughnuts, and some commercially baked goods. All of these foods contain unhealthy chemicals that may disrupt your body's functions, particularly the production of brain chemicals that influence your mood.

Replace these foods with healthier choices such as fruits, vegetables, soy foods, and starches such as pasta, rice, cereal grains, breads, and legumes. These are complex carbohydrates, which are necessary for energizing the body and creating a sense of well-being.

Herbal Medicine

St. John's wort has a long-standing reputation as a treatment for depression. It is widely used in Europe as an antidepressant, and it's gaining popularity in the United States as well. But it's gotten mixed reviews in studies to date, producing either remarkable results or no effect at all. Most likely, the response simply varies from person to person. Because St. John's wort can interfere with certain prescription medications, be sure to talk with your doctor before you try it.

For clients with depression, some herbalists recommend a tea made from a combination of herbs such as St. John's wort, peppermint, and lavender. These herbs are readily available in health food stores. To make a tea, steep 1 teaspoon of dried lavender flowers, 1 teaspoon of dried peppermint leaves, and 2 teaspoons of dried St. John's wort in a cup of boiling water for 15 minutes. Strain the herbs and allow the tea to cool. Drink 1 cup, three times a day.

Hypnotherapy

The goal of hypnotherapy is to overcome old, unhealthy patterns of thinking, so you can function more positively and effectively, with less fear, pain, and/or distraction. Hypnotherapy is especially effective for alleviating stress and anxiety, both of which are symptoms of depression.

To locate a qualified hypnotherapist in your area, visit the Web site of the American Society of Clinical Hypnosis at www.asch.net or the National Guild of Hypnotists at www.ngh.net.

Nutritional Supplements

Certain nutritional supplements support the production and function of neurotransmitters in the brain, which help to relieve depression.

- Multivitamin/mineral supplement: Take as directed on the label. Helps to maintain proper nutrient levels.

- B-complex vitamins: Take as directed on the label. Improves energy, concentration, and mental function and reduces fatigue by helping to coordinate the activity of certain brain chemicals that transmit messages throughout the nervous system.

- 5-HTP: 150 milligrams daily, in divided doses of 50 milligrams. Works as an antidepressant. 5-HTP is a precursor to serotonin, the neurotransmitter that has a direct, positive effect on mood.

- SAMe (S-adenosyl-methionine): Start with 200 milligrams three times daily and work up to 400 milligrams three times daily; then, after several weeks, taper to 200 milligrams daily. SAMe is a quick-acting antidepressant; taken with the B-complex vitamins, it can help relieve severe depression.

Reiki

Reiki is a gentle but powerful therapeutic discipline that works on four levels of a person's being: physical, emotional, psychological, and spiritual. It restores the flow of the body's natural healing energy and provides an outlet for the release of old emotional patterns. It also reduces stress and promotes relaxation.

In a Reiki session, a practitioner may use light touch or no touch at all, simply placing his or her hands above the affected area. This technique releases old energy while channeling new energy into the body's cells. This fresh energy, in turn, revitalizes and strengthens each cell, stimulating the body's systems and normalizing functions.

Many hospitals sponsor community programs to educate the public about Reiki. You also might find a practitioner by looking in the Yellow Pages under terms such as "Reiki," "Holistic Centers," or "Holistic Practitioners." To learn more about the discipline itself, you can visit the Web site for the Reiki Alliance at www.reikialliance.com.

Relaxation/Meditation

Excess stress and anxiety may cause blood sugar to rise drastically or drop precipitously, which can lead to mood swings. Further, people who are stressed or anxious may struggle to maintain a healthy lifestyle, especially eating nutritiously and exercising regularly. So make time in your daily routine to practice techniques that can help alleviate stress and anxiety, which in turn can relieve symptoms of depression and improve your general sense of well-being. Among the techniques that may be beneficial are biofeedback, yoga, meditation, qigong, tai chi, visualization, and deep breathing.

To try deep breathing, lie flat on your back on the bed or the floor. Place both hands on your abdomen. Slowly inhale through your nose, pushing your abdomen upward as though inflating a balloon. Then slowly exhale through your mouth, feeling your abdomen deflate. Repeat 8 to 10 times. Focusing on your breathing in this way can slow your heart rate and take your mind off any stress or anxiety.

Therapeutic Massage

Besides reducing levels of stress hormones, massage releases endorphins, the neurotransmitters that help improve mood. Regular massage treatments also ease muscular tension and help quiet the mind.

To find a certified massage therapist, visit the Web site of the National Certification Board of Therapeutic Massage and Bodywork at www.ncbtmb.com.

Lifestyle Recommendations

Stay active. Exercise can play a role in relieving mild to moderate depression by triggering the release of endorphins and other brain chemicals that boost mood. A long period of moderate physical activity can be just as beneficial as a short burst of intense exercise.

Avoid alcohol. Alcohol blocks the absorption of B vitamins, which are essential for proper cognitive function.

Diabetes

Diabetes, sometimes called diabetes mellitus, is a disease characterized by impaired production of the hormone insulin or by cells' resistance to the actions of insulin. Secreted by the pancreas, insulin affects the metabolism of blood sugar, or glucose, the basic fuel source for all cells. In people with diabetes, glucose accumulates in the bloodstream, a situation that has the potential to compromise health. A number of medical conditions are associated with diabetes, including vision loss (diabetes is the leading cause of adult blindness), kidney disease, and leg amputations.

People with diabetes face short-term health problems as well, some of which may be serious or even life-threatening. For example, if blood glucose levels climb too high, they can lead to diabetic ketoacidosis, which involves the buildup of dangerous substances known as ketones in the blood. High blood glucose can occur in people who are unaware that they have diabetes or who don't use their diabetes medi-

cations correctly. It also can affect people with diabetes who are on high-dose steroid medications, who have an infection such as a cold or flu, or who drink large amounts of alcohol. Even stress may cause blood glucose to rise.

Sometimes blood glucose can drop too low. This condition, known as hypoglycemia, can occur when someone with diabetes skips a meal, exercises more than usual, or takes an incorrect dose of diabetes medication.

Diabetes is very common in the United States, affecting some 17 million Americans—including about 15 percent of those over age 60. It's on the rise, too, with the incidence climbing by about 6 percent each year.

Causes and Risk Factors

Generally, diabetes is diagnosed as either type 1 or type 2. In type 1 diabetes, the body destroys the pancreatic cells that manufacture insulin. As a result, the pancreas makes little if any of the hormone on its own. Type 1 diabetes usually begins in childhood—hence its former name, juvenile-onset diabetes—though 25 percent of cases are diagnosed after age 35. It accounts for 5 to 10 percent of all diabetes diagnoses. Though the cause of type 1 diabetes remains unknown, genetic factors are believed to play a major role.

In type 2 diabetes—which is far more common than type 1, accounting for 90 to 95 percent of cases—the pancreas is able to produce insulin, but not as much as it should. Further,

A Quick Guide to Symptoms

☐ **Increased thirst**
☐ **Frequent urination**
☐ **Weight loss or weight gain**
☐ **Blurred vision**
☐ **Flulike symptoms**
☐ **Frequent infections**
☐ **Gums that are red, swollen, and tender**

the body's cells are resistant to the hormone, keeping it from ushering glucose through the cell walls. Until recently, type 2 diabetes was thought of as primarily a disease of adulthood. Now it's turning up in children and adolescents, too.

A number of lifestyle factors can make a person more likely to develop type 2 diabetes, with overweight being the most significant. People who carry excess weight in the abdominal region are at higher risk. The more fatty cells the body has, the more resistant to insulin the cells may become.

Other factors that raise the risk of type 2 diabetes are aging and inactivity. People over age 45 are at increased risk, as are those who lead relatively sedentary lives. Physical activity uses up glucose, which not only makes cells more sensitive to insulin but also improves circulation and increases bloodflow.

As with type 1 diabetes, type 2 has a strong association with genetics and family history. For 39 percent of patients diagnosed with type 2 diabetes, at least one parent also has the disease. Ethnic background plays a role, too: While type 1 diabetes is more common in white people, type 2 more often is found in African Americans, Latinos, and Native Americans (an alarming half of all adults in the Pima Tribe of Arizona have type 2 diabetes). Newly emigrated Asians are at high risk for type 2 diabetes, as they forgo the traditional Asian diet for an American diet. With weight gain and reduced physical activity, Asians tend to develop type 2 diabetes at lower weights than other ethnic groups.

Certain medical conditions can raise a person's risk for developing type 2 diabetes. These include pancreatitis (inflammation of the pancreas), hypertension, and hepatitis C. The incidence of diabetes is higher among people who've undergone pancreatic surgery as well as those who've been exposed to certain industrial chemicals. Some medications—including beta-blockers, corticosteroids, and phenytoin—may trigger diabetes, though it usually goes away once drug therapy stops.

Signs and Symptoms

The symptoms of type 1 diabetes tend to come on fairly quickly. For this reason, the disease tends to be diagnosed quite readily. With type 2 diabetes, symptoms develop more slowly. It's possible to have high blood glucose for years before a diagnosis is made.

For both types of diabetes, the two most common symptoms are increased thirst and frequent urination. This is because the excess glucose in your blood draws water from your tissues. As a result, you feel dehydrated, so you drink more fluids. Of course, this means you'll need to urinate more often.

Other diabetes symptoms include weight loss or weight gain, blurred vision, flulike symptoms, frequent infections, and gums that are red, swollen, and tender. Men may experience erectile dysfunction.

There are kits on the market that allow you to self-test for diabetes. If you use such a kit and the test results suggest the presence of diabetes, or you simply suspect diabetes based on your symptoms, you need to see your doctor as soon as possible for proper testing and diagnosis.

Diabetes complications cause their own set of symptoms. For example, if your glucose drops below 60 milligrams per deciliter of blood (mg/dL), you may experience sweating, shakiness, hunger, dizziness, weakness, and nausea. Blood glucose below 40 mg/dL can lead to slurred speech, drowsiness, or confusion. If blood glucose drops too low, it can cause loss of consciousness and even what's known as a diabetic coma, a condition that's potentially life-threatening.

Too-high blood glucose—300 mg/dL or above—can cause excessive thirst, increased urination, weakness, confusion, leg cramps, and convulsions. As with low blood glucose, a diabetic coma may occur if glucose levels don't return to normal.

The symptoms of diabetic ketoacidosis resemble the flu: loss of appetite, nausea, vomiting, stomach pain, and fever. Your breathing may be abnormally deep and rapid, with fre-

Studies have shown that adults with type 2 diabetes who also take an ACE inhibitor appear to have greater protection from proteinuria, a kidney disease that's a potential diabetes complication.

quent sighing, and your breath may smell sweet and fruity. Diabetic ketoacidosis is a very serious condition that can lead to coma and death. If you're having symptoms of this or any of the above diabetes complications, you need to seek medical attention without delay.

Conventional Treatments

If you are an adult at midlife or older and you've recently been diagnosed with diabetes, you more than likely have type 2. Your treatment may begin with dietary changes and an exercise program. If you weigh more than you should, your doctor may instruct you to slim down as well. He or she may suggest meeting with a nutritionist and/or a diabetes educator to help create a diabetes management plan just for you.

Sometimes these lifestyle adjustments are enough to rein in wayward blood glucose levels. With blood glucose under control, you're less likely to develop diabetes complications such as heart and circulatory problems and nerve, eye, and kidney damage.

If your blood sugar doesn't stabilize despite your best efforts to modify your lifestyle, then the most likely next step is to add medication to your self-care plan.

Medications

Doctors use a number of medications to help manage diabetes. Which one your doctor prescribes for you depends on how the disease has manifested and how you've responded to the lifestyle modifications mentioned above.

Besides insulin, a number of oral diabetes medications are available. Often the two are used in combination.

Alpha-glucosidase inhibitors. Alpha-glucosidase inhibitors such as acarbose (Precose) and miglitol (Glyset) prevent enzymes in your gastrointestinal tract from breaking down carbohydrates. This slows the rate at which glucose enters your bloodstream. Potential side effects associated with this class of drugs are abdominal bloating, gas, and diarrhea, especially after a meal that is high in carbohydrates. In high doses, alpha-glucosidase inhibitors may cause liver damage.

Biguanides. Biguanides are considered especially useful for people with diabetes who are markedly obese. They work by inhibiting the production and release of glucose from the liver. Perhaps the best known of the biguanides is metformin (Glucophage, Glucophage XR). Among the potential side effects of these medications are loss of appetite, nausea, vomiting, a metallic taste in the mouth, abdominal bloating and pain, gas, and diarrhea. Taking biguanides with food seems to reduce these side effects, which normally diminish over time.

A rare but much more serious potential side effect of the biguanides is the buildup of lactic acid in the body, a condition known as lactic acidosis. Symptoms of lactic acidosis include muscle aches, weakness, fatigue, and drowsiness. You are at increased risk for lactic acidosis if you have congestive heart failure or kidney or liver disease. If you are experiencing symptoms of lactic acidosis, you need to seek medical attention without delay. Untreated, the condition has a 50 percent fatality rate.

Insulin. Anyone with type 1 diabetes must use insulin. It also is prescribed for some people with type 2 diabetes, in order to replace the insulin that the body is unable to make.

The insulin used to treat diabetes is known as synthetic human insulin. Though it is manufactured, it is chemically identical to the natural hormone.

Since stomach enzymes break down insulin, the hormone must be injected with a syringe or an insulin pen injector. If you require a continuous supply of insulin, your doctor may suggest an insulin pump. About the size of a deck of cards, an insulin pump is worn outside the body. A tube from the pump carries insulin to a catheter under the skin of the abdomen. The pump may be adjusted to administer a larger or smaller amount of insulin.

Meglitinides. Meglitinides, such as repaglinide (Prandin) and nateglinide (Starlix), are another class of medications commonly used to treat type 2 diabetes. Though chemically similar to sulfonylureas (described next), they are less likely to trigger low blood glucose. They also seem to be a better alternative for those with kidney problems. Potential side effects include headache, diarrhea, and a slightly elevated risk of cardiac events.

Sulfonylureas. Sulfonylureas prompt the pancreas to release more insulin. They work only if your body is able to make some insulin on its own. Examples of this class of medications are glipizide (Glucotrol, Glucotrol XL) and glyburide (DiaBeta, Glynase PresTab, Micronase).

The most common side effect of sulfonylureas is low blood glucose, which is most likely to occur during the first few months of treatment or if a patient is suffering from impaired liver or kidney function. Other potential side effects include weight gain and water retention.

These medications are not appropriate for people who are allergic to sulfa drugs. Since they may interact with other drugs, be sure to tell your doctor about all of the medicines—prescription and over-the-counter—that you're taking.

Thiazolidinediones. Also called TZDs or glitazones, thiazolidinediones make the body's tissues more sensitive to insulin, thereby improving their utilization of glucose. This class of medications includes rosiglitazone (Avandia) and pioglitazone (Actos).

Among the potential side effects of the TZDs are weight gain, swelling, fatigue, and anemia. They also may cause liver damage, which is why if your doctor prescribes a TZD, he or she should be checking your liver function every 2 months for the first 12 months of treatment. Further, if you experience any symptoms of liver damage (nausea, vomiting, abdominal pain, loss of appetite, dark urine, and yellowing of your skin and the whites of your eyes), you should see your doctor as soon as possible.

When compared to a placebo, rosiglitazone (Avandia) has been associated with a significant increase in the risk of heart attack as well as a borderline significant increase in the risk of death from cardiovascular causes. Additional studies are necessary to draw definitive

If you are experiencing low blood glucose, you need to eat or drink something that contains a good deal of sugar, such as hard candy or fruit juice. If you are on insulin, you should carry a syringe containing glucagon, a hormone that stimulates the release of glucose into the bloodstream. Teach your family members and close friends how to give you the injection, in case you aren't able to do so.

conclusions about the drug's safety. You may want to discuss these risks with your doctor if he or she prescribes rosiglitazone for you.

Monitoring Blood Glucose Levels

Once you're diagnosed with diabetes, your doctor will give you very specific instructions for monitoring your blood glucose levels. Generally, glucose tends to be more stable in people with type 2 diabetes, compared to those with type 1. So if you have type 2, you may need to check your blood glucose only once or twice a day—unless you're taking insulin, in which case your doctor may recommend more frequent monitoring.

A number of different kinds of monitoring devices are available. Ask your doctor for his or her opinion on which might be best for you.

Your doctor also may ask you to measure your glycosylated hemoglobin (HbA1c), considered to be a highly accurate indicator of overall diabetes control. Generally, the goal is to keep glycosylated hemoglobin below 7.0. Approved home testing kits are available for this purpose.

In a study involving patients with type 1 diabetes, researchers sought to compare the outcomes of intensive treatment versus conventional treatment. With intensive treatment, patients checked their blood glucose levels four times each day and adjusted their insulin based on their glucose readings. The goal was to keep blood glucose as close to normal as possible. Conventional treatment was less rigorous, with the objective of simply preventing glucose levels from rising too high or falling too low. The researchers found the prevalence of cardiovascular disease to be much lower in the group practicing intensive treatment. Based on this finding, it appears that keeping blood glucose as close to normal as possible can have long-term cardiovascular benefits.

Complementary Treatments

Like conventional medicine, complementary medicine advocates dietary modification and exercise as the primary strategies for both managing and preventing type 2 diabetes. Certain herbs, supplements, and relaxation techniques may be beneficial as well.

Ayurveda

The ancient Indian discipline known as Ayurveda takes a whole-body view of diabetes. A typical Ayurvedic "prescription" might include dietary changes, herbal remedies, relaxation techniques, and physical activities such as walking and yoga.

Gymnema (*Gymnema sylvestre*) is one of several herbal remedies used in Ayurveda to treat elevated blood glucose. Others include guggul, which has been successful in improving insulin function; and banaba, an herb native to India, Southeast Asia, and the Philippines that has proven effective in lowering blood glucose in people with type 2 diabetes.

If you'd like to explore what Ayurveda has to offer, your best bet is to consult an Ayurvedic practitioner, who will create a treatment plan specific to your diabetes. The Ayurvedic Institute may provide names of practitioners in your area. Visit the institute's Web site at www.ayurveda.com.

Diet

Diet is so critical to proper diabetes management that, as mentioned earlier, it's best to work with a nutritionist to create an eating plan that is specific to your health status and your dietary needs and preferences. A nutritionist also will take into consideration lifestyle factors such as your work schedule and your physical activity level. With this information, he or she can formulate dietary recommendations to support optimal blood glucose control.

The basic dietary advice for diabetes is to eat a proper balance of complex carbohydrates and protein. Complex carbs—which include whole grains, fruits, and vegetables—help regulate both insulin and blood glucose. Further, these foods are good sources of fiber, which not only helps control blood glucose but also lowers blood cholesterol.

In a diabetes diet, very few calories come from simple carbohydrates—that is, sugar. While fruit is good for you, eating too much of the extra-sweet varieties, such as pears and bananas, may not be. The reason: They contain quite a bit of concentrated sugar. The same is true for dried fruit and fruit juices.

Cold-water fish such as salmon, mackerel, and herring can be beneficial for diabetes because of their abundant supplies of essential fatty acids. These good fats, which include the omega-3 fatty acids, help protect the heart and blood vessels. This is important, since diabetes raises the risk of heart disease. If you aren't fond of fish, you can get your essential fatty acids from walnuts, flaxseed oil, evening primrose oil, and black currant seed oil.

On the subject of fats, do your best to steer

clear of trans fatty acids, which are common in packaged and processed foods. These bad fats contribute to diabetes as well as heart disease.

Garlic and onions help manage blood sugar by slowing the pace at which the body uses insulin. Garlic also is good for the heart, and it helps prevent yeast infections. Since yeast thrives in high-sugar environments, yeast infections are common in people with diabetes.

The trace mineral chromium helps insulin shuttle glucose into cells, where it can be used as fuel. In this way, chromium can help lower blood sugar. It also appears to reduce sugar cravings. Food sources of chromium include brewer's yeast, whole-wheat bread, and wheat bran.

The mineral zinc plays a role in insulin metabolism. To ensure that you're getting enough of this mineral in your diet, focus on food sources like pumpkin seeds, sunflower seeds, wheat germ, whole grains, brown rice, barley, and corn.

You may want to talk with your nutritionist about switching to a vegetarian diet. According to some recent research, this sort of diet can be very effective for managing diabetes and preventing its complications.

Exercise

As mentioned earlier, exercise is an important component of any diabetes management plan. It improves circulation, as well as the way in which the body uses insulin and burns fat. It also offsets stress and lowers blood pressure.

Exercising with diabetes does require a few precautions. Begin with a visit to your doctor, who can assess your fitness level and rule out any other underlying health issues, such as heart disease. If you have been relatively sedentary, don't try to do too much too soon. A daily 10-minute walk is a good starting point; over time, you can increase the duration and intensity of your workouts. You can vary your activities as well.

Just be careful not to overdo. Avoid prolonged or intense exercise, which actually may increase blood glucose. Also steer clear of activities that involve heavy lifting, which may raise blood glucose as well as blood pressure.

Before every exercise session, you'll need to check your blood glucose level. If it's below 100 mg/dL, eat a snack before you begin. If it is above 300 mg/dL, postpone your workout until later. Try to exercise with a buddy whenever possible, and always wear a medical ID bracelet.

Herbal Medicine

A number of herbs support insulin production, lower blood sugar, and help protect against diabetes complications. Always check with your doctor before adding any herb to your self-care regimen, to rule out potential interactions with any medication you may be taking.

Agave nectar. This natural sweetener is a derivative of the agave plant, a cactus native to Mexico. Because it is slowly absorbed into the bloodstream, it won't spike blood glucose levels. For this reason, agave nectar often is recommended as a sugar substitute for people with diabetes.

American ginseng. In recent studies, people with type 2 diabetes experienced smaller surges in blood glucose after taking 1 to 3 grams of American ginseng in capsule form 40 minutes before mealtime. It's believed that the ginsenosides in ginseng may stimulate the pancreas to make more insulin, which would help account for the effects on blood glucose. The typical dose of American ginseng is 200 milligrams daily of an extract standardized to 7 percent ginsenosides.

Bilberry. This herb helps protect against retinopathy and diabetes-related cataracts, perhaps by helping to normalize blood glucose levels. The recommended daily dose is one 100-milligram capsule, standardized to 25 percent anthocyanosides, three times a day.

Cinnamon. Research suggests that taking 1, 3, or 6 grams of cinnamon in capsule form per day can reduce blood glucose, triglycerides, LDL cholesterol, and total cholesterol in people with type 2 diabetes.

Pine bark extract. Also known as pycnogenol, this herb—which comes from the French maritime pine—appears to help heal diabetic ulcers. In studies, the people who were taking pycnogenol showed greater improvement in their ulcers than those whose ulcers were only washed and disinfected. Take 80 milligrams daily, in divided doses of 40 milligrams.

Stevia. Stevia, or sweet leaf, comes from a plant that is native to Brazil and Paraguay. Because it is highly concentrated, it is much sweeter than sugar. Just a small amount can satisfy sugar cravings and therefore reduce sugar consumption.

You can find stevia in health food stores and some supermarkets. Try to limit total daily intake to 1 gram or less.

Naturopathy

Naturopathic doctors (NDs) advocate a holistic approach to managing diabetes. Their recommendations may include dietary modifications, nutritional supplements, and herbal remedies, along with exercise and other lifestyle strategies. To find a naturopath in your area, visit the Web site for the American Association of Naturopathic Physicians at www.naturopathic.org.

Nutritional Supplements

Many nutritional supplements have proven effective in helping to manage diabetes and protect against diabetes complications.

- B-complex vitamins: Take as directed on the label. Support sugar metabolism; necessary for ensuring normal nerve function and protecting against nerve damage (diabetic neuropathy).

- Vitamin C: 1,000 milligrams daily, in divided doses of 500 milligrams. Improves the body's ability to use glucose. It also fights infection and heals wounds.

- Vitamin D: 800 IU daily. In one recent study, the combination of vitamin D and calcium (on page 72) lowered diabetes risk by 33 percent in the study participants, who were tracked over a 20-year period.

- Vitamin E: 400 IU daily. Improves glucose tolerance.

- Alpha-lipoic acid (ALA): 600 milligrams daily, in divided doses of 300 milligrams. Studies have linked ALA to a significant reduction in the severity of pain associated with diabetic neuropathy.

- Calcium: 1,200 milligrams daily. As mentioned on page 71, taking calcium along with vitamin D appears to protect against type 2 diabetes.
- Chromium: 200 micrograms daily. Improves glucose tolerance, lowers insulin levels, reduces fasting glucose levels, lowers triglycerides and total cholesterol, and increases HDL cholesterol.
- DHEA: 25 milligrams daily. Increases insulin sensitivity and improves blood vessel function.
- Magnesium: 500 milligrams daily. Magnesium deficiency is common among people with diabetes. In the case of type 2 diabetes, running low on this mineral may interfere with blood sugar control.
- Zinc: 30 milligrams daily. Supports insulin metabolism.

Relaxation/Meditation

Excess stress and anxiety may cause blood glucose to rise dramatically or fall precipitously. Further, people who are stressed or anxious may struggle to stick with the dietary and lifestyle strategies that are necessary for optimal diabetes management.

Many physicians recommend relaxation techniques to patients with diabetes to help offset the effects of stress, balance their emotions, and lower their blood pressure. Disciplines such as deep breathing, meditation, visualization, and yoga are excellent for promoting relaxation; you can use them whenever you need them for stress reduction. Other effective techniques include biofeedback, qigong, and tai chi.

Here's a deep breathing exercise that you can try on your own. Begin by lying flat on your back, either on the bed or on the floor. Slowly inhale through your nose, pushing up your abdomen as though inflating a balloon. Then slowly exhale, allowing your abdomen to "deflate" as you do. Repeat the entire cycle 8 to 10 times. Practice this exercise as necessary.

Traditional Chinese Medicine

Traditional Chinese medicine (TCM) has a good track record for treating diabetes. Practitioners focus on the three Gs—great thirst, great hunger, and great urination, all of which are diabetes symptoms. They also consider emotional factors when creating a diabetes management plan.

Acupuncture is very effective for treating diabetes, though improvements come about very slowly. It works best when used in conjunction with conventional treatments.

Besides acupuncture, a TCM practitioner likely will recommend a nutritious diet and proper rest. Herbal remedies can help alleviate diabetes symptoms, as well as stress and anxiety.

To find a TCM practitioner in your area, visit the Web site of the National Certification Commission for Acupuncture and Oriental Medicine at www.nccaom.org or the American Association of Acupuncture and Oriental Medicine at www.aaaomonline.org.

Lifestyle Recommendations

Because of the risk of complications, people with diabetes need to closely monitor certain aspects of their health—in particular, their blood pressure and their eyes, feet, and gums. There are other lifestyle strategies to consider, too.

Get regular dental checkups. People with diabetes are more likely to develop gum infections. This is important, since research now suggests that gum disease has a direct link to cardiovascular disease, which often occurs in tandem with diabetes. Visit your dentist regularly for professional cleanings and exams. Practice good home care, too: Brush and floss at least twice a day. If your gums ever appear red and swollen, make an appointment to see your dentist as soon as possible.

Schedule annual eye exams. If you have diabetes, you should be getting annual screenings for retinal damage, cataracts, and glaucoma. People with diabetes are at increased risk for eye problems.

Tend to your feet. Diabetes can damage the nerves in your feet, thus reducing your ability to feel pain in the event of an injury. And since diabetes reduces bloodflow to the feet, wounds and sores may not heal properly.

To protect your feet, wash them and dry them thoroughly, then check for sores. Do this every day. Also wear good-fitting shoes at all times. You're less likely to injure your feet if you don't go barefoot.

Don't forget your vaccinations. Diabetes can weaken your immune system, leaving you more vulnerable to influenza and pneumonia. Be sure to get your vaccinations every year. Stay up-to-date on your tetanus booster shots, too.

If you smoke, quit. People with diabetes who smoke are three times more likely to die from cardiovascular disease or stroke. Smoking also increases your chances of developing kidney disease or nerve damage.

Check your blood pressure. Because people with diabetes are at increased risk for high blood pressure, you should see your doctor regularly for blood pressure screenings. You also might wish to invest in a blood pressure monitor (or sphygmomanometer) to track your readings at home.

Preventive Measures

Researchers have yet to find a way to prevent type 1 diabetes. On the other hand, since type 2 diabetes is largely a lifestyle disease, you can take steps to reduce your risk.

Overhaul your eating habits. According to an article that appeared in a 2002 issue of *Annals of Internal Medicine*, the typical Western diet—consisting of fatty meats, high-fat dairy products, sugar and refined grains, and fried foods increases diabetes risk by 60 percent. Try to weed these foods from your diet, replacing them with lots of fruits, vegetables, whole grains, and nuts. This change alone can go a long way toward protecting against diabetes.

Get moving. People who exercise regularly are less likely to develop type 2 diabetes. Aim for at least 30 to 45 minutes of physical activity at least 5 or 6 days each week.

Slim down, if necessary. In light of the strong correlation between overweight and type 2 diabetes, it's in your best interest to get rid of any extra pounds that you may be carrying. This is especially true if those pounds have accumulated in your abdominal region, which is a risk factor for diabetes as well as heart disease.

Diverticulosis/Diverticulitis

In diverticulosis, small bulging pouches called diverticula develop in the colon—usually along the left side, above the rectum, in what's known as the sigmoid colon. Diverticulosis is an extremely common medical condition. But since the diverticula usually don't cause any problems, most people are unaware that they have them.

For about 15 to 20 percent of people with diverticulosis, a diverticulum becomes infected or inflamed. This condition, called diverticulitis, may be caused by a small piece of stool lodging in the pouch and hindering bloodflow, or by a small tear in the pouch. Generally, the infection or inflammation remains localized around the diverticulum.

On occasion, small holes or perforations may develop in the infected diverticulum, and pus may leak through the holes into the abdomen. In rare instances, the diverticulum ruptures and intestinal waste enters the abdominal cavity. This may lead to inflammation of the lining of the abdominal cavity, a condition known as peritonitis. Peritonitis is a medical emergency that requires immediate care.

Causes and Risk Factors

Diverticula often occur after years of straining to pass stool. This can cause the colon wall to develop a weak spot, which eventually gives way to a bulge. Another potential contributor to diverticulosis is the typical American diet, which tends to have too little fiber. In the absence of fiber, stool becomes small, hard, and difficult to pass. This increases pressure inside the sigmoid colon.

The most significant risk factor for diverticulosis is age. In fact, by the time you reach 80, you're almost certain to have diverticula. As you get older, the outer, muscular colon wall begins to thicken, in turn narrowing the colon's inside passageway. The subsequent rise in pressure inside the colon increases the likelihood of pouch formation. It also slows the passage of food through the colon; the extra transit time places even more pressure on weak areas in the colon walls.

Signs and Symptoms

As mentioned earlier, in many cases diverticulosis produces no symptoms. Sometimes there's rectal bleeding, most likely because a weakened blood vessel in a diverticulum has burst. You may see dark blood in the stool or bright red blood in the toilet bowl. Generally, bleeding from a pouch lasts just a short time and stops without medical intervention.

You can buy home testing kits to detect rectal bleeding, but they aren't very reliable. If you suspect that you have diverticulitis, consult your doctor for a proper diagnosis.

Diverticulitis can produce severe symptoms such as pain, abdominal tenderness, constipation, diarrhea, nausea, and fever. Less common are rectal bleeding, frequent or painful urination, difficulty urinating, bloating, and vomiting. In the event of a flare-up of diverticulitis, you should seek medical attention right away, as it can lead to an intestinal obstruction. Once you've had one flare-up, there's a 30 percent chance of recurrence.

Conventional Treatments

For diverticulosis without symptoms, the standard treatment is a high-fiber diet. A flare-up of diverticulitis requires a few days of bed rest, along with a restricted diet (such as liquid or low fiber). This will reduce contractions in the colon and give it a chance to heal.

About half of all cases of diverticulitis require hospitalization. For example, if you are very nauseated or vomiting continuously, your doctor may advise you to not consume anything by mouth. Instead, you'll be given fluids intravenously. As your symptoms subside, you'll be able to reintroduce solid foods gradually.

To prevent a recurrence of diverticulitis, your doctor or nutritionist will provide instructions for increasing the amount of fiber in your diet.

Medications

If you know you have diverticulosis and you're prone to constipation, your doctor may rec-

ommend an over-the-counter stool softener. Diverticulitis may require a mild pain reliever, plus an antibiotic to kill any bacteria that are causing infection. Be sure to follow your doctor's prescription to the letter; if you're given an antibiotic, for example, take it as directed and complete the entire course. Patients with more complicated cases of diverticulitis may be given antibiotics intravenously.

Surgery for Diverticulitis

Ordinarily, dietary changes and medications work well to treat a first attack of diverticulitis. They aren't as effective for recurrences. In this case, your doctor may recommend surgery to remove the diseased section of the colon.

Approximately 20 percent of diverticulitis

A Quick Guide to Symptoms

Diverticulosis
☐ Rectal bleeding

Diverticulitis
☐ Pain
☐ Abdominal tenderness
☐ Constipation or diarrhea
☐ Nausea
☐ Fever
☐ Rectal bleeding
☐ Frequent or painful urination
☐ Bloating
☐ Vomiting

Surgery for Peritonitis

If the infection from diverticulitis leaks into the abdominal cavity—causing a condition known as peritonitis—it will require immediate surgery. An emergency situation like this almost always requires traditional surgery rather than a laparoscopic procedure. The goal of surgery is to identify and treat any infection or obstruction. Untreated, peritonitis can be fatal.

patients require surgery. The most common procedures are bowel resection with colostomy and primary bowel resection.

Bowel resection with colostomy. If you have extensive inflammation, you may need a bowel resection with colostomy. In this procedure, the surgeon removes the diseased section of the colon and makes a hole in the abdominal wall. The colon is connected to the hole, or stoma, and stool passes through the stoma into a bag attached to the abdomen.

Not all colostomies are permanent. Sometimes after a period of healing, the surgeon is able to reconnect the colon with the rectum, and the external bag no longer is necessary.

Primary bowel resection. In this procedure, which may be done traditionally or laparoscopically, the diseased portion of the colon is removed and the healthy sections are reconnected to each other. A traditional resection requires a long incision in the abdomen; for a laparoscopic resection, the surgeon makes several smaller incisions. Generally, patients recover much more quickly from the laparoscopic procedure than from the traditional surgery.

Complementary Treatments

Because diverticulosis is so closely linked to diet and lifestyle, changes in these areas may be enough to treat a mild case of the disease. Complementary therapies can help alleviate any symptoms that may arise, particularly pain from inflammation and gas.

Diet

A few key dietary strategies can help reduce pressure inside the colon. Begin by gradually increasing your consumption of fiber-rich foods such as fruits, vegetables, and whole-grain products. The word *gradual* is critical; by adding too much fiber too quickly, you raise your risk of uncomfortable gastrointestinal symptoms such as diarrhea, gas, bloating, and cramping.

Also be sure to get enough fluids. A good benchmark is eight 8-ounce glasses of water or other noncaffeinated, nonalcoholic beverages per day.

Herbal Medicine

Chamomile, ginger, peppermint, and slippery elm. Chamomile soothes and relaxes, which is beneficial for an agitated gastrointestinal tract. Ginger, a carminative (digestive aid), helps relieve gas; peppermint reduces intestinal spasms; and slippery elm protects the bowel lining. All of these herbs are readily available as prepared tea bags in health food stores and some supermarkets. Drink the tea of your choice as often as you wish, particularly after meals and before bedtime.

Garlic. Garlic fights infection through its antiseptic properties. The recommended dose for the fresh herb is two or three cloves per day, while the dose for supplements is 500 milligrams per day. If you have a choice, select fresh garlic over supplements; the supplements contain concentrated extracts, which may raise the risk of excessive bleeding. For this same reason, you should consult your doctor before using garlic supplements if you're on a blood-thinning medication (including aspirin), taking the herb ginkgo, or about to undergo surgery.

Nutritional Supplements

To increase your fiber intake, you might ask your doctor whether you could benefit from adding a natural fiber supplement containing psyllium seeds (such as Metamucil or Citrucel) to your self-care regimen. Follow the directions on the product label. The added bulk from the fiber stimulates intestinal contractions, softens stools, and supports proper digestive function.

If you do decide to try a fiber supplement, be sure to drink plenty of water. Otherwise, you may become constipated.

The following supplements also support optimal gastrointestinal function.

• *Lactobacillus acidophilus:* 200 milligrams daily. These beneficial bacteria help maintain intestinal health and combat yeast infections resulting from frequent antibiotic use. Look for a product that mentions "live" or "active" cultures on the label, with 1 billion to 2 billion organisms per capsule.

• L-glutamine: 400 milligrams three times daily, between meals. Necessary for proper intestinal function.

• Omega-3 fatty acids: 1,000 milligrams as fish oil daily. May help reduce inflammation associated with diverticulitis.

Lifestyle Recommendations

Regular exercise reduces pressure inside the colon and promotes normal bowel function. Try to set aside at least 30 minutes every day for physical activity. Any activity that gets you moving will be beneficial, so choose one that you enjoy and that you can easily fit into your schedule.

If you have been relatively sedentary, walking might be a good "starter" activity for you. It requires no equipment other than a pair of good-fitting shoes, and it can be done just about anywhere. Begin with an easy 10-minute walk, and gradually increase the intensity and duration of your workouts.

If you have access to a heated pool, you might try walking in water. It offers a great cardiovascular workout while increasing your muscle strength and improving flexibility.

Fiber Content of Selected Foods

Use the following table to calculate the amount of fiber in your current diet and to increase your intake as needed.

Food	Serving Size	Fiber Content
Fruit		
Apple, fresh	1 medium	4 g
Peach, fresh	1 medium	2 g
Pear, fresh	1 medium	4 g
Tangerine, fresh	1 medium	2 g
Nonstarchy Vegetables		
Acorn squash, fresh	½ cup, cooked	7 g
Asparagus, fresh	½ cup, cooked	1.5 g
Broccoli, fresh	½ cup, cooked	2 g
Brussels sprouts, fresh	½ cup, cooked	2 g
Cabbage, fresh	½ cup, cooked	2 g
Carrot, fresh	1 medium, cooked	1.5 g
Cauliflower, fresh	½ cup, cooked	2 g
Romaine lettuce	1 cup	1 g
Spinach, fresh	½ cup, cooked	2 g
Tomato, fresh	1 medium, raw	1 g
Zucchini, fresh	1 cup, cooked	2.5 g
Starchy Vegetables		
Black-eyed peas, fresh	½ cup, cooked	4 g
Kidney beans, fresh	½ cup, cooked	6 g
Lima beans, fresh	½ cup, cooked	4.5 g
Potato, fresh	1 medium, cooked	3 g
Grains and Grain Products		
Bread, whole-wheat	1 slice	2 g
Cereal, bran flake	½ cup	5 g
Oatmeal, plain	½ cup, cooked	3 g
Rice, brown	1 cup, cooked	3.5 g
Rice, white	1 cup, cooked	1 g

Source: United States Department of Agriculture Web site, USDA National Nutrient Database for Standard Reference.

The warm water is soothing and causes less muscular contraction.

Over time, you might incorporate other activities into your exercise program. Consider bicycling, dancing, or yoga.

Preventive Measures

Don't ignore your bowel. Delaying a bowel movement will leave stool harder and more difficult to pass. This adds to the pressure inside the colon.

Get more fiber. Just as increasing fiber intake can help treat diverticulosis, it also can help prevent it. The American Dietetic Association recommends consuming 20 to 35 grams of fiber each day. The average American doesn't get nearly that much.

To add fiber to your diet, build your meals around fiber-rich fruits, vegetables, and whole grains. Meanwhile, cut back on processed foods, which tend to have too little fiber.

You may experience some bloating as your body adjusts to your new, high-fiber eating habits. To reduce your risk of bloating, increase your fiber intake very gradually, over a period of 6 to 8 weeks.

Drink plenty of fluids. Fiber absorbs water to create soft, bulky stool. If you do not replenish your body's fluids, you may become constipated. Try to drink at least 2 quarts—that's eight 8-ounce glasses—of water or other noncaffeinated, nonalcoholic beverages each day.

Emphysema

Emphysema is a form of chronic obstructive pulmonary disease (COPD) in which the air sacs, or alveoli, in the lungs lose their elasticity and their walls begin to break down. The air that is trapped inside overinflates the alveoli and causes them to rupture, thereby reducing the amount of surface area. The damage to the alveoli is permanent and irreversible; it prevents a person with emphysema from inhaling an adequate amount of oxygen and exhaling an adequate amount of carbon dioxide. As the disease progresses, the flow of air in and out of the lungs becomes more limited.

Emphysema is a fairly widespread health problem, affecting almost 2.8 million Americans—more men than women. People with emphysema are at greater risk for a number of other medical conditions, including asthma, acute and chronic bronchitis, pneumonia, and other respiratory problems.

Causes and Risk Factors

The vast majority of emphysema cases result from smoking—especially cigarettes, though smoking cigars and pipes also causes the disease. Smoking disrupts the chemical balance within the lungs, robbing the lungs of their ability to protect themselves against damage. People over age 40 who have smoked 20 cigarettes per day for 20 or more years are most likcly to develop emphysema.

There is good evidence that long-term exposure to secondhand smoke may raise a person's risk for this condition. Exposure to air pollution, fumes, and dust (often on the job) also may play a significant role.

A far smaller number of emphysema cases are associated with an inherited disorder in which people are born with a deficiency of alpha-1-antitrypsin (AAT), a protein that protects against the damage caused by smoking or other pollutants. This may lead to an illness known as AAT-deficiency-related emphysema, which usually is diagnosed between ages 20 and 40. Most of those with AAT deficiency are of Northern European descent.

Signs and Symptoms

The first symptom of emphysema usually is an acute chest illness characterized by increased coughing, sputum, wheezing, and shortness of breath. As the disease progresses, shortness of breath may become more frequent; you may breathe harder than usual when you are exercising or running up stairs. Eventually, you will experience bouts of difficult breathing, with your exhalations taking twice as long as your inhalations.

Other common symptoms of emphysema include anxiety, weight loss, fatigue, and swelling of the legs, ankles, and feet. In addition, there may be an increase in the diameter of your chest, a condition known as barrel-shaped chest.

If you develop shortness of breath, you should see your doctor—especially if you are a smoker or you have a family history of the genetic form of emphysema. Shortness of breath is a symptom of a number of health problems and so requires proper medical evaluation.

Conventional Treatments

If you smoke, the first and most important step in treating emphysema is to quit. In addition, try to avoid exposure to secondhand smoke.

Medications

Antibiotics. Having emphysema places you at increased risk for respiratory infections, which will worsen your symptoms. Your doctor probably will recommend treating any infection with a course of broad-spectrum antibiotics, such as cephalosporin, ampicillin, tetracycline, or erythromycin.

Anti-inflammatory drugs (corticosteroids). To reduce inflammation in your lungs, your doctor may prescribe an anti-inflammatory medication such as prednisone. While these medicines are quite good at healing the delicate lining of the lungs, they can have a number of negative side effects, especially when used for an extended period. These include osteoporosis (in both men and women), weight gain, loss of lean body mass, and elevated blood pressure and blood sugar. Since inhaled steroids tend to have fewer side effects, they may be a better option than oral steroids.

Bronchodilators. Your treatment plan probably will include a bronchodilator, which relaxes the muscles around the airways.

A Quick Guide to Symptoms

- ☐ Onset of acute chest illness characterized by increased cough, sputum, wheezing, and shortness of breath
- ☐ Bouts of difficult breathing
- ☐ Anxiety
- ☐ Weight loss
- ☐ Fatigue
- ☐ Swelling of the legs, ankles, and feet
- ☐ Barrel-shaped chest

Examples of bronchodilators are albuterol, terbutaline, ipratropium bromide, and theophylline. Generally, these medications have few side effects.

Oxygen Therapy

If emphysema has severely impaired your lung function, and you are unable to obtain a sufficient amount of oxygen through normal respiration, your doctor may suggest oxygen therapy. It's helpful in treating shortness of breath and also may prevent heart failure.

Protein Therapy

If your emphysema is the result of an AAT deficiency, you might benefit from weekly intravenous infusions of the protein. This treatment may slow damage to your lungs.

Pulmonary Rehabilitation Program

A treatment plan for emphysema often includes participation in a pulmonary rehabilitation program. These programs combine education about emphysema with smoking cessation, nutrition counseling, physical activity, psychosocial support, and training in special breathing techniques. If you are interested in such a program, you should ask your doctor for a referral.

Surgery

For certain patients with emphysema, surgery may be necessary. Usually it involves one of two procedures: lung volume reduction surgery and transplant surgery.

Lung volume reduction surgery. This procedure may eliminate the need for supplemental oxygen. Once a CT scan has determined the location of the damaged lung tissue, the surgeon makes two or three small incisions in the chest, through which he threads a tiny camera to view the inside of the lungs. An instrument removes small wedges of damaged tissue—usually between 20 and 30 percent of each lung. Since there is less lung, there is less pressure on the diaphragm, and the remaining lung is able to return to a normal position. After this procedure, the contraction and relaxation of the diaphragm—and your breathing—should improve.

One study compared the outcomes of lung volume reduction surgery to those of medical management of emphysema. Though surgery did not affect overall mortality, the patients who'd undergone surgery showed improvement in their exercise capacity.

Transplant surgery. Because of the serious shortage of transplantable lungs as well as

the invasiveness and high risk associated with the procedure, doctors generally recommend transplant surgery only as a last resort. It may be appropriate for younger patients who have no other serious health problems.

Complementary Treatments

For people with emphysema, practitioners of complementary therapies will focus their efforts on improving breathing and relieving any discomfort.

Diet

Eat smaller but more frequent meals. With emphysema, obstructed air may become trapped in the enlarged lungs and push down on the abdominal area. Since less oxygen makes its way to the stomach, digesting large meals is harder.

Try to avoid foods that produce gas, such as legumes, cabbage, onions, broccoli, and radishes. These foods cause the abdomen to distend, which may hinder breathing. Likewise, steer clear of foods that produce excess mucus, such as dairy products and anything fried. People who have emphysema tend to collect mucus in their airways.

Remember, too, that drinking lots of fluids will help thin mucus secretions. Aim for at least eight 8-ounce glasses of water and other non-caffeinated, nonalcoholic beverages per day.

Herbal Medicine

Garlic. An antioxidant, garlic helps fortify the immune system and is effective for all chronic respiratory conditions, particularly for preventing pneumonia. The recommended dose of fresh garlic is two or three cloves per day, while the dose for supplements is 500 milligrams per day. If you have a choice, select fresh garlic over supplements, which contain concentrated extracts and so may increase the risk of excessive bleeding.

Mullein, coltsfoot, wild cherry bark, and peppermint. This blend of herbs may assist in loosening mucus and eliminating phlegm. To make a tea, fill a saucepan with water and add the herbs in equal amounts. Use 1 tablespoon of each herb per 1 cup of water. Bring the tea to a boil, then turn off the burner and allow to steep for at least an hour before straining. Drink 2 cups of the tea each day.

Nutritional Supplements

Antioxidant nutrients are helpful for strengthening lung tissue and detoxifying the body after exposure to harmful substances, including cigarette smoke and environmental pollutants.

- Multivitamin/mineral: Take as directed on the label. Look for a supplement product that contains the minerals magnesium, potassium, selenium, and zinc, which often are deficient in people with emphysema.

- Vitamin A: 10,000 IU daily. Aids in repairing lung tissue.

- Vitamin C: 2,000 milligrams daily, in divided doses of 1,000 milligrams. Heals inflamed lung tissue.

- Vitamin E: 400 IU daily. Delivers oxygen throughout the body.

Lifestyle Recommendations

Watch your weight. If you weigh more than you should, your body must work even harder to obtain extra oxygen.

Take a walk. While people with emphysema tire easily, any amount of walking is better than none at all. It will improve your endurance and build your muscle strength.

Practice breathing exercises. The following exercises can be beneficial in cases of emphysema, though you may wish to consult a respiratory therapist to learn proper technique.

Begin with diaphragmatic breathing. Lie on your back, with pillows under your head and knees for support. Position your fingertips on your abdomen, below your rib cage, so that you can feel your diaphragm lift with each inhalation. As your chest fills with air, push your abdomen against your hand. Slowly inhale through your mouth for a count of three, then exhale through pursed lips for a count of six.

Practice this technique until you are able to complete 10 to 15 cycles of inhaling and exhaling. Then try it while lying on your left and right sides in turn. Next perform the exercises while sitting in a chair, standing, and walking. Eventually, you should be able to do diaphragmatic breathing while you are climbing the stairs.

Along with diaphragmatic breathing, work on deep breathing. Sit or stand comfortably and inhale deeply. Hold your breath for a slow count of five while arching your chest. Then contract your abdominal muscles and force out the air. Repeat 10 times. Practice deep breathing once a day.

Alleviate stress. Studies have shown that stress increases the body's demand for oxygen. To help unwind and reduce your stress level, try relaxation techniques that incorporate deep breathing, such as meditation, tai chi, and yoga. Listening to music or a relaxation CD also can help relieve tension and anxiety.

Avoid wearing restrictive clothing and accessories. Because emphysema interferes with breathing, the chest and abdomen must be able to expand freely.

Protect your respiratory system from cold air. If you have emphysema, your respiratory tract is very sensitive to cold. Cover your face with a mask or scarf when heading outside in cold weather.

Reduce your exposure to air pollution. Inhaling airborne pollutants will only aggravate your condition. Pay attention to daily air quality reports, and stay inside as much as possible when the air quality is compromised.

Address respiratory infections. Because any type of respiratory infection will aggravate emphysema symptoms, you should contact your doctor at the first signs of a respiratory illness, such as a cold or the flu. Your doctor may be able to suggest medication that will reduce the severity of your symptoms.

Seek support from others. Emphysema is an emotionally difficult disease that can take a serious toll on you and your family. A few sessions with a counselor or therapist may help you better cope with your situation. So may joining a support group, in which you can commiserate with and learn from others who are facing similar challenges.

Set priorities. Don't expect your life to be the same as it was before emphysema. Learn to control what you can physically, emotionally, and psychologically. Continue to pursue the activities that are important to you, but with adjustments so that they require less effort.

Preventive Measures

Don't smoke, and if you do smoke, stop. Smoking is the primary cause of emphysema. Smokers are 10 times more likely than nonsmokers to develop the disease. The risk is even higher for smokers with an AAT deficiency.

Since it's possible to develop emphysema from exposure to secondhand smoke, try to steer clear of smoky environments, too.

Erectile Dysfunction

Erectile dysfunction, the current term of choice for what long was known as impotence, refers to the inability to obtain an adequate erection for sexual performance and satisfaction. Erectile dysfunction, or ED, is thought to be quite common, affecting between 20 million and 30 million American men (and their partners). An estimated 620,000 men between ages 40 and 70 have a bout of erectile dysfunction each year.

Causes and Risk Factors

Aging is the most significant risk factor for erectile dysfunction. Though study results tend to vary, a significant number of men over age 50 are believed to have the disease to some degree.

A number of physical conditions can make a man more likely to develop ED. For example, chronic disease of the kidneys, heart, liver, thyroid, lungs, or nerves can contribute to ED, as can multiple sclerosis, epilepsy, Parkinson's disease, stroke, and endocrine disorders such as diabetes. Atherosclerosis—that is, the accumulation of fatty deposits in the arteries—may impede bloodflow to the penis. Other possible medical causes include surgery to the pelvic area or spinal cord and surgery for rectal, bladder, or prostate cancer. A deficiency of the male hormone testosterone can be a risk factor, too.

Certain medications identify ED as a possible side effect. Among these are medicines for high blood pressure (especially diuretics and beta-blockers), cancer, and pain, as well as antidepressants, antihistamines, tranquilizers, sleeping pills, and antifungal drugs, particularly ketoconazole (Nizoral).

Chronic excessive alcohol consumption can contribute to ED, as can illegal drugs such as marijuana, heroin, and cocaine. Smoking can damage penile arteries. Sometimes men who ride their bicycles for prolonged periods experience temporary ED.

About 10 to 15 percent of all ED cases are believed to have a psychological cause, such as depression, anxiety, or stress. Often multiple psychological causes occur at once, or psychological causes occur along with physical ones. For example, a physical condition may lead to ED, the onset of which can trigger anxiety that only aggravates ED.

ED and Heart Disease

According to one study that tracked 9,500 men—all over age 55—for 5 years, erectile dysfunction (ED) may be a harbinger of future cardiovascular disease. The men who had ED at the beginning of the study, as well as those who developed ED during the study, were at higher risk for cardiovascular disease than those who did not have ED. Any man with ED should talk with his doctor about the possibility of heart trouble.

Signs and Symptoms

With erectile dysfunction, you are unable to have an erection or to maintain an erection for a sufficient amount of time to have sex.

Every man should expect an occasional bout with erectile dysfunction, especially as he gets older. You should consult your doctor if ED persists for more than 2 or 3 months.

Conventional Treatments

Medications

Most men with ED will see improvement with one of the following medications.

Alprostadil. A synthetic version of the hormone prostaglandin E, alprostadil relaxes the smooth muscle in the penis, thereby enhancing bloodflow as necessary for an erection. The medication is available in several forms.

With injectable alprostadil (Edex, Caverject), you administer the medicine directly into the side of the penis using a fine needle. It produces an erection within 5 to 20 minutes, and the erection will last for about an hour. The pain from the injection is minimal,

though you may experience other side effects such as prolonged erection, the formation of fibrous tissue in the penis, or bleeding at the site of the injection. Some doctors recommend using injectable alprostadil in combination with other prescription drugs such as phentolamine (Regitine) or papaverine. Do not inject yourself with alprostadil more than once a day or three times a week.

Alprostadil also is available as a tiny suppository that is inserted into the tip of the penis. The erectile tissue absorbs the drug, which increases bloodflow. The trade name for this delivery system is medicated urethral system for erection (MUSE). Possible side effects include minor bleeding in the urethra, pain, dizziness, and the formation of fibrous tissue in the penis. Do not use MUSE more than twice a day.

Then there is the topical cream form of alprostadil, sold under the brand names Topiglan and Alprox-TD. The cream is rubbed directly on the penis 15 minutes before intercourse.

Alprostadil is not appropriate for men who have severe circulatory or nerve damage or bleeding abnormalities, who take blood-thinning medication, or who have penile implants. Some female partners of men using alprostadil experience vaginal itching or burning. If this happens, try using a condom.

Sildenafil. Most people will recognize sildenafil by its brand name: Viagra. It works by increasing bloodflow to the genital area, producing an erection within 30 to 60 minutes after a pill is taken.

A Quick Guide to Symptoms

- ☐ **Unable to have an erection**
- ☐ **Unable to maintain an erection for a sufficient amount of time to have sex**

Not all men are good candidates for sildenafil. For example, anyone taking a nitrate or a nitrate-containing medication (including nitroglycerin) should not use sildenafil. Combining these medications—both of which dilate blood vessels—may cause low blood pressure, dizziness, and heart and circulatory problems.

Common side effects of sildenafil include headaches, indigestion, nasal congestion, dizziness, flushing, and blurred vision. About 2.5 percent of men who take sildenafil report seeing a blue haze or increased brightness, or briefly losing their vision, after taking sildenafil. Fortunately, these side effects appear to be temporary.

Sildenafil is best taken on an empty stomach, as combining it with food will diminish its effectiveness. Do not use it more than once a day, and do not combine it with other medications for erectile dysfunction. Likewise, sildenafil should not be taken at the same time as certain antibiotics, such as erythromycin, or certain acid blockers, such as cimetidine (Tagamet).

Vardenafil and tadalafil. While sildenafil probably has received the most media attention, there are other oral medications for erectile dysfunction. Two of them, vardenafil (Levitra) and tadalafil (Cialis), seem to work in much the same way as sildenafil. But they do vary in dosage, duration of effectiveness, and possible side effects. As with sildenafil, neither of these drugs should be taken in combination with nitrate medications. Any man with a history of cardiac problems should use vardenafil or tadalafil with care.

Psychological Counseling

In the absence of any physical cause for ED, your doctor may recommend counseling. Ask for a referral to a professional with training and experience in addressing sexual issues. Generally, the goal of such treatment is to reduce any anxiety associated with sex.

Surgery

Penile implants. This procedure involves the surgical placement of implants on two sides of the penis. The implants may be some sort of inflatable devices, or somewhat rigid rods made from silicone or polyurethane. While the procedure generally is safe, there is a small risk of infection.

Vascular surgery. If erectile dysfunction is a result of damage to the arteries or other blood vessels, your doctor may recommend surgery. The two most common surgical procedures for ED are revascularization (bypass) and venous ligation.

During revascularization, the surgeon removes an artery from the leg and surgically connects it to the arteries in the back of the penis. This circumvents any arterial blockage and restores normal bloodflow. Sometimes a penile vein is used to create the bypass; this procedure is known as deep dorsal vein arterialization.

In cases where the penis isn't able to store enough blood to maintain an erection, doctors may opt for venous ligation. In this procedure, any veins that are causing too much blood to drain from the erection chambers are either tied off or removed. A related procedure, known as venous ablation, involves injecting ethanol into the deep dorsal vein, which is the primary vein for draining blood from the penis. This causes scarring, which closes smaller veins and stops blood from leaking.

Testosterone Replacement Therapy

If your doctor concludes that an inadequate amount of testosterone may be responsible for your ED, he or she may recommend treatment to increase blood levels of the hormone.

Vacuum Devices

Vacuum devices consist of an external vacuum and one or more tension rings (rubber bands). A hollow plastic tube is placed over the penis, and then a pump is used to create a vacuum inside the tube. This pulls blood into the penis. Once an erection occurs, usually in 3 to 5 minutes, a tension ring is placed around the base of the penis. This should sustain the erection long enough to have sexual intercourse.

Potential side effects of the vacuum devices include blocked ejaculation, minor bruising, and mild discomfort from both the pump and the tension ring. If you decide to use a vacuum device, ask your doctor to recommend one that has been medically approved. Those that aren't may not have the necessary safety elements, and so raise the risk of injury.

Venous Flow Controllers

If you are able to achieve an erection but it doesn't last, you may be a candidate for a venous flow controller. It's a simple constricting device with rings made from rubber or silicone, which are placed at the base of the penis to "trap" an erection. One example of a venous flow controller is Actis, a product made by the Vivus Corporation.

To avoid causing damage to the penis due to lack of oxygen, refrain from using one of these devices for more than 30 minutes at a time. They are not appropriate for men who have bleeding problems or who are taking blood-thinning medications.

Complementary Treatments
Acupuncture

Numerous studies have confirmed the benefits of electro-acupuncture for the treatment of erectile dysfunction. In electro-acupuncture, a mild electric current is run through the needles to help stimulate the appropriate acupuncture points.

To locate an acupuncturist in your area, visit the Web site of the National Certification Commission for Acupuncture and Oriental Medicine at www.nccaom.org.

Diet

Build your meals around fruits, vegetables, and whole grains. These foods support a healthy vascular system, which is essential for proper bloodflow to the penis. A diet of these nutritious foods also can help melt away extra pounds—an important benefit, since overweight is a risk factor for ED. Aim for at least four servings of fruits, five servings of vegetables, and six servings of whole grains per day.

As you shift your dietary focus to fresh, whole foods, you may be less inclined to eat anything fatty or sugary. That's a good thing, since these unhealthy foods not only contribute to weight gain, they also interfere with the absorption of essential nutrients. Also steer clear of anything containing caffeine. Though caffeine is a central nervous system stimulant, it actually relaxes muscles and may interfere with normal genital function.

The mineral zinc is necessary for your body to produce testosterone. Even a mild zinc deficiency can play a role in ED. Good food sources of zinc include pumpkin and sunflower seeds.

Herbal Medicine

The following herbs may be helpful for treating ED.

Asian ginseng. Asian ginseng helps maintain an erection and improves male potency. It is available in tea or capsule form. The recommended daily dose of Asian ginseng is 100 to 200 milligrams, standardized to 4 to 7 percent ginsenosides. The herb is not appropriate for anyone with high blood pressure, heart trouble, or hypoglycemia.

Damiana. This herb has a long history as an aphrodisiac, able to increase libido and calm jangled nerves. Damiana capsules generally contain 3 to 4 grams of the powdered leaves; take two capsules twice a day. When using damiana tincture, add 3 to 4 milliliters to an 8-ounce glass of water or juice and drink twice a day.

If you prefer, you can brew a tea from dried damiana leaves, which are available in some health food stores and organic grocery stores. Place 2 to 3 grams of dried leaves in a cup of boiling water and steep for 10 minutes, then strain and allow to cool. Drink 2 to 3 cups per day.

Garlic. The use of garlic as a medicinal herb dates back thousands of years. Studies have shown the herb to be effective for improving circulation. Fresh garlic works best; if you tolerate the herb well, try to eat one whole clove every day.

For garlic supplements, look for enteric-coated tablets or capsules with standardized allicin potential. Take 400 to 500 milligrams, once or twice per day, to provide up to 5,000 micrograms of allicin.

Garlic has anticoagulant properties, so if you are taking any blood-thinning medication, be sure to talk with your doctor before using the herb therapeutically. Also inform your doctor that you're taking garlic if you require any sort of surgery. You may need to discontinue treatment for at least 2 weeks prior to your procedure.

Ginkgo biloba. Ginkgo improves blood-flow to the penis as well as throughout the entire body. It is sold raw or in capsule form. The recommended dose is 120 milligrams, twice a day, of an extract standardized to 24 percent flavone glycosides and 6 percent terpene lactones. The terpene lactones are responsible for ginkgo's effect on circulation, while the flavone glycosides have antioxidant properties.

If you are taking any blood-thinning medication, be sure to consult your doctor before adding ginkgo to your self-care regimen.

Maca. Grown at elevations of 12,000 feet and higher in its native Peru, maca belongs to the same plant family as turnips and radishes. It is known for treating ED because of its ability to increase sexual desire and performance. It also is quite nutrient dense, which is beneficial for physical vitality, endurance, and stamina.

Maca is available in capsule form. The recommended dose is 550 milligrams, twice a day.

Sarsaparilla. In Central and South America, sarsaparilla has been used for centuries as an impotency treatment and as a general tonic. It is known for restoring the male reproductive organs.

You can buy packaged sarsaparilla tea in health food stores and organic grocery stores. Drink 1 cup of tea two or three times daily.

Siberian ginseng. Siberian ginseng increases energy and stamina. Look for the herb in capsule form, standardized to at least 0.8 percent eleutherosides. Take 100 to 300 milligrams daily.

Because of the herb's stimulant properties, avoid taking Siberian ginseng within 1 hour of going to bed. Anyone with hypertension should not use this herb.

Hypnotherapy

Hypnotherapy is beneficial for ED that is psychological rather than physical in origin. To learn more about hypnotherapy and to locate a practitioner in your area, visit the Web site of the American Society of Clinical Hypnosis at www.asch.net.

Kegel Exercises

Studies have shown that men who practice Kegels—which involve contracting and relaxing the muscles around the scrotum and penis—experience improvement in erectile function, if not a return to normal function. To try Kegels, you first need to identify your pelvic muscles, which can be done by slowing or stopping the urine flow while you are urinating. The muscles that allow you to do this are the same ones that you need to strengthen. Try to perform 5 to 15 Kegels, three to five times daily. Hold each Kegel for a count of 5 to start, and gradually work your way to a count of 10.

Nutritional Supplements

The following nutrients are necessary for normal sexual function in men.

- B-complex vitamins: Take as directed on the label. May help relieve anxiety.

- DHEA: 50 milligrams daily. Reduces the incidence of ED.

- L-arginine: 1,000 to 2,000 milligrams daily. Necessary for the body to produce nitric oxide, which is vital to a normal erection.

- Zinc: 30 milligrams daily. Supports normal sexual function in men.

Lifestyle Recommendations

Check your medications. As mentioned earlier, ED is a common side effect of medications. Read the labels or the product inserts of any medicines that you may be taking. If you see ED listed as a potential side effect, you might want to ask your doctor about reducing your dosage or switching to another medication.

Control your cholesterol. Studies have shown that high cholesterol may raise a man's risk of erectile dysfunction.

Adopt a healthy lifestyle. Beyond the dietary changes suggested starting on page 88, other lifestyle strategies can help treat ED. Increase your physical activity. Get enough sleep. Cut back on caffeine and alcohol.

Reduce stress. Since stress may contribute to ED, find ways to relax and unwind. Even 10 minutes a day of uninterrupted "quiet time" can help. Just close your eyes, empty your mind, and breathe deeply.

Communicate. If you have been experiencing bouts of ED, you need to talk about it with your partner. Your chances of overcoming ED are much greater if the two of you work together.

Preventive Measures

The following lifestyle strategies can reduce your chances of experiencing ED.

Get regular exercise. Men in midlife who are in good physical shape are less likely to develop ED. Exercise not only increases testosterone but also improves oxygen and blood flow to the penis. Focus on activities that improve circulation, such as walking, running, and swimming.

Address emotional issues. Stress, anxiety, and depression contribute to ED. To help keep them in check—and thus avoid erectile issues—practice relaxation techniques such as deep breathing, guided imagery, and/or visualization.

Limit alcohol consumption. You're more likely to develop ED if you drink in excess. In fact, having more than one alcoholic beverage per day may depress your central nervous system and impair sexual function.

Quit smoking. Smokers are more likely than nonsmokers to develop ED.

Essential Tremor

As its name suggests, essential tremor involves abnormal shakiness. While it may manifest in any part of the body, it most often affects the head, voice box (larynx), hands, or arms. When essential tremor occurs in more than one member of a family, it is referred to as familial tremor.

Essential tremor is the most common movement disorder, affecting as many as 5 million Americans. Though it sometimes is confused with Parkinson's disease, it is an entirely different disorder and, in fact, is far more prevalent than Parkinson's.

Essential Tremor versus Parkinson's Disease

The symptoms of essential tremor differ from those of Parkinson's disease. With essential tremor, the symptoms tend to appear when you are using a particular part of your body, such as your hands. There is obvious shaking when you pick up a glass, for instance. In Parkinson's, the symptoms are most noticeable when you are resting. Also, essential tremor does not cause other medical conditions, while Parkinson's is known to contribute to problems such as rigid limbs, stooped posture, and slow movement.

Causes and Risk Factors

Essential tremor is the result of abnormal communication between different portions of the brain, including the cerebellum, thalamus, and brain stem. The two primary risk factors for the disorder are genetics and age.

Researchers believe that about half of all cases of essential tremor can be traced to genetic mutations. If one of your parents has the genetic mutation for essential tremor, you have a 50-50 chance of developing the disorder. Two genes—designated as ETM1 and ETM2—have been linked to essential tremor, though other genes may be involved as well. In imaging studies, people with essential tremor show increased activity in certain parts of the brain, such as those responsible for relaying pain and other sensory messages.

The risk of essential tremor rises as we get older. Though the mean age of onset is 45, the disorder is particularly common among those over age 60. It affects men and women about equally, though women appear more likely to develop essential tremor of the head.

Certain lifestyle factors may trigger essential tremor. Chief among these are tobacco use, excessive caffeine consumption, and alcohol withdrawal. The disorder can be a side effect of certain medications, such as some asthma, antidepressant, and antiseizure drugs, as well as lithium. It also is associated with medical conditions, including pheochromocytoma (a tumor of the adrenal glands), Wilson's disease (a rare condition in which copper accumulates in the brain and liver), and hyperthyroidism.

Signs and Symptoms

The most common symptom of essential tremor is trembling (or up-and-down movement) of the hands—or, in rare instances, of just one hand. You may have difficulty writing, holding a glass of water, or threading a needle. As mentioned earlier, essential tremor also may affect the head, voice box (larynx), arms, and on occasion other parts of the body. The tremors occur at a rate of 6 to 10 per second.

Fatigue, anxiety, and extreme temperatures tend to worsen symptoms. Conversely, symptoms tend to diminish with adequate rest.

Conventional Treatments

In many cases of essential tremor, there is no formal course of treatment. Doctors simply advise patients to avoid stressful situations and to limit consumption of caffeinated foods and beverages. If essential tremor is interfering with day-to-day living, however, treatment may be necessary.

Medication

Medications provide relief for about 40 to 60 percent of people with essential tremor. Any of the following may be prescribed.

Antiseizure medications. These medicines—an example is Mysoline—may be helpful in cases of essential tremor that do not respond to beta-blockers (discussed next). Potential side effects include drowsiness, difficulty concentrating, nausea, poor gait, and flulike symptoms.

Beta-blockers. Beta-blockers are best known for treating high blood pressure, but they also have proven effective for about 50 percent of those with essential tremor. One commonly prescribed beta-blocker is propranolol (Inderal). Potential side effects of this class of drugs include dizziness, fatigue, nausea, erectile dysfunction, shortness of breath, nasal stuffiness, and—in some older adults—confusion and memory loss. Generally, anyone with asthma, type 1 diabetes, or certain heart problems should not use beta-blockers.

Botulinum toxin injections. Perhaps best known by their brand name, Botox, these injections not only erase wrinkles, they also alleviate certain types of essential tremor—especially tremor of the head or larynx. The injections work by blocking neuromuscular transmissions. Because they can cause weakness in the fingers, Botox injections generally are not used to treat tremor of the hands.

It is important to note that although these injections minimize tremors, they do not improve a patient's functioning.

Bronchodilators. In one study, researchers found that the bronchodilator theophylline reduced essential tremor as well as propranolol and significantly better than a placebo. No side effects were reported.

Tranquilizers. If anxiety seems to play a role in your tremors, your doctor may suggest taking a tranquilizer such as diazepam (Valium) or alprazolam (Xanax). Among the potential side effects of these drugs are memory loss and confusion.

Physical Therapy

Ask your doctor to refer you to a physical therapist, who can teach you exercises that will promote stability in your hands and wrists. After a few sessions, you will be able to practice the exercises at home, on your own.

Psychotherapy

Some people with essential tremor may struggle to cope with the disorder, experiencing emotional effects such as embarrassment and depression. In these cases, psychotherapy—which focuses on healing the mind and emotions—may prove helpful.

Your primary-care physician or your local hospital should be able to provide a referral to a trained psychotherapist. You also might try visiting the Web sites for the following professional organizations: the American Psychiatric Association (www.psych.org), the American Psychological Association (www.apa.org), and the National Association of Social Workers (www.naswdc.org).

Surgery

If your symptoms of essential tremor are severe or disabling, and they haven't responded to treatment with medication, you may require surgery. Here are two procedures that your doctor may recommend.

Deep brain stimulation (DBS). This procedure involves the surgical implantation of a device known as a thalamic stimulator in the thalamus of the brain. Then a pacemaker-like chest unit sends electrical pulses to the implant through a wire. These pulses stop the signals from the thalamus that cause the tremors. This procedure is not as risky as a thalamotomy (described next), and since it may be used on both sides of the thalamus, it may control tremors on both sides of the body.

Stereotactic thalamotomy. In this procedure, a small section on one side of the thalamus is destroyed. If the surgery is effective, as it is in about 70 to 80 percent of patients, it will relieve tremors on the opposite side of the body. Since operating on both sides of the thalamus poses a risk of speech loss and other complications, surgeons usually operate on only one side.

Complementary Treatments

Depending on the cause of the essential tremor, complementary treatments may be useful in reducing symptoms of this disorder.

Biofeedback

Biofeedback involves using an electric monitoring device, which provides data on certain of the body's vital signs, such as heart rate and blood pressure. In a biofeedback session, you will learn how to alter or slow these signs through the use of relaxation techniques. In cases where essential tremor is triggered or aggravated by nervousness, excitement, or tension, biofeedback may help control it.

Various health care professionals use biofeedback in their practices, including psychiatrists, psychologists, social workers, nurses, physical therapists, occupational therapists, speech therapists, respiratory therapists, exercise physiologists, and chiropractors. Try to find someone who has been certified through the Biofeedback Certification Institute of America. For help in locating a biofeedback instructor in your area, visit the BCIA Web site at www.bcia.org or contact your local hospital for a referral.

Lifestyle Recommendations

If you smoke, quit. Smoking may trigger episodes of essential tremor.

Avoid caffeine. Caffeine tends to make your body produce more adrenaline, which may intensify the tremors.

Don't use alcohol as medication. Many people with essential tremor report that their symptoms improve when they drink alcoholic beverages. But using alcohol as a treatment for essential tremor is dangerous and could lead to addiction.

Be safe. If your tremors are severe or not well controlled, take care when holding containers of hot liquid, for example.

Avoid heavy physical exertion. Intense physical activity can aggravate essential tremor. Try not to overdo it.

Reduce stress. Since emotional stress may worsen essential tremor, you need to find ways to offset stress and promote relaxation. Techniques such as deep breathing, guided imagery, and visualization can help alleviate tension and anxiety.

Join a support group. People who are unable to control their tremors often isolate themselves socially, leaving their jobs and spending most of their time at home. A support group not only provides much-needed social interaction and engagement, it also offers a setting in which you can share information and ideas and learn from the experiences of others.

Participate in a clinical trial. If you are having trouble controlling your symptoms, you might want to enroll in a clinical trial for testing of new medications, surgical procedures, and other treatments. Discuss your options with your doctor.

Gastroesophageal Reflux Disease (GERD)

In people with gastroesophageal reflux disease (GERD; also known as acid reflux), the lower esophageal sphincter (LES), which controls the passage of food from the esophagus into the stomach, fails to function properly. As a result, stomach acids travel back into the esophagus, a process called reflux. Without the thin layer of mucus that protects the stomach from these acids, esophageal tissue may be injured and symptoms develop, most often heartburn (a burning feeling in the chest and throat). The regurgitation, or acid reflux, into the esophagus may cause coughing and leave an unpleasant taste in your mouth.

People who suffer from GERD may develop an inflammation of the esophagus known as esophagitis. As time passes, esophagitis may further erode the esophagus and cause bleeding and difficulty in swallowing. In about 10 percent of the people who have GERD, scar tissue forms in the lower esophagus. The scar tissue results in a narrowing of the food pathway and may cause swallowing problems. Because stomach acid has the potential to erode esophageal tissue, it may lead to the formation of painful ulcers, open sores that may bleed and make swallowing difficult.

Just about everyone has occasional bouts of heartburn and acid reflux. However, when these symptoms occur repeatedly over an extended period of time, they are classified as GERD. GERD is a relatively common disorder: It affects at least 5 percent of the world's population. Yet, it is frequently unrecognized and undiagnosed.

Barrett's esophagus, a potentially serious complication of GERD, occurs in about 5 percent of those who are affected. In this disorder, the normally pink-colored stratified squamous epithelium tissue of the lower esophagus changes to an intestinal-type epithelium, which is a salmon color. People with Barrett's esophagus are 30 to 125 times more likely to develop esophageal cancer.

GERD is associated with an increased risk for certain other medical problems. For example, people who have GERD frequently also have asthma and other respiratory disorders, such as chronic bronchitis, chronic sinusitis, and recurrent pneumonia. And because of the acid backing up into the mouth, people with GERD tend to have erosion of dental enamel.

Causes and Risk Factors

There are a number of factors that increase the risk for developing GERD. Though people of any age may develop GERD, about half of those diagnosed with GERD are between the ages of 45 and 64. To determine if there is a relationship between body mass index (BMI) and GERD, more than 10,000 women were studied. A strong positive association was found between the symptoms of GERD and BMI. In subjects who were normal weight and overweight, the risk of GERD symptoms increased with a rising BMI. Symptoms increased as the percentage of body fat increased. Some research has shown that obese people have higher levels of acid in the esophagus, which increases the chance for GERD.

Family history is also thought to play a role. Do you have close family members with this disease? If you do, you probably have a higher risk. People who have a hiatal hernia (a protrusion of part of the stomach into the lower chest so that the diaphragm no longer supports the LES) are more vulnerable. Smoking and drinking excess amounts of alcohol are known to raise the risk.

Signs and Symptoms

In addition to heartburn, GERD may cause a number of other symptoms, including difficulty swallowing, chest pain, nausea, belching, and acid regurgitation. You might also have throat problems, such as chronic sore throats, and you may need to clear your throat frequently.

Symptoms are more frequent at night. Further, they may appear when you are engaging in the following activities: lifting, lying down on your back, and bending over. Symptoms are also more likely to occur after a heavy meal.

Although Barrett's esophagus may cause precancerous changes in the esophagus, it may cause few symptoms. On the other hand, some people have severe heartburn without any damage to the esophagus.

Conventional Treatments

Conventional treatment for GERD may involve a number of approaches, among them lifestyle changes, a variety of medications, and surgery.

Lifestyle Changes

Treatment for GERD normally begins with several lifestyle changes. These include eating smaller meals, sitting or standing after you eat, limiting your consumption of fatty foods, avoiding foods and drinks that tend to be more problematic (chocolate, onions, citrus fruits, coffee, and carbonated beverages), wearing more comfortable clothing that is not tight around your stomach, losing weight, avoiding or limiting your consumption of alcohol, and raising the head of your bed. You may also be advised to

A Quick Guide to Symptoms

☐ **Heartburn**
☐ **Difficulty swallowing**
☐ **Chest pain**
☐ **Nausea**
☐ **Belching**
☐ **Acid regurgitation**
☐ **Throat problems (chronic sore throats or needing to clear the throat frequently)**

stop smoking and make time for relaxation.

Medication may be another factor that contributes to GERD. Your doctor will want to review all your medications, as you may be taking a medication that tends to exacerbate GERD. These include nonsteroidal anti-inflammatory drugs (NSAIDs) such as aspirin, ibuprofen, naproxen, and ketoprofen; sedatives and tranquilizers; potassium tablets; vitamin C tablets; calcium-channel blockers (often prescribed for high blood pressure); anticholinergics (medications that relax smooth muscle, such as those used for chronic obstructive pulmonary disease); theophylline (an asthma drug); quinidine (used to treat heart arrhythmia); and alendronate (for osteoporosis). Don't discontinue any of these medications without consulting your doctor.

Medications

If you have not achieved sufficient relief from lifestyle changes and a medication review, your doctor may suggest medication. There are a number of different types that may be used.

Acid blockers. Acid blockers, which are also called H-2 blockers, reduce the secretion of stomach acid. They last longer than antacids and may prevent acid reflux and heartburn in about half the people who have GERD. Some acid blockers are available over-the-counter; others are sold by prescription only. The over-the-counter acid blockers have half the strength of those sold by prescription. Well-known examples are cimetidine (Tagamet HB) and famotidine (Pepcid AC). On occasion, these medications may have side effects such as dry mouth, dizziness,

drowsiness, and bowel changes. Be sure to ask your doctor if they may interfere with other medications you are taking.

Antacids. Over-the-counter antacids, which neutralize gastric acid, are probably better for occasional heartburn than for GERD, but you may wish to see if they help you. Though they do not cure GERD, they may relieve your symptoms. Common examples are Tums and Rolaids. When antacids are consumed frequently, they may sometimes trigger constipation or diarrhea. Some antacids may interfere with other medications, particularly those for kidney and heart disease. Frequent use of antacids that contain calcium may place you at risk for kidney stones. Further, antacids that contain aluminum, calcium, or magnesium are known to interfere with the absorption of some medications, such as ciprofloxacin (Cipro), tetracycline, and propranolol (Inderal). To prevent these interactions, take these medications either 1 hour before or 3 hours after the antacid.

Proton-pump inhibitors (PPIs). Proton-pump inhibitors (PPIs), such as lansoprazole (Prevacid), omeprazole (Prilosec, Zegerid), and pantoprazole (Protonix), are the most effective medications for GERD. These medications block the production of acid, giving the tissue time to heal. But they may have potential side effects, such as diarrhea, headaches, flatulence, loose stools, and stomach or abdominal pain.

Surgery

The effectiveness of GERD medications has reduced the need for fundoplication surgery, but sometimes surgery may be the most reasonable course of action. Your doctor may recommend surgery if you have a large hiatal hernia, repeated narrowing of the esophagus, Barrett's esophagus, severe esophagitis (particularly with bleeding), or lung problems caused by the acid reflux. A study demonstrated that surgery does not eliminate the need for acid-reducing medications in all patients. In addition, the procedure does not lower the risk for esophageal cancer in patients with GERD and Barrett's esophagus. Surgery corrects about 85 percent of GERD-related respiratory symptoms.

Laparoscopic fundoplication. The open Nissen fundoplication (see below) has now largely been replaced with the laparoscopic fundoplication, in which only tiny incisions are made in the abdomen. The surgeon wraps the upper part of the stomach around the esophagus, creating the same collarlike structure that is found in the open Nissen fundoplication. Because of complications, in about 8 percent of the cases, the surgeon must discontinue the laparoscopic procedure and switch to the open Nissen fundoplication. Your chances of having a successful laparoscopic fundoplication procedure are greatly improved if you select a highly experienced surgeon.

Postoperative problems may include a delay in intestinal functioning, which may result in vomiting, gagging, and bloating. Typically, this lasts for no more than a few weeks. Though uncommon, there may be complications such as bowel obstruction; wound infection; respiratory problems, such as a collapsed lung; muscle spasms after food is swallowed; and an excessively wrapped

Self-Testing

There is no specific self-test for GERD. However, if you suspect that you may have GERD, the American College of Gastroenterology suggests that you ask yourself the following questions. If you answer "yes" to two or more of the questions, you may have GERD.

1. Do you frequently have one of the following:
   ☐ An uncomfortable feeling behind the breastbone that seems to be moving upward from the stomach?
   ☐ A burning sensation in the back of the throat?
   ☐ A bitter acid taste in your mouth?

2. Do you often experience these problems after meals?

3. Do you have heartburn or acid indigestion two or more times per week?

4. Do you find that antacids provide only temporary relief from your symptoms?

5. Are you taking prescription medication to treat heartburn symptoms but still having symptoms?

fundus that causes difficulty swallowing or gas, bloating, or the inability to burp.

Open Nissen fundoplication. Until the early 1990s, open Nissen fundoplication was the surgery most often used for GERD. After making wide surgical incisions, the surgeon wraps the upper part of the stomach around the esophagus, thus forming a collarlike structure. By putting pressure on the LES, reflux is prevented. With this surgery, hospital stays average 6 to 10 days. Failure rates range from 9 to 30 percent. When the procedure fails, it needs to be repeated.

Repairing the lower esophageal sphincter (LES). Using endoscopy, physicians may repair the lower esophageal sphincter (LES). This may be accomplished in a number of ways. In the Bard Endoscopic Suturing System (Endocinch), a tiny "sewing machine" stitches weakened areas of the LES. In the Stretta System, radio-frequency energy heats and melts tissue in the malfunctioning valve and the area connecting the esophagus to the stomach. The scar tissue seems to tighten the valve. With both surgeries, it is possible to return home the same day. There may be some chest, stomach, or throat pain. You should not have either procedure if you have a hiatal hernia or Barrett's esophagus.

Complementary Treatments

Complementary approaches treat the symptoms of GERD, address the underlying cause, and promote dietary and lifestyle changes that are helpful in reducing or eliminating this problem.

Herbal Medicine

Chamomile and ginger. Chamomile, which has an antispasmodic effect, and ginger, a carminative (helps to relieve gas), may be taken as a tea three or four times a day between meals. Chamomile and ginger are readily available in prepared tea bags.

Coriander. Coriander, a stomachic (stimulates digestion) herb, has also been used for the relief of GERD. Steep 2 teaspoons of dried seeds in 1 cup of boiling water for 15 minutes. Drink 1 cup daily.

Devil's claw. Devil's claw is considered a bitter herb that helps neutralize stomach acid. It is available in a tincture, tea, or capsule. As a tea, 1 to 2 grams of the dried powdered root is steeped in a cup of boiling water for 5 to 10 minutes. Drink 3 cups per day. With a tincture, take 1 teaspoon three times a day. In capsule form, 400 milligrams is the recommended daily dose. (There is no standardization of devil's claw.)

Fennel seeds. Chewing fennel seeds can help reduce the burning sensation associated with GERD.

Licorice. Deglycyrrhizinated licorice (DGL) is an anti-inflammatory and helps coat the esophagus. Chew one or two 380-milligram wafers three times daily.

Turmeric. Turmeric reduces acid and breaks down fatty foods. It has long been used in India as a remedy for heartburn. To make a tea, pour 1 cup of boiling water over 1 teaspoon of powdered turmeric and let steep for 5 minutes. Strain well and drink 2 or 3 cups daily.

Hydrotherapy

Prior to eating, place an ice pack over your stomach for 5 minutes. This may reduce the probability of acid reflux.

Nutritional Supplements

Bromelain and quercetin help promote healing of GERD. You may wish to purchase a supplement that contains both bromelain and quercetin.

- Bromelain: 150-milligram capsule three times a day between meals. Anti-inflammatory digestive enzyme that enhances the action of quercetin. Take together.

- Quercetin: 500-milligram capsule three times a day between meals. Anti-inflammatory flavonoid that accelerates healing.

Lifestyle Recommendations

Change your nighttime routine. Since a large percentage of people who suffer from GERD have nighttime symptoms, consider some of these suggestions.

- Avoid bedtime snacks. In fact, don't eat for at least 2 hours before going to bed; 3 hours is even better.

- Take an after-dinner walk, or at least sit upright after eating.

- In bed, lie on your left side. When you sleep on your right side, the stomach is higher than the esophagus, which may put pressure on the LES.

- To raise the entire top half of your body, elevate the head of your bed with 4- to 6-inch blocks or a wedge support. This will help keep stomach acids in the stomach.

Don't attempt to accomplish this goal with pillows—that raises only the head and increases your risk of reflux.

Preventive Measures

Make dietary changes. Avoid or reduce your consumption of chocolate, caffeine, spearmint, peppermint, alcohol, carbonated drinks, tomatoes, onions, garlic, and citrus fruits, all of which lower LES pressure. At the same time, increase your intake of whole grains, protein, and non-acidic fruits and vegetables. Remember to eat slowly and in a relaxed environment.

Quit smoking and reduce alcohol. If you smoke, quit. Also, reduce your consumption of alcoholic beverages. Both smoking and alcohol lower LES pressure, making acid reflux more likely to occur. Quitting smoking and reducing alcohol consumption are thought to be key elements in the prevention of GERD.

Reduce stress. Participating in regular exercise and relaxation techniques such as yoga, tai chi, qigong, and meditation may help reduce stress and improve digestion and other bodily functions.

Reduce your waistline. Large waistlines seem to increase the risk of acid reflux symptoms among white adults, according to a study of more than 80,000 members of the California Health Plan.

Glaucoma

In almost all forms of glaucoma, an abnormally high pressure inside the eyeball causes damage to the optic nerve. If the optic nerve is impaired, you will develop blind spots and suffer the loss of peripheral (side) vision. By the time you experience these symptoms, significant damage has occurred.

At present, there are no known means to correct the damage once it has occurred. Luckily, there are now easy methods to detect glaucoma early, and there are a number of treatments.

Because of internal pressure in the eye, known as intraocular pressure (IOP), the eye is able to function properly and keep its shape. Aqueous humor, a type of eye fluid, is key to this process. In a healthy eye, aqueous humor is produced and drained continuously through what is called the trabecular meshwork (or drainage angle). This process maintains normal pressure within the eye. If eye fluid is unable to drain properly, eye pressure builds and the optic nerve may be damaged, as it is in glaucoma.

In open-angle glaucoma (also known as primary open-angle glaucoma), the eye's means of drainage remains open, but the aqueous humor is draining too slowly. As a result, the fluid backs up and the IOP rises. Acute closed-angle glaucoma (also known as angle-closure glaucoma) is far less common than open-angle glaucoma, but is potentially more serious. In this type of the disease, part of the iris (the colored area of the eye around the pupil) pushes against the lens, closing off the drainage angle and leading to a rapid increase in IOP.

It is possible to have glaucoma without an increase in IOP, a condition known as normal-tension glaucoma. Or you may have a higher-than-normal IOP without injury to the optic nerve. So, in contrast to the prevailing perception that a high IOP is synonymous with glaucoma, a high IOP is actually only one possible component of a glaucoma diagnosis.

Affecting about 3 million Americans, glaucoma is a very common disorder. Almost all of those who have glaucoma have a chronic form of the most common type of glaucoma, open-angle glaucoma.

Causes and Risk Factors

It is believed that open-angle glaucoma is genetically linked. Thus, people with close relatives who have been diagnosed with glaucoma are at greater risk. Also, the incidence increases with age. Open-angle glaucoma is rarely seen among those under the age of 40. Once you turn 50, your risk for open-angle glaucoma doubles about every 10 years. Approximately 14 percent of people who are 80 years old have glaucoma.

African Americans are three to four times more likely than whites to have glaucoma, and they tend to develop glaucoma at younger ages. Asian Americans and Hispanic Americans are also at greater risk. Other factors that increase the risk include medical conditions such as diabetes, high blood pressure, heart disease, retinal detachment, hypothyroidism, eye tumors, and eye inflammation. People who have suffered trauma to the eye as well as those who are profoundly nearsighted are also more vulnerable. Eye abnormalities and prolonged use of corticosteroids also increase the chance that you will develop glaucoma.

Signs and Symptoms

A large number of people with glaucoma do not realize they have a problem. The symptoms of open-angle glaucoma tend to be subtle and do not become more apparent until there is serious damage to the optic nerve. During this time, people lose more and more of their peripheral vision. Open-angle glaucoma tends to affect both eyes, though usually not at the same time. Other symptoms of open-angle glaucoma include problems with night vision, sensitivity to glare and lights, and an inability to distinguish differing shades of light and dark. It is not uncommon for people with open-angle glaucoma to require frequent changes in eyeglass or contact lens prescriptions.

With a rapid rise in eye pressure, closed-angle glaucoma develops quickly. Symptoms include severe eye pain, headache, eye redness, "halos" around lights, blurred vision, and nausea and vomiting. Closed-angle glaucoma requires immediate attention. In only a few hours, there can be permanent vision loss, and blindness may occur in a day or two.

Conventional Treatments

There is no cure for glaucoma, and none of the treatments is able to reverse the damage caused by the disease. Yet, glaucoma may be controlled. If you have been diagnosed with glaucoma, you will need to become more aware of your vision, and you will become a more frequent visitor to your eye care specialist. Conventional treatments for glaucoma include medication and surgery. Recommendations vary according to the type of glaucoma as well as the individual's particular needs.

Medications for Open-Angle Glaucoma

To prevent further damage of the optic nerve, your eye care professional will probably prescribe medication in the form of eye drops; sometimes, he or she may advise more than one type of eye drop. These are designed either to reduce the amount of aqueous fluid produced by the eye or allow better drainage of the fluid

A Quick Guide to Symptoms

Open-Angle Glaucoma
☐ Loss of peripheral vision
☐ Problems with night vision
☐ Sensitivity to glare and lights
☐ Inability to distinguish differing shades of light and dark
☐ Frequent changes in eyeglass or contact lens prescriptions

Closed-Angle Glaucoma
☐ Severe eye pain
☐ Headache
☐ Eye redness
☐ "Halos" around lights
☐ Blurred vision
☐ Nausea and vomiting

If you are experiencing any of the symptoms of open-angle glaucoma and believe that you may have the disease, visit an eye care professional for testing. If you think you may be having symptoms of closed-angle glaucoma, seek medical help immediately.

in the eye. It is very important to administer these drops exactly as your doctor advises.

Beta-blockers. Beta-blockers reduce the production of aqueous humor. The most common beta-blocker is timolol (Betimol, Timoptic). Timolol is long acting and has excellent efficacy for the treatment of glaucoma. It also has few ocular side effects. Though generally used without any problems, beta-blockers must be taken with caution by anyone with a breathing or heart problem.

Carbonic anhydrase inhibitors. Carbonic anhydrase inhibitors reduce the production of aqueous humor and are available in oral and eye drop forms. Dorzolamide (Trusopt) is an example of a carbonic anhydrase inhibitor. When taken orally, some common potential side effects are frequent urination and tingling in the fingers and toes. Depression, stomach problems, fatigue, weight loss, and sexual dysfunction have also been noted from the oral form. Since carbonic anhydrase inhibitors are a form of sulfa medication, people who are allergic to sulfa drugs should not take them.

Prostaglandin analogues. These hormone-like medications increase the outflow of aqueous humor. Latanoprost (Xalatan) is an example of a prostaglandin analogue. They have the potential to cause allergic reactions, inflammation within the eye, blurred vision, fatigue, and headache. In some people, they cause blue, green, or hazel eyes to permanently change to brown, and they cause eyelashes to grow longer.

Miotics. By reducing the size of the pupil and pulling the iris away from the drainage network, miotics allow better drainage of fluid. But they also cause a dimming of vision and problems seeing at night or in a darkened room. Other potential side effects include allergic reactions, teary eyes, and eye pain. Pilocarpine (in Piloptic and other medications) is an example of a miotic.

Alpha-2 adrenergic agonists. These agents reduce the production of aqueous humor and increase its outflow. Apraclonidine (Iopidine) is an example of an alpha-2 adrenergic agonist. While their most common potential side effects are dry mouth and altered sense of taste, they may also cause an allergic reaction, with red and itching eyes and lids.

Medications for Acute Closed-Angle Glaucoma

As has been noted, acute closed-angle glaucoma is an emergency situation. Doctors generally administer medications to reduce eye pressure. After that, surgery is normally required.

Medications for Normal-Tension Glaucoma

Since the IOP does not rise to an abnormal level with this form of glaucoma, this is a more challenging situation for eye care professionals and their patients. However, it has been determined that the usual IOP-reducing medications do slow the development and progression of the disease.

Surgery for Open-Angle Glaucoma

If the medications are poorly tolerated or ineffective, your eye care professional may recommend surgery. Types of surgery for open-angle glaucoma include laser trabeculoplasty and conventional incisional surgery. It should be noted, however, that while surgery may be helpful, it does not actually cure glaucoma. More than half of the patients who undergo surgery require medication within 2 years. None of these surgeries are without risk, and there may be complications. Selecting a highly trained and experienced eye surgeon may reduce the risk of these.

Conventional incisional surgery. This procedure is also referred to as trabeculectomy or filtering surgery. After you receive medication to help you relax, eye drops, and an anesthetic injection to numb your eyes, your physician uses an operating microscope to open a small hole in the sclera or white part of the eye. Fluid is able to drain from the small bubble, or bleb, that forms over this opening. Filtering blebs are at risk for leaking and infection, and retinal swelling may blur or reduce vision.

If there is scar tissue from the glaucoma, a physician may prefer an alternative surgical technique in which a plastic valve is implanted. This provides a means by which eye fluid may drain. After this procedure, expect several follow-up visits. About one-third of the people who have this type of surgery develop cataracts within 5 years, but it is not certain whether or not the cataracts are related to the surgery.

Laser trabeculoplasty. In a trabeculoplasty, a physician uses a laser to burn tiny spots in the trabecular meshwork, a drainage area located in the front of the eye. These spots tend to improve the eye's ability to drain. With improved drainage, the damage to the optic nerve may be halted.

Before the office procedure, which requires less than 30 minutes, the doctor numbs the eye with drops. During the surgery, you sit at a slit lamp and are fitted with a special eye lens. The doctor aims the laser beam through the lens. You may see flashes of green or red light. One or two hours after the surgery, the doctor checks your eye pressure. For a few days after the procedure, you may have blurred vision and a sensitivity to light, but there should be no pain. Anticipate follow-up appointments to check eye pressure. Unfortunately, the benefits of a trabeculoplasty may be limited: There's evidence that in more

Tips for Using Eye Drops

The eye is able to hold only about 20 percent of the amount of fluid in a standard eye drop. Therefore, put only one eye drop in your eye at a time. If you have been instructed to use more than one eye drop, wait about 5 minutes between the drops. This will allow more of the drops to be absorbed and will reduce waste.

To minimize the amount of eye drops absorbed into your bloodstream, after putting the drops in your eyes, close your eyes for a minute or two. While your eyes are closed, lightly touch the corner of your eyes closest to your nose. This will help close the tear ducts, which keeps the drops from getting into your nose and being absorbed through the blood vessels in the nasal mucosa. End the process by wiping excess eye drops from your eyelid.

than half of all cases, the eye pressure rises to an unsafe level within 2 years of surgery.

Surgery for Acute Closed-Angle Glaucoma

This condition is a medical emergency. If you have symptoms of acute closed-angle glaucoma, seek help from an eye care professional immediately. In an attempt to lower the eye pressure as quickly as possible, the physician will probably administer several medications. Then, the eye surgeon will make a tiny opening in the eye's iris, thereby enabling the aqueous fluid to flow more freely. This may be done either with a laser (iridotomy) or conventional surgery (iridectomy). Since it is likely that if you have acute glaucoma in one eye the other eye will also develop this disorder, physicians generally recommend surgery in the second eye as well. Recovery may take up to 8 weeks, and during this time your vision may be blurred.

Complementary Treatments

By using dietary measures, lifestyle changes, and herbal medicine, practitioners of complementary medicine can boost the body's natural healing powers. A number of nutrients also hold promise for people with glaucoma.

Diet

Studies have shown that people with glaucoma may be deficient in certain vital nutrients, such as vitamins A, B_{12} (cobalamin), C, and E, plus the minerals magnesium and selenium. These substances are essential for protecting the optic nerve, reducing eye pressure, and preventing vision loss.

Vitamin A may be found in yellow, orange, and dark green vegetables and fruits, such as carrots, broccoli, spinach, winter squash, sweet potatoes, and cantaloupe. Further, it is found in liver, eggs, cheese, and butter. Vitamin B_{12} is best obtained from animal-based food such as meat, fish, livers, eggs, milk, and oysters. Vitamin C is found in all fruits and vegetables, such as those that contain vitamin A. Good sources of vitamin E include green leafy vegetables, liver, whole-grain cereals and breads, and dried beans.

Magnesium is found in virtually all raw, green leafy vegetables, as well as in almonds, cashews, soybeans, most seeds, and whole grains. You may obtain selenium from seafood, chicken, meat, whole-grain cereals, egg yolks, and garlic.

Increasing your intake of foods rich in these nutrients may aid in reducing the effects of glaucoma. Dark green, leafy vegetables such as spinach, kale, and broccoli contain phytochemicals known as carotenoids, including beta-carotene, lutein, and zeaxanthin, which play an important role in eye health. The body converts beta-carotene into vitamin A, the "eye vitamin." Studies have shown that lutein and zeaxanthin in particular slow vision loss associated with glaucoma and even help improve eyesight. A healthy diet that includes lots of whole grains, vegetables, and fruits may help to avoid many of the risk factors associated with glaucoma, such as diabetes, high blood pressure, and heart disease.

Studies have shown that coffee may reduce bloodflow to the retina. If you presently have retinal damage, you may want to reduce your consumption of coffee or eliminate it altogether. Moreover, drinking a quart or more of any liquid within a half-hour period should be avoided. People with glaucoma should drink lots of fluids, but not a lot at any given time; just drink smaller amounts throughout the day.

Herbal Medicine

Ginkgo and bilberry are two promising herbal remedies for the treatment of glaucoma.

Bilberry. Bilberry acts as an antioxidant. By stabilizing collagen, decreasing capillary fragility, and improving the delivery of oxygen to the eyes, bilberry has a protective effect. Bilberry extract is available as a dietary supplement. The recommended dose is 100 milligrams of bilberry extract (standardized to 25 percent anthocyanosides), three times a day.

Ginkgo biloba. Ginkgo contains a variety of bioflavonoids and also acts as an antioxidant. It increases the oxygen supply to the eyes, assists in improving circulation to the optic nerve, and reduces oxidative damage. One study found that people with decreased ocular bloodflow experienced a mild improvement after taking 160 milligrams of ginkgo extract (standardized to 24 percent flavone glycosides and 6 percent terpene lactones) for 4 weeks, then 120 milligrams a day for an indefinite period of time. However, a dose as low as 40 milligrams per day is often recommended. The flavone glycosides give ginkgo its antioxidant benefits; the terpene lactones increase circulation and have a protective effect on nerve cells. You should not use ginkgo if you are taking a blood-thinning medication. Consult with your doctor.

Hydrotherapy

Alternating hot and cold compresses over the eyes for a short period of time may help to increase circulation in the eyes. Hot compresses relax the nervous and circulatory systems; cold compresses stimulate the circulation in the eyes. Begin with 2 minutes using a hot compress, then follow that with 1 minute using a cold compress. This procedure may be repeated two or three times, but always end the treatment with a cold compress.

Nutritional Supplements

The following nutrients decrease IOP and protect the optic nerve by neutralizing free radicals and aid in maintaining healthy eyes.

- Vitamin A: 10,000 IU daily. Reduces visual impairments such as night blindness, an early symptom of open-angle glaucoma.

- Vitamin B_{12}: 100 micrograms daily. Protects the optic nerve and prevents visual loss. One Japanese study reported that people with glaucoma who took 1,500 micrograms of B_{12} daily over a 5-year period regained some sight and showed no visual deterioration.

- Vitamin C: 1,000 milligrams daily in divided doses of 500 milligrams each. Antioxidant that helps prevent cell damage. Do not take with selenium.

- Vitamin E: 400 IU daily. Neutralizes free radicals and protects optic nerve.

- Beta-carotene: 25,000 IU daily. Aids in maintaining healthy eyes.

- Fish oil (essential fatty acid): 3,000 milligrams daily in divided doses of 1,000 milligrams. Reduces inflammation.

- Magnesium: 500 milligrams daily. Increases blood supply to the optic nerve.

- Selenium: 200 micrograms daily. Decreases IOP and protects the optic nerve. Take with vitamin E for better absorption.

Traditional Chinese Medicine

Practitioners of traditional Chinese medicine have used acupuncture, tai chi, and herbal medicine (particularly the herb *Salvia miltiorrhiza*) to lower IOP. In Chinese medicine, the eyes are a reflection of the strength of the liver. The acupuncture treatment is focused on nourishing and strengthening that organ. Acupuncture is very effective in treating the early stages of glaucoma. It is also useful in treating other symptoms associated with glaucoma, such as headaches and vomiting. To locate a practitioner trained in traditional Chinese medicine, visit the Web site of the National Certification Commission for Acupuncture and Oriental Medicine (NCCAOM) at www.nccaom.org or the American Association of Acupuncture and Oriental Medicine at www.aaaomonline.org.

Lifestyle Recommendations

Aerobic exercise appears to be a factor in the control of IOP. Studies have shown that people with glaucoma who take a brisk, 40-minute walk 5 days a week are able to reduce their eye pressure by 2.5 milliliters, which is equivalent to the reduction expected from beta-blockers. When exercise is discontinued, the pressure increases. This form of exercise also aids in lowering cholesterol, reducing high blood pressure, and improving circulation to the retina.

Preventive Measures

Limit your intake of coffee. One study found that coffee produced a reduction of up to 13 percent in the retinal bloodflow. This is particularly damaging to those who are already in the process of losing vision.

Protect your eyes. Wear a protective hat and sunglasses that block out 100 percent of the sun's ultraviolet-A (UVA) and ultraviolet-B (UVB) rays and filter out at least 85 percent of blue-violet rays.

Quit smoking. If you smoke, quit. And avoid exposure to secondhand smoke. Smokers have an increased risk for developing glaucoma. If you have glaucoma and you smoke, your disease will probably progress more rapidly. Studies have shown that retinal bloodflow is reduced by 16 percent by the nicotine in cigarettes.

Reduce stress. It is believed that stress may trigger acute closed-angle glaucoma. Relaxation and meditation involve deep-breathing exercises, muscle relaxation, and focused attention, all of which work together toward shutting down the anxiety-producing "fight-or-flight" response of the body and reducing IOP. Some of these techniques include tai chi, yoga, biofeedback, and various forms of meditation.

Watch what you eat. Eliminate trans fatty acids and avoid refined foods such as white sugar and white bread and saturated fats. This type of diet can lead to diabetes, a condition that can then lead to glaucoma.

Watch your blood pressure. Elevated blood pressure is a risk factor for developing open-angle glaucoma.

Gout

Recognized as an illness for more than 2,000 years, gout (also known as acute gouty arthritis) is an arthritic condition that causes inflammation of the joints. When the body has more uric acid than it can manage, it may convert some of it into needlelike crystals (tophi). These may then be stored in the joints. But elevated uric acid alone does not cause gout. Many people with elevated levels never have this disorder.

Uric acid is a by-product of the breakdown of purine, a substance that is part of human tissue and is found in a number of foods, among them organ meats, sardines, anchovies, and meat gravies. Normally, uric acid is dissolved in the blood and eliminated from the body via urine or broken down in the gut and eliminated via the stool. If the body starts to produce excess amounts of uric acid, if the kidneys fail to eliminate sufficient amounts, or if you start to eat large amounts of food with high amounts of purine, levels of uric acid in the blood may rise. This is a condition known as hyperuricemia. Then, if uric acid forms crystals that collect in joint spaces, you may develop gout. Once in the joints, the crystals may cause inflammation, including swelling, redness, and intense pain. Under the skin, the collection of crystals may look like lumps.

Because uric acid crystals may collect in the kidneys, if you have gout, there is a 10 to 40 percent chance that you will also develop kidney stones. About 25 percent of people who have chronic hyperuricemia develop progressive kidney disease. People with gout frequently have cardiovascular problems such as high blood pressure, coronary artery disease, and congestive heart failure, and they have higher rates of cataracts and dry eye syndrome.

Gout is a relatively common disorder: More than 2 million Americans have it. It affects more men than women (especially men 40 and older).

Causes and Risk Factors

A number of factors are believed to play a role in the development of gout. Family history (genetics) helps determine your risk. Do you have family members with this disorder? If you do, you may be at increased risk. In some cases, there is an enzyme defect that interferes with the way the body breaks down purines. Because people who are overweight have more tissue to turn over and break down, excess weight is associated with an increased risk. Also, alcohol interferes with the removal of uric acid from the body, so drinking too much alcohol raises your risk. Lead in the environment may trigger gout, and there is some evidence that people with thyroid problems are at greater than normal risk.

Some medical conditions raise the risk of gout, including hypertension (high blood pressure), hyperlipidemia (high levels of fat in the blood), and arteriosclerosis (narrowing of the arteries). Uric acid levels in the body may rise because of surgery, immobility due to bed rest, and severe or sudden illness. As chemotherapy treatments break down abnormal cells, they may cause purine to be released into the blood and increase the risk of gout.

Certain medications interfere with the body's ability to remove uric acid, so they increase the amount of uric acid in the body. These include diuretics (taken for hypertension, edema, and heart disease) and anti-inflammatory medicines made from salicylic acid, such as aspirin. Other suspect medicines include niacin, levodopa (used for Parkinson's disease), and cyclosporine (which suppresses the body's immune system and is given to recipients of an organ transplant). That explains why people who have undergone organ transplantation are at greater than normal risk for gout.

Signs and Symptoms

The majority of people first realize that they may have gout when they have excruciating pain in the great toe or knee. Gout is less likely to occur initially in the ankle, wrist, finger, elbow, or instep. There are four basic stages of the disease.

1. In the first stage, known as asymptomatic hyperuricemia, you have an elevated uric acid level, but experience no symptoms. During this time, you will not know that you have gout. For a fortunate few, the disease never advances beyond this stage.

2. With the second stage, known as acute gout or acute gouty arthritis, you have uric acid deposits in the joints. You will experience a sudden (between 8 and 12 hours) onset of intense pain and swelling in (usually) one joint, which tends to be warm and tender. The skin over the area may be taut, red, and shiny, and, after a few days, it may peel. There also may be chills and a mild fever. You may not want to eat, and you may feel generally ill. Acute attacks tend to occur at night and may be triggered by stress, alcohol, drugs, or another illness. The pain may be so severe that you are unable to endure the weight of your blanket on your toe. Most early attacks subside within 3 to 10 days, even without treatment. It may be months or years before another attack.

3. Most people with untreated gout will have a second attack within 2 years. With time, attacks last longer and occur more often. The period between acute attacks is known as intercritical gout.

4. The final stage of gout, known as chronic tophaceous gout, develops over an extended period of time. However, gout that is properly treated may not advance to this stage. In chronic tophaceous gout, the intercritical periods become shorter and the attacks longer. There is permanent joint dam-

age, chronic low-grade pain, and mild to acute inflammation. Several joints may be affected. Knobby crystal deposits may appear on the curved ridge on the edge of the ear, the forearms, elbows, knees, hands, feet, and (rarely) around the heart and spine. If you have chronic tophaceous gout, the cartilage and bone at the affected joints may be destroyed. Tophi may grow as large as handballs. Though it is rare, if the crystals lodge in the spine, there may be serious damage.

Conventional Treatments

Designed to relieve pain, reduce inflammation, and prevent damage to the affected joints, there are several treatments for an acute attack of gout. Conventional treatment for gout includes resting and protecting the affected joint with a splint. Applying ice packs four times a day for 30-minute intervals may bring quite a bit of relief. Whenever possible, treatment should begin at the very first sign of an attack. It is always advisable to keep a supply of your medication on hand, as you never know when you might have an attack.

Since asymptomatic hyperuricemia doesn't always lead to gout, it is not normally treated. However, treatment may be recommended if very high uric acid levels pose a threat to the kidneys.

Medications

During the intercritical period between acute attacks and to prevent further attacks, your doctor may recommend low doses of either

A Quick Guide to Symptoms

☐ Excruciating pain in the great toe or knee
☐ Taut, red, and shiny skin over the affected area
☐ Chills and a mild fever

anti-inflammatories or colchicine. Antihyperuricemic drugs help reduce the amount of uric acid.

Antihyperuricemic drugs. Because your doctor may want to reduce the amount of uric acid, a drug classified as an antihyperuricemic may be prescribed. These drugs dissolve monosodium urate (MSU) crystals and tophi. They are more likely to be recommended if you have had two or more acute gout attacks, if your x-rays show damage from gout, if your gout attacks are severe, if more than one joint is affected, if you are considered at risk for tophaceous gout, or if your hyperuricemia is caused by an identified inborn metabolic deficiency. Still, if you do not have normal kidney function, you should not take these drugs.

Before prescribing an antihyperuricemic drug, your doctor will want to determine if your high levels of uric acid are caused by an overproduction of uric acid or by your body's failure to eliminate a sufficient amount of uric acid. To do this, your doctor may ask you to collect your urine for 24 hours. If you produce too much uric acid, you may be prescribed allopurinol (Zyloprim); if you excrete too little uric acid, you may be prescribed a uricosuric (probenecid or sulfinpyrazone).

Before you begin antihyperuricemic therapy, your doctor will want to have your most recent attack of gout under complete control. The joints should no longer be inflamed. Some doctors advise waiting a month.

Anti-inflammatory drugs. Younger people with no serious health problems are typically started on high doses of nonsteroidal anti-inflammatory drugs (NSAIDs), such as indomethacin (Indocin) and naproxen (Anaprox, Naprosyn). NSAIDs reduce inflammation caused by the uric acid crystals, but they do nothing to alter the amount of uric acid in the body. COX-2 inhibitors may also be effective medications to reduce the inflammation during an acute attack. If you are unable to tolerate the gastrointestinal side effects of NSAIDs, then oral corticosteroids may be recommended or a steroid preparation may be injected into the affected joint. The most frequently prescribed oral corticosteroid is prednisone.

When taken over an extended period of time, these medications are likely to cause gastrointestinal side effects. Other possible side effects include increased blood pressure, dizziness, ringing in the ears, headache, skin rash, and depression. If you experience any of these problems, you should report them to your doctor.

Be aware, too, that NSAIDs—particularly aspirin and other salicylate drugs—diminish the effectiveness of uric acid medications.

Colchicine. In some cases, if you do not respond to NSAIDs or corticosteroids, your doctor may consider colchicine. This is a urate blocker that is most useful when taken within the first 12 hours of an attack. It is not recommended for adults who have kidney or liver problems. Possible side effects include nausea, vomiting, diarrhea, and blood and/or kidney problems.

Surgery

On occasion, large tophi are surgically removed. But it is rarely necessary to replace a joint.

Complementary Treatments

Complementary medicine treatments focus on removing excess uric acid from the body. Nutrition and herbal medicine are the main approaches to reduce and eliminate the symptoms of gout.

Diet

Purine is a compound in the body that breaks down to form uric acid. Eating foods high in purine may raise the levels of uric acid in the body, causing gout in people who are susceptible to this condition. The following foods are high in purine and should be eliminated from the diet: organ meats, anchovies, sardines, mackerel, herring, fish roes, and meat extracts. Because they have moderate amounts of purine, limit your consumption of other meats and fish as well as lentils, whole-grain cereals, beans, peas, asparagus, cauliflower, mushrooms, and spinach.

To lower your uric acid levels and prevent an attack, eat a half pound of fresh or frozen cherries every day for 2 weeks. The antioxidants that they contain have been shown to be effective in lowering uric acid levels. Other beneficial antioxidants are hawthorn berries, blueberries, strawberries, and other dark red-blue berries. Noncitrus juices and vegetable juices such as celery, parsley, and carrot juice are also recommended. Vegetables such as cabbage, kale, and other green leafy vegetables may be valuable.

Herbal Medicine

Bilberry and grape seed extract. Bilberry and grape seed extract, also referred to as pro-anthocyanidin (PAC) bioflavonoids, are both antioxidants that are useful in the relief of gout. Bilberry eliminates uric acid, and grape seed extract reduces inflammation. The recommended daily dose of bilberry is one 100-milligram capsule, standardized to 25 percent anthocyanosides, three times a day. Take one daily 100-milligram capsule of grape seed extract, standardized to contain 95 percent procyanidolic oligomers (PCOs).

Devil's claw. Devil's claw, which is an anti-inflammatory agent, relieves joint pain and reduces uric acid levels. It is available in a tincture, tea, or capsule. As a tea, 1 to 2 grams of the dried powdered root is steeped in a cup of boiling water for 5 to 10 minutes. Drink 3 cups per day. With a tincture, take 1 teaspoon three times a day. In capsule form, 400 milligrams is the recommended daily dose.

(There is no standardization of devil's claw.)

Flaxseed and charcoal poultice. Another useful herbal remedy is a poultice made of flaxseed and charcoal. To prepare, combine equal amounts of flaxseed powder and activated charcoal powder. Both of these are available in health food stores. Gradually add hot water until a paste is formed. Place the paste on the afflicted joint and cover it with plastic wrap. This will draw out toxins. Replace the poultice every 2 to 4 hours.

Juniper berries and nettle. Juniper berries and nettle are two diuretic herbs, effective in reducing uric acid. Juniper berries are available in tincture form; take 0.5 to 1.0 milliliter, three times a day. It should be noted that due to their stimulating effect on the kidneys, juniper berries should be avoided by people with kidney disease. Stinging nettle supports kidney function. The recommended daily dose for nettle is 250 milligrams.

Nutritional Supplements

Nutritional supplementation aids in maintaining proper levels of nutrients, prevents the production of uric acid, and has anti-inflammatory effects.

- Multivitamin/mineral: Take as directed on the label. Ensures proper levels of essential nutrients.

- B-complex vitamins: Take as directed on the label. Assist in proper digestion.

- Bromelain: 200 to 400 milligrams three times a day between meals. Anti-inflammatory. Often found in capsules with quercetin as they should be taken together for better absorption.

- Folic acid: 5 milligrams daily. Helps inhibit the production of uric acid.

- Omega-3 fatty acids: 1 tablespoon of flax-seed oil daily. Decreases inflammation and tissue damage of gout.

- Quercetin: 250 to 500 milligrams three times a day between meals. Bioflavonoid that inhibits the enzyme that produces uric acid and prevents release of inflammatory compounds.

Lifestyle Recommendations

Elevate the painful joint. During an attack, keep the painful joint elevated.

Lose weight. If your doctor has indicated that excess weight is contributing to your gout, you need to lose some of the pounds. Ask your doctor for some suggestions or a referral to a weight-loss program.

Preventive Measures

Sip coffee. Canadian researchers found that coffee consumption, both caffeinated and decaffeinated, lowered uric acid levels, which reduces the risk of gout.

Don't smoke. Smoking increases blood pressure and cholesterol, two risk factors of gout.

Drink nonalcoholic and noncaffeinated fluids. Drink plenty of nonalcoholic and non-caffeinated fluids throughout the day. Fresh juices made from raw fruits and vegetables are best, particularly during an attack. Juices made with blueberries, carrots, celery, cherries, parsley, strawberries, and any other dark red-blue berries are most beneficial, as all of these help to neutralize uric acid. This dilutes and promotes the excretion of uric acid in urine. You also need to keep your fluid intake up in order to avoid dehydration, which can trigger a gout attack.

Exercise. Exercising and stretching regularly increase circulation, which helps to remove uric acid and other excess toxins from the body. Any type of exercise that does not irritate the affected joint is beneficial. Swimming, walking, and bicycling are all recommended. Tai chi, yoga, and qigong are other forms of exercise that increase circulation and remove excess uric acid.

Reduce alcohol consumption. Reduce your consumption of alcohol. Studies have shown that a daily glass of red wine may provide some health benefits without increasing the risk of gout or an attack as compared to consuming beer or hard liquor.

Gum Disease

Gum disease is an infection of the gums or the tissues that surround and support the teeth. It is caused by plaque, a sticky film of bacteria, which may harden into a substance called tartar (calculus). Toxins emitted by the bacteria damage the gums.

In the early stage of gum disease, which is called gingivitis, the gums tend to be red and swollen, and they may bleed easily. Still, this type of gum disease is reversible. In the more advanced forms of gum disease (periodontitis), the inner layer of the gum and bone recede and form pockets, called periodontal pockets. Spaces between the teeth and gums have the tendency to collect debris and become infected. Gums and the bones supporting the teeth become profoundly damaged. Teeth may fall out or require extraction by a dentist.

In addition to harming your teeth and their supporting bones, periodontal (gum) disease places you at increased risk for other medical problems. For example, if you have periodontal disease, you have a greater risk for respiratory infection. Moreover, people with periodontal disease are almost twice as likely to have coronary artery disease, and there is also an association between gum disease and stroke.

Gum disease is extremely common. It has been estimated that more than 75 percent of Americans over the age of 35 have some level of this disorder.

Causes and Risk Factors

While gum disease may be caused by inadequate oral hygiene, there are also a number of other factors that may play a role. One of the key causes is the use of tobacco. People who smoke are far more likely than nonsmokers to have gum disease. Moreover, smoking reduces the likelihood that any treatment will be effective. Other possible contributing factors are hormonal fluctuations, stress, poor nutrition, poor-fitting fillings and crowns, anatomical tooth abnormalities, illness, and clenching and grinding of the teeth.

People who are living with HIV/AIDS or autoimmune conditions such as rheumatoid arthritis and Crohn's disease are known to have higher rates of gum disease, as do those who have inadequate amounts of vitamin C in their diet. Diabetics are more likely to suffer from periodontal disease. Likewise, people with diabetes who have periodontal disease experience increases in their blood sugar, which means they have a greater risk for complications.

Since saliva is protective of the teeth and gums, medications that reduce the levels of saliva in the mouth may foster gum disease. The antiseizure medication diphenylhydantoin (Dilantin) and the drug nifedipine (Nimotop, a calcium-channel blocker used to treat cardiovascular disease) may cause gum tissue to grow abnormally.

Your risk for gum disease increases as you

age. More than half of those over age 55 have periodontitis. Furthermore, it is believed that up to 30 percent of the American population may have a genetic tendency for gum disease. Those who are predisposed may be up to six times more likely to develop some level of gum disease than those who do not have this predisposition.

Signs and Symptoms

Even if you don't notice symptoms, you still may have gum disease. That is one of the reasons that regular visits with a dentist are so important. However, many people with gum disease do have symptoms. These may include receding gums; gums that bleed during and/ or after brushing the teeth; frequent bad breath or bad taste in the mouth; red, swollen, or tender gums; loose or shifting teeth; abscesses; deep pockets or pus between teeth and gums; and changes in your bite or the fit of your partial dentures.

Conventional Treatments

The goal of treatment is to stop the progression of gum disease and control infection. Your dentist will suggest how often you should brush and floss your teeth. Since brushing removes only the plaque from the outside of the teeth, flossing is very important. It gets under the gumline and between the teeth. In some instances, to obtain a better cleaning, your dentist may advise using a special toothbrush that has motorized heads.

During a checkup, your dentist or dental hygienist will remove plaque and tartar that are above and below the gumline. If there is evidence of gingivitis, more frequent cleanings will most likely be advised. Your dentist may also suggest that you use a toothpaste or mouthwash that is FDA-approved for gingivitis. Colgate Total, which contains the mild antimicrobial triclosan, has received FDA approval for that use. You will need a prescription from your dentist for a mouthwash that contains chlorhexidine, which has received similar approval.

If your dentist determines that there has been bone loss and your gums have receded, you will probably be referred to a periodontist, a dentist who specializes in gum disease and dental implants. It is at the periodontist's office that you will have a more intensive, deep clean-

A Quick Guide to Symptoms

☐ Receding gums
☐ Gums that bleed during and/or after brushing the teeth
☐ Frequent bad breath or bad taste in the mouth
☐ Red, swollen, or tender gums
☐ Loose or shifting teeth
☐ Abscesses
☐ Deep pockets or pus between teeth and gums
☐ Changes in your bite or the fit of your partial dentures

ing, which is called a scaling and root planing (or SRP). To reduce the discomfort, before the procedure, you will be given a local anesthetic. During a scaling, the periodontist performs a deeper scraping of the plaque and tartar above and below the gumline. Root planing smoothes the roots of the teeth and aids in the removal of bacteria. With a smooth, clean surface, gums are better able to reattach to the teeth.

In conjunction with an SRP, you will probably be given a prescription for doxycycline hyclate (Periostat), an oral medication. It curtails the action of collagenase, an enzyme that is instrumental in the destruction of teeth and gums.

Surgery

If you have significant gum disease, surgery may be advised. Surgery allows for a more extensive deep cleaning of the root surface as well as the removal of diseased tissue. Bones, gum, and tissues supporting the teeth may be repositioned and shaped.

Bone grafting. If there has been severe bone loss, it may be useful to attempt to encourage the regrowth and restoration of bone tissue. During a bone-grafting procedure, either your bone or bone from a donor (decalcified freeze-dried bone allografts or DFDBAs) is used to replace lost bone and stimulate new bone growth.

Gingivectomy and gingivoplasty. In a gingivectomy, a periodontist removes gum tissue. This procedure is followed by a gingivoplasty, in which gum tissue is reshaped. Since the size of the periodontal pockets is significantly

Choosing Floss

Avoid using very thin floss, which may cut the gum. Fortunately, it has become increasingly more difficult to locate. If you have little room between your teeth, try a floss made of Gore-Tex. It will slide more easily and not tear as quickly. If you have bridgework, you may want to consider a floss threader, a device that resembles a needle with a large loop. After floss is threaded into the loop, it may be placed between the bridge and the gum. It may then clean under the false tooth and along the sides of the adjacent teeth. A Proxabrush, a tiny narrow brush, is also useful for cleaning areas under bridges.

reduced, bacteria have a less desirable environment in which to grow, and the gums may be restored to good health.

Guided-tissue regeneration. In the beginning of this procedure, which is used to stimulate bone and gum tissue growth, the root surfaces and diseased bone are carefully cleaned. Special absorbable or nonabsorbable fabrics are used to cover any holes in the

If you have a history of mitral valve prolapse or rheumatic heart disease, tell your dentist. You may be prescribed an antibiotic before you undergo any dental work. This is done to prevent bacterial endocarditis, a life-threatening illness in which there is a bacterial infection in the heart valves.

bone. Gum is sewn over the fabric. In about 4 to 6 weeks, the nonabsorbable fabric must be removed.

Implants. Some patients who have lost teeth as a result of periodontal disease want dental implants. Endosteal implants are the most common type; they are positioned in the jawbone. Subperiosteal implants are placed on the jaw and are used when there is minimal bone height, due to age or disease.

Open flap curettage. During this procedure, small incisions are made in the gums, and the gums are lifted away from the teeth and bone. The diseased root surfaces are curetted (cleaned and scraped), and the pocket depth is minimized. Bone may be recontoured. Gum tissue is then positioned into the proper place.

Medications

After periodontal procedures, your dentist or periodontist may recommend continued treatment with antibiotics or other medications. Some antibiotics or other medications are applied directly to the gums; other antibiotics are taken orally.

Agents applied directly to the gums. Actisite is a thin strip that resembles dental floss, but contains tetracycline hydrochloride, an antibiotic to kill bacteria. Threads are generally inserted between a tooth and the gum and secured with dental adhesive, a type of glue. Steady concentrations of tetracycline are released into the gum. After 10 days, the threads are removed.

While the Actisite is in place, avoid foods that may loosen or dislodge the strips. These include peanuts, raw vegetables, crusty breads, and sticky items. When brushing or flossing your teeth, avoid the areas with Actisite. Also, be aware that tetracycline medication increases your sensitivity to the sun. So, as long as you are using it, be sure to wear sunscreen and, during the sunniest times of the day, try to stay out of the sun.

Other products include Atridox, which conforms to the surface of the gums and solidifies and releases antibiotics, and PerioChip, a chip that is placed inside the gum pocket after it is scaled. It releases the powerful bacteria-killing antiseptic chlorhexidine. Elyzol is either a gel or strip that is placed on the gum. It contains metronidazole, which is useful against bacteria and parasites. Since they only work locally and do not affect other areas of the body, topical products are generally the preferred method.

Oral antibiotics. A 10-day course of treatment with doxycycline (Periostat) has been found useful for acute inflammation and infection. Sometimes, a low-dose form of doxycycline is prescribed for a number of weeks. Though the dose is too low to fight bacteria, it blocks the actions of collagenase, the enzyme that harms the connective tissues that hold the teeth. Taking a nonsteroidal anti-inflammatory drug (NSAID) such as aspirin or ibuprofen (Advil) with doxycycline appears to improve the effectiveness of doxycycline.

There is also evidence that chronic periodontal disease responds to a combination of metronidazole and amoxicillin. These are administered for 1 week per month for 4 months. Potential side effects include yeast overgrowth, stomach upset, allergic reactions, and sensitivity to sunlight.

Complementary Treatments

By addressing the underlying causes, complementary medicine has been successful in providing approaches that stop the progression of gum disease and control gum infection.

Ayurveda

Because of its strong antibacterial and anti-inflammatory properties, Ayurvedic practitioners often recommend the use of neem powder to fight gum disease. In addition, neem prevents plaque and is an excellent agent in fighting periodontal disease. Neem is available as a toothpaste, as a mouthwash, and as a gum.

Biofeedback

Biofeedback uses an electric monitoring device to obtain data on vital body functions. During a session, you will be taught ways to use relaxation techniques to alter or slow the body's signals. Biofeedback has been shown to be valuable for people who have gum disease caused by clenching or grinding their teeth. Various health care professionals incorporate biofeedback into their practice, including psychiatrists, psychologists, social workers, nurses, physical therapists, occupational therapists, speech therapists, respiratory therapists,

Oral treatments, or medications you ingest by mouth, have the potential to cause side effects such as gum redness, swelling, pain, aching, throbbing, soreness, and bleeding. If you are experiencing more than mild discomfort, you should contact your dentist or periodontist.

exercise physiologists, and chiropractors.

It is recommended that you seek a health care practitioner who has been certified through the Biofeedback Certification Institute of America (BCIA). To locate a practitioner in your area, look on the BCIA Web site at www.bcia.org, check your local hospitals and medical clinics, or check the Yellow Pages under the practitioners mentioned above.

Diet

Gums and teeth always benefit from a healthier diet. The absence of antioxidants in your diet can lead to an increase in free radicals, which increase bacteria and inflammation of the gums. Be sure to include lots of fruits and vegetables that contain vitamin C, such as broccoli, brussels sprouts, cantaloupe, grapefruit, oranges, and strawberries. Deficiency in vitamin C is directly linked to gum disease. Additionally, many smokers have lower levels of vitamin C, which may increase the risk of developing gum disease even further. Limit your intake of processed foods and foods that are high in sugar and saturated fat. An unbalanced, poor diet may weaken the immune system, which may cause receding gums and bone loss.

Herbal Medicine

Herbs may be found in all dental care products, such as toothpaste, mouthwash, dental floss, dental picks, and lip balm. Because of their antiseptic and antibiotic properties, there are many herbs that are helpful in treating gum disease. Others are used for their invigorating and fresh taste. They safely and effectively provide the same benefits as ingredients found in conventional dental products. Instead of artificial flavors and sweeteners, such as saccharine or glycerine, natural toothpaste may freshen breath with natural ingredients such as fennel or peppermint. Peppermint also has antiseptic and antibiotic properties that treat gum infections. Clove is useful in relieving toothaches and is invigorating to the mouth and gums, as is ginger. Chamomile has anti-inflammatory properties that soothe the mucous membranes in the mouth. Eucalyptus is a germicide, antiseptic, and astringent; myrrh repairs painful bleeding gums; and calendula eases toothache pain.

Aloe vera. To help reduce pain and inflammation, rub a small amount of aloe vera gel directly on the gums. Aloe vera is available as a prepared ointment, a liquid drink, or a gel. To accelerate the healing of irritated gums, the natural gel or prepared ointment should be rubbed directly on the gums.

Echinacea and goldenseal. When used in mouthwashes, echinacea and goldenseal are as effective against germs as are conventional mouthwashes that contain alcohol.

Horsetail and bloodroot. Horsetail and bloodroot have been found to be extremely helpful in preventing and treating gum disease. The gel from the silica of the horsetail plant is particularly effective for periodontal disease caused by years of smoking. It also protects against bacteria, fungi, and viruses. Bloodroot has been shown to inhibit oral bacteria, diminish plaque, and stimulate the flow of saliva. The enzyme in the saliva breaks down plaque and flushes out food particles, so bloodroot is useful in the treatment of gingivitis.

Sage. Because of its antiseptic and astringent properties, sage is another herb that is beneficial in mouthwash.

Tea tree oil. Tea tree oil is a powerful antiseptic, germicide, and fungicide commonly found in dental products. It is particularly useful for combating bacteria that cause gum disease.

Nutritional Supplements

Deficiency in essential vitamins and minerals can increase the risk for periodontal disease.

- Multivitamin/mineral: Take as directed on the label. Should contain 200 IU of vitamin D for its anti-inflammatory effects, which can help reduce susceptibility to gum disease.

- Vitamin C: 1,000 milligrams daily in divided doses of 500 milligrams each. Deficiency leads to gum disease.

- Calcium: 1,000 milligrams daily in divided doses of 500 milligrams each. Needed for strong teeth.

Lifestyle Recommendations

Check your town's fluoride levels in drinking water. A study reported in the April–June 2007 issue of the *Indian Journal of Dental Research* stated that when excess fluoride was added to the drinking water, incidence of gum disease increased. Interestingly, for the study, fluoride levels were brought up to the level commonly used in many US cities, 4 ppm (parts per million).

Choose natural dental care products. Natural ingredients are able to perform the same functions as the chemicals and additives found in conventional dental products. Calcium carbonate (natural chalk) polishes teeth without harsh abrasives. In addition to cleaning and whitening, by hardening the tooth enamel, baking soda remineralizes and strengthens the teeth as effectively as fluoride. Sea salt also remineralizes the teeth and makes them stronger. Peroxide is particularly useful for fighting gingivitis.

Drink sufficient water. Drink at least eight 8-ounce glasses of water every day. That will enable your mouth to produce sufficient amounts of saliva, which reduces mouth inflammation. This becomes increasingly more important as one ages. In addition, an adequate amount of daily water may reduce bad breath, tooth decay, and infection.

Replace your toothbrush about once a month. Brushes that are worn are less effective in removing plaque. Look for an American Dental Association (ADA) seal on your toothbrush and always choose a toothbrush with a soft head.

Use correct brushing technique. Begin by brushing your teeth with a dry brush for about 1$\frac{1}{2}$ minutes. Brush where the gum meets the tooth. The bristles should rest at a 45-degree angle to the teeth. Brush the inside of the bottom teeth first, and then the inside of the top teeth and the outside of the teeth. Don't forget also to brush the biting surfaces of the teeth. After applying a paste to the toothbrush, repeat the entire process. Conclude the process by brushing the tongue for about 30 seconds. Thoroughly rinse your toothbrush and follow the brushing with flossing.

In choosing a toothbrush, it is important that you find the right one for you. There are scores of different options. Experiment with the various shapes, and replace the brush when the bristles become frayed. You do not need to brush hard.

Use correct flossing technique. In spite of the proven benefits, about two-thirds of people do not floss. Yet, flossing is one of the most important things you can do for your teeth. Begin with about 18 inches of dental floss. Wind it around the middle fingers of both hands. Holding the floss between your thumbs and forefingers, glide it gently back and forth between your teeth. At the gum line, curve it around each tooth and slide it against the gum. Then, rub it up and down the teeth.

Preventive Measures

Brush often. Brush your teeth at least twice a day. Use a soft-bristled toothbrush that is in good condition and toothpaste and mouth-washes containing natural ingredients that strengthen teeth and prevent decay. At least once each day, clean between your teeth with floss or an interdental cleaner.

Cut down on sugar. Sugar helps the bacteria that create plaque to multiply.

Get outside. Vitamin D, which is absorbed through direct sunlight, is needed for healthy gums. Try to get 15 minutes of sun per day to give your body an adequate amount of vitamin D.

Get regular dental checkups. Keep regular visits with your dentist. This will improve the chances that problems will be caught early, when they are easiest to treat. Also, professional cleanings are vital in the prevention of periodontal disease.

Massage the gums. To help strengthen your gums and improve their overall health, use a sulcus brush, which is a toothbrush with a stimulator. These are sold wherever toothbrushes are sold. The brush should be used without toothpaste to massage the gums. By stimulating lymphatic flow, this will improve circulation and help remove waste products. It is recommended that you do this 2 to 3 minutes every day.

Another option is to massage your gums with the tip of a finger onto which you have applied a small amount of eucalyptus or witch hazel. Massage in a circular motion for 5 minutes each day.

Reduce stress. Take measures to reduce stress and to deal with the stress that you cannot avoid. Excess stress and worry may lead to higher levels of the stress hormone cortisol in the saliva. Cortisol lowers immunity, which in turn may lead to gum disease.

Stop smoking. If you smoke, stop. Smoking contributes to gum disease. Studies have shown that smoking is the number one cause of periodontal disease. More than half of periodontal cases are linked to smoking.

Use a tongue scraper. Remove as much bacteria from your tongue as you can. The tongue is a breeding ground for bacteria. In fact, 90 percent of bad breath is from bacteria on the tongue. To combat the buildup of bacteria, you may wish to use a tongue scraper. It removes bacteria from the tongue crevices. To avoid gagging, start at the tip of the tongue and gradually work your way to the back, scraping toward the tip.

Take your time to brush. The American Dental Association recommends brushing your teeth for 2 minutes to ensure adequate removal of plaque. Plaque is a thick, sticky substance similar to peanut butter. If you try to wipe peanut butter from your counter surface, you will find that it does not remove with one easy swipe of a paper towel or sponge. Many toothbrushes, both manual and electric, have built-in timers that beep to let you know when you have reached 2 minutes.

Hearing Loss

Hearing loss is the diminished ability to hear sounds in one or both ears. It's hardly surprising that so many of us experience hearing loss as we age. After all, hearing is a complicated and delicate affair. The ear is divided into three components: the outer ear (auricle and external ear canal), the middle ear (eardrum, middle ear bones, and middle ear space), and the inner ear (the cochlea, semicircular canals, and internal auditory canal). Sound waves are trapped by the auricle and channeled through the external ear canal to the eardrum. The sound waves cause the eardrum to vibrate, leading to motion in the middle ear bones. This motion triggers fluid waves within the cochlea, which are then transformed into nerve impulses in the auditory nerve. The auditory nerve transmits these impulses to the brain, where the messages are organized into sounds.

Hearing loss is generally classified as either sensorineural or conductive in origin. Sensorineural hearing loss is due to problems in the inner ear or auditory nerve. This form of hearing loss, which may be the result of head injury, tumors, illness, the use of certain prescription drugs, poor circulation, stroke, high blood pressure, or birth defects, may not be reversible. Conductive hearing loss is due to problems in the outer or middle ear that block or limit sounds from the tympanic membrane (eardrum) from reaching the inner ear. Blockage may be caused by the presence of fluid in the middle ear, abnormal bone growth, earwax in the ear canal, or a middle-ear infection.

Conductive hearing loss is often correctable.

The most common type of hearing loss in aging adults is presbycusis, which is sensorineural in origin and is caused by changes in the inner ear (the cochlea and semicircular canals). As we age, hair cells in the cochlea die and are not replaced. As a result, there is a reduced transmission of electrical messages from the outer ear to the brain. Hair cells that receive high-frequency sounds are the first to deteriorate.

Tinnitus is another common form of hearing loss, which is usually sensorineural in origin. With tinnitus, you hear ringing, roaring, or other sounds inside your ears. The condition may be caused by a number of factors, such as the overuse of aspirin, the use of antibiotics, earwax, an ear infection, or a nerve disorder. However, doctors are frequently unable to locate a cause. The progression of tinnitus is variable: It may stop entirely, periodically reappear, or remain more or less constant.

Though statistics vary, it has been estimated that tinnitus may affect as many as 50 million Americans. About 10 million are so disturbed by the condition that they seek medical care. Of these, about 2.5 million people are seriously disabled.

Hearing loss is quite common. A total of about 28 million Americans of all ages have some degree of hearing loss. By the age of 55, about 20 percent of all Americans are affected. A decade later, at the age of 65, that figure climbs to 33 percent.

Causes and Risk Factors

The process of aging increases your risk for hearing loss. Genetics is also believed to play a role, and environmental factors are extremely important. Those who have been exposed to loud sounds for extended periods of time are at greatly increased risk.

An increasingly common cause of hearing loss is the exposure to loud noise, a sensorineural condition that is called noise-induced hearing loss. While this may be due to sudden exposure to loud noise such as an explosion, noise-induced hearing loss is most often seen in people who are exposed to persistent loud sounds, such as those who work (or previously worked) in noisy environments. Musicians, construction and airport workers, and tree cutters are among those particularly prone to noise-induced hearing loss.

Tinnitus may be the result of jaw joint (temporomandibular) disorders, the stiffening of the bones in the middle ear (otosclerosis), and (rarely) head and neck tumors. Because of the abrupt change in atmospheric pressure, people who scuba dive may experience tinnitus. If you already have tinnitus, your symptoms may worsen if you have earwax buildup, an ear infection, or a rupture of your eardrum.

Medications That May Cause Hearing Loss

The following are some of the prescription medications that may cause hearing loss.

☐ Beta-blockers such as metoprolol (Lopressor) and propanolol (Inderal), which are frequently used for high blood pressure

☐ Aminoglycoside antibiotics, such as gentamicin (Geramycin, G-Mycin, Jenamicin 2), neomycin, and tobramycin (Nebcin)

☐ Diuretics such as furosemide (Lasix, Myrosemide) and ethacrynic acid (Edecrin), prescribed for high blood pressure and congestive heart failure

☐ Chloroquine, a malaria drug (the hearing loss is usually reversible)

☐ Aspirin (the hearing loss is usually reversible)

☐ Quinidine (Cardioquin, Quinaglute, Quinidex, Quin-Release), used to treat irregular heartbeat

☐ Cisplatin (Platinol), a cancer chemotherapy agent

Signs and Symptoms

If you have hearing loss, you are having difficulty hearing what other people say. You may have a problem hearing the other person on the telephone. It may seem as if others are mumbling or the radio or television volume is too low. You may have trouble hearing when there is noise in the background. If more than two people are talking at the same time, you may be unable to follow a conversation. You may have tingling or ringing in your ears.

Do you often misunderstand what people are saying? Do others tell you that the TV or radio volume is too loud? Are you finding that you are frequently asking others to repeat what they just said? These are all signs of hearing loss.

Conventional Treatments

If your doctor determines that your hearing loss is caused by an ear infection, then the appropriate antibiotic may be prescribed. Similarly, if the loss is from impacted earwax, your doctor will remove it. This process begins with putting a few drops of baby oil, mineral oil, or glycerin into the affected ear to loosen the wax. Then, using a bulb syringe, your doctor squirts warm water into your ear. On occasion, the procedure needs to be repeated several times before the wax falls out. At times, a doctor may use a suction device or a small instrument known as a curette to scoop out the wax.

Other treatments for hearing loss, depending on their cause and nature, may include the use of hearing aids and surgery.

Hearing Aids

The vast majority of adults with age-related hearing loss benefit from wearing a hearing aid. It is important to remember that hearing aids make sounds louder, but they do not make them any clearer. However, you don't want the hearing aid to make sound too loud, which could further damage your ears. So, take care to find a reputable dealer; ask your doctor to recommend one. Allow yourself at least 4 to 6 weeks to adjust to a hearing aid.

The following is a brief outline of the main types of available hearing aids.

- Completely in-the-canal (CIC): The size of a jellybean, this is the smallest and least visible style. It fits into the ear canal. This type of hearing aid is useful for mild to moderate hearing loss. Since the volume is preset, you may need to return to the dealer several times for adjustments. Also, this type is not for people with a lot of earwax.

A Quick Guide to Symptoms

- ☐ **Difficulty hearing what other people say**
- ☐ **The radio or television volume seems too low**
- ☐ **Trouble hearing when there is noise in the background**
- ☐ **Tingling or ringing in your ears**

- In-the-canal (ITC): This type of hearing aid fits into the opening of the ear canal. It is useful for people with moderately severe hearing loss. Though the volume control device is small and may be difficult to use for someone who has arthritis in the fingers, the user may adjust the volume. As with CIC devices, these hearing aids are not for people with a lot of earwax or fluid that drains from the ear.

- In-the-ear (ITE): While far more noticeable than the previous two types of hearing aids, these have controls that are easier to adjust. They are also the smallest type that may be used by people who have a buildup of earwax or fluid in the ears. They are useful for people with moderately severe hearing loss.

- Behind-the-ear (BTE): These are the largest and most powerful type of hearing aid. They may be useful for people with severe hearing loss. It is easy to change the batteries and adjust the volume controls.

- Implantable bone-conducting hearing aids: For people who are unable to use any of the previously noted hearing aids, this type is another option. With this type, a metal screw is implanted into the skull behind the ear. The hearing aid may then be attached to the protruding metal. Unlike the other types of hearing aids that amplify sound, these devices conduct sound into the inner ear by vibrating against the mastoid bone. Implantation requires two surgical procedures.

In addition to selecting a style of hearing aid, be prepared to choose a type of circuitry.

Self-Testing

If you suspect that you have a diminished ability to hear, ask yourself the following questions. Positive answers may mean that you have lost some of your hearing.

☐ Do you find yourself straining to understand conversations, especially if several people are talking?
☐ Do you find yourself having trouble hearing people on the telephone?
☐ Do you seem to hear better in one ear than the other?
☐ Are you misunderstanding what other people are telling you?
☐ Have other people told you that the radio or TV is too loud?
☐ Do you sometimes fail to hear your telephone ringing?
☐ Do you frequently ask people to repeat what they have said?
☐ Do you work or have you worked in a noisy environment?
☐ Do you have a great deal of difficulty hearing the voices of women and children?
☐ Have you found yourself avoiding social situations because of communication problems?

Circuitry determines the quality of sound that you will obtain from your hearing aid. The oldest type, analog circuitry, amplifies all the sounds. It is better for people who are home more and who tend to have one-on-one conversations. Programmable circuitry is more flexible and is a better choice for someone who lives in a variety of sound environments. The newest circuitry is digital circuitry, which provides the best sound but is also the most expensive.

Surgery

If your hearing loss has been caused by abnormal bone growth or trauma to the ear, it may be corrected by surgery. You will need to consult with an otolaryngologist, a physician specializing in disorders of the ear, nose, and throat, who will be able to determine if you would benefit from a surgical intervention.

Adults with severe sensorineural hearing loss who have obtained little or no benefit from hearing aids may wish to consider a cochlear implant. A cochlear implant consists of a microphone, speech processor, transmitter and receiver/stimulator, and electrodes. During the procedure, an otolaryngologist makes an incision behind the ear and mastoid on one side of the head. Some bone is removed and electrode wires are inserted through the middle ear into the cochlear or inner ear. About 6 weeks after the surgery, you will be fitted with the remaining parts. The small microphone picks up sounds from the environment and the speech processor, then selects and arranges the sounds. A transmitter and receiver/stimulator converts signals from the speech processor into electric impulses, and the electrodes collect impulses from the stimulator and send them to the brain.

Since the procedure requires surgery under general anesthesia, you should be in overall good health. Once you have a cochlear implant, you will need to work with an audiologist to learn how to interpret the sounds. Rehabilitation for an adult may take 6 months to a year.

Complementary Treatments

Individuals suffering from hearing loss should seek the care of a specialist. Complementary medicine treatments may be used as an adjunct to this care and are generally concerned with the moving of blockages, such as fluid, mucus, or earwax, and with stimulation of the auditory nerve. Lifestyle changes with diet, nutrition, and herbs may be beneficial.

Acupuncture

Acupuncture improves the flow of stagnant *qi* (life energy), which is associated with hearing loss. Specialized treatments may decrease the symptoms of tinnitus and remove blockages to the middle ear. To locate an acupuncturist in your area, visit the Web site of the National Certification Commission for Acupuncture and Oriental Medicine (NCCAOM) at www.nccaom.org.

Alexander Technique

Keeping the head in the correct position in relation to the spine may improve circulation to the inner ear and has been shown to ease the symptoms of tinnitus, such as dizziness and nausea. A practitioner trained in the Alexander Technique may teach you the proper method. To locate an Alexander Technique teacher, visit the Web site of the American Society for the Alexander Technique at www.alexandertech.org.

Chiropractic

Chiropractic adjustment and manipulation of the neck and spine may increase circulation to the inner ear and relieve blockages affecting the nerves that supply the inner ear. To locate a chiropractor, visit the Web site of the American Chiropractic Association (ACA) at www.amerchiro.org.

Craniosacral Therapy

Imbalances and discrepancies in the rhythm of the cerebrospinal fluid lead to impaired body functions, which may result in chronic ear infection and hearing loss. The practitioner works to reestablish a balanced rhythm and normal function of the cerebrospinal fluid. To search for a qualified therapist in your area, visit the Web site of the International Association of Healthcare Practitioners at www.iahp.com.

Diet

Preliminary studies have shown that deficiency in folate (folic acid or B_9) and B_{12} contributes to age-related hearing loss. Good sources of folate are cooked asparagus, black beans, black-eyed peas, chickpeas, kidney beans, lentils, baby lima beans, navy beans, and cooked spinach. B_{12} is found mostly in meat, fish, and eggs, and some breakfast cereals are fortified with B_{12}. Since the B vitamins work best when taken together, taking a B-complex supplement is recommended.

Eating plenty of raw fruits and vegetables may help clear mucus that is clogging the ears. Garlic, which dilates tiny capillaries, including those that supply the inner ear, should be eaten freely.

Since it causes retention of water in the middle ear, which may cause hearing loss, you should avoid or greatly reduce your consumption of sodium (salt). Saturated fats, processed meats, and other meats place stress on the body and constrict the arteries. Sugar narrows the blood vessels of the inner ear. As a result, these foods should be avoided. Also, dairy products have been linked to recurrent middle-ear infections, which may cause hearing problems.

If you have Ménière's disease or tinnitus, avoid caffeine, chocolate, alcohol, salt, and sugar. This may help reduce the frequency of attacks.

Herbal Medicine

A number of herbs have been shown to be useful for hearing loss.

Black cohosh. Black cohosh has been shown to be effective in decreasing the symptoms of tinnitus. It is available in capsule form. The recommended daily dose is 20 milligrams, twice a day, of standardized extract containing 1 milligram of deoxyactein per tablet.

Echinacea and goldenseal. Echinacea and goldenseal are antioxidant herbs that fight infection, which may reduce the dizziness often associated with hearing loss. These may be taken in capsule form, but a tincture of echinacea with goldenseal is also available. The recommended daily dose is 500 milligrams of standardized extract per day. If taken in liquid extract form, 1 teaspoon, three times each day, is the recommended dose.

When taking an echinacea and goldenseal tincture combination, follow the directions recommended on the label. To avoid building up immunity to the herbs, they should be used for relatively short periods of time, such as 2 weeks. Take them when you have symptoms or when you believe that your immune system has been compromised.

Ginger. Ginger improves circulation and bloodflow to the ear and aids in reducing nausea from tinnitus and Ménière's disease. It is advised that you consume a ¼-inch slice of fresh ginger each day. It may be grated over a salad or added to a stir-fry or any other meal where the flavor would work well. Ginger is also available in tincture form as well as tea bags. For the tincture, follow the directions on the label.

Ginkgo biloba. Ginkgo is an antioxidant that supports circulation, increases bloodflow to the inner ear, and relieves dizziness. It is available in capsule form. However, if you are taking prescription blood-thinning medication, be sure to consult your doctor before taking the ginkgo supplements. The recommended daily dose is 120 milligrams, twice a day, of extract standardized to 24 percent of flavone glycosides and 6 percent terpene lactones. The flavone glycosides give ginkgo its antioxidant benefits, while terpene lactones increase circulation and have a protective effect on nerve cells.

Nutritional Supplements

Deficiency of certain vitamins can lead to hearing loss. Supplementation also supports ear function and reduces symptoms associated with hearing loss.

- Vitamin A: 10,000 IU daily. Stimulates auditory nerve and aids in proper functioning of the cochlea.

- B-complex vitamins: Take as directed on the label. Deficiency linked to ear problems. Reduces tinnitus and stabilizes fluid in inner ear.

- Vitamin B_{12}: Injections or a 1,000-microgram sublingual tablet daily. Deficiency found in many individuals with hearing loss. Injections of B_{12} have been more effective with this condition.

- Vitamin D: 400 IU daily. Supports the cochlea, prevents damage to bones of the middle ear, and may restore some hearing loss.

- Zinc: 30 milligrams daily. May restore some hearing and control symptoms of tinnitus.

Lifestyle Recommendations

It is important to minimize loud background noise as it can cause hearing loss. For example, when mowing the lawn, use adequate hearing protection.

Be observant. Acute hearing loss caused by loud noise, such as from a concert or parade, should go away within 2 days. If your hearing loss persists, consult your doctor.

Exercise. Regular aerobic exercise may improve circulation, boost the immune system, and disperse blockages.

Fluid drainage. If fluid starts to drain from an ear, let it flow; this is a good sign and a natural process, which indicates that the excess buildup of fluid may be releasing.

Reduce noise exposure. Reduce background noise. At home, turn off the TV and/or radio when you are not watching or listening. When dining outside the home, try to sit in the least busy/noisy area of the restaurant.

Communicate more effectively. When you are speaking with others, face them directly and ask them to speak directly to you. That should improve your ability to hear what is being said. Further, so that facial expressions and gestures may be observed, it is useful to have good lighting.

Tell people not to shout at you. Rather, tell them to lower the pitch of their voices—high-pitched sounds are more difficult to hear. Because it makes you raise the tone or pitch of your voice, talking loudly is often counterproductive. Also, ask people to speak at a normal speed. It is not necessary to speak slowly.

Watch what you eat. Pass up foods and drinks that contain caffeine, chocolate, alcohol, salt, and sugar to reduce the frequency of attacks of Ménière's disease and tinnitus.

Preventive Measures

Protect your hearing. Much of hearing loss is permanent and can't be restored. If you work in a noisy environment, wear sound-reducing earmuffs or earplugs, which can help prevent hearing damage. After all, hearing damage can occur at noise levels of just 85 decibels. For comparison, a normal conversation is around 60 decibels, while a chain saw operates at approximately 100 decibels.

Quit smoking. Studies have shown that there is a direct correlation between smoking and an increased risk of hearing loss.

Heart Palpitations

Heart palpitations are the sensation that your heart is beating irregularly, forcefully, or rapidly. Normally, you are unaware of your heart beating. Palpitations may be associated with a heart that beats faster than 100 beats per minute or a heart with a normal rate that has an occasional early beat. They may be felt in the throat, chest, or neck.

Heart palpitations are very common. One study found that 16 percent of outpatient internist or cardiologist patients reported experiencing palpitations.

Causes and Risk Factors

Heart palpitations may be caused by a number of different medical conditions, including anemia, anxiety, fever, hyperthyroidism, problems with the heart's nervous system, and mitral valve prolapse (mild deformity in a valve of the heart). Other things that might trigger heart palpitations include caffeine in foods such as soda, tea, and coffee, as well as the nicotine in cigarettes. Exercising too strenuously may result in palpitations. Some diet pills and decongestants may have stimulants that trigger them. Higher than needed doses of thyroid hormone medications as well as certain antidepressants may cause palpitations, as may the illegal drug cocaine. In addition, palpitations may be seen in individuals with depression and panic disorder. Palpitations are more common in people over age 40.

Signs and Symptoms

If you are experiencing palpitations, your heart feels as if it is pounding or racing. It might also seem as if your heart is fluttering, thumping, or jumping around in your chest. You may feel as if you have butterflies in your chest. The symptoms may last for a few seconds or continue for as long as a few minutes.

Conventional Treatments
Addressing the Underlying Cause

Heart palpitations are generally treated by addressing the underlying cause. If your palpitations are from a stimulant in a medication, your doctor may recommend an alternative medication. If you have been taking too high a dose, your doctor may recommend a lower dose. If the cause is anxiety, you may be advised to take anti-anxiety medications and undergo psychotherapy. Relaxation techniques such as meditation are also useful. If you have anemia, your doctor will want to determine the source. If you have an overactive thyroid, you will require treatment for that condition.

If there is a problem with the heart's nerve

A Quick Guide to Symptoms

- ☐ Heart feels as if it is pounding
- ☐ Heart feels as if it is racing, fluttering, thumping, or jumping around the chest
- ☐ Feel butterflies in chest

conduction system, then further evaluation and testing are needed. These should be conducted by an electrophysiologist, who finds or "maps" the nerve that is causing the problem. When that location is determined, then radiofrequency ablation (radio waves) will be used to destroy the specific site of the conduction problem.

Medications

If you have been diagnosed with an abnormal heart rhythm, you may be treated with an anti-arrhythmic medication such as a beta-blocker or a calcium-channel blocker.

Anticlotting medication. If you have a type of abnormal heart rhythm known as atrial fibrillation, your doctor may recommend that you take low-dose aspirin or another anticlotting medication. Aspirin inhibits the activity of blood platelets, thereby helping to prevent blood from clotting. Still, you should realize that the prolonged use of aspirin may increase your risk for gastrointestinal ulcers and bleeding. Other medications that suppress the activity of blood platelets include clopidogrel (Plavix) and ticlopidine (Ticlid).

Beta-blockers. Beta-blockers reduce the heart rate and lower arterial pressure. Some examples are propranolol (Inderal), atenolol (Tenormin), and carvedilol (Coreg). Potential side effects include moderate lowering of levels of high-density lipoproteins (HDL or "good" cholesterol), fatigue, and lethargy. There have been reports of unusually vivid dreams, nightmares, memory loss, sensations of cold in the extremities, and depression. Some people experience a diminished capacity for exercise, decreased heart function, sexual dysfunction, or gastrointestinal upset.

Calcium-channel blockers. Calcium-channel blockers reduce the heart rate and dilate the blood vessels. Some examples are verapamil (Calan, Isoptin), nifedipine (Adalat, Procardia), nicardipine (Cardene), diltiazem (Cardizem, Tiazac), and amlodipine (Norvasc). Do not mix them with grapefruit juice, which may increase their effects.

> **If, during a single episode,** you experience heart palpitations for an extended period of time or if your palpitations are accompanied by chest pain, sweating, fainting, shortness of breath, or dizziness, you may be having a heart attack or another serious heart event. Call 911 or seek emergency assistance immediately.

Complementary Treatments

When addressing the underlying cause of heart palpitations, complementary medicine offers a number of treatment options.

Diet

Many processed and refined foods contain a high level of preservatives, artificial colors and flavors, saturated fats, caffeine, and other chemicals that may lead to heart palpitations. It is best to eat a healthy diet that is as close to nature as possible. Your diet should include lots of fruits, vegetables, whole-grain foods, and foods that are high in fiber. Try to include a minimum of five servings of vegetables, four servings of fruit, and six servings of whole grains each day.

Self-Testing

Though there are no self-tests for heart palpitations, you will probably know if you are having them. Keep a record of all your episodes. Note how long they last, and list what you were doing when they occurred. Were you experiencing any unusual stress? Were you exercising? What other symptoms did you have? Also, note any medications that you were taking and what you had been eating and drinking.

Be sure to wash fruits and vegetables carefully to remove pesticides and other chemicals that may have been used. Better yet, buy organic products that have been grown without the use of pesticides and chemicals. If you consume animal-based foods such as poultry, pork, or red meat, select organically raised, free-range varieties.

Potassium is a nutrient that is essential for healthy heart rhythm. It is found in many fruits, vegetables, and whole grains. If you consume a diet that contains plenty of these foods, you will eat sufficient amounts of potassium. Since it may affect the potassium level in your body, be sure to limit your salt intake.

Herbal Medicine

Because it strengthens the action of the heart and helps to alleviate sleeplessness due to anxiety, hawthorn is particularly good for heart palpitations. It is available in tea and capsule form. To make tea, steep 2 teaspoons of the herb in a cup of boiling water for 10 minutes and drink slowly. Drink 2 cups of tea each day. Hawthorn is also available in capsule or tincture form, standardized to 2.2 percent total bioflavonoid content. The recommended dose of hawthorn capsules varies widely, ranging from 100 to 300 milligrams, two or three times per day. Be aware that higher doses may significantly lower blood pressure, which may cause you to faint. In tincture, the recommended dose of hawthorn is 4 to 5 milliliters, three times per day. It may take up to 2 months before you see the effects of this herb.

Nutritional Supplements

The following nutrients are effective in reducing or eliminating heart palpitations.

- Multivitamin/mineral: Take as directed on the label. Ensures proper levels of essential nutrients.

- Calcium: 1,000 milligrams daily in divided doses of 500 milligrams. Helps with the absorption of magnesium.

- Magnesium: 500 milligrams daily. Essential for normal heart function and regulates heart rhythm.

- Potassium: Before taking potassium supplements, consult with your doctor. Effective for reducing or eliminating heart palpitations.

Relaxation/Meditation

If you find that your heart palpitations are triggered by anxiety, stress, or other emotional issues (such as anger), it is important to find some coping mechanism. Any practice that addresses the mind/body connection may be useful. These techniques assist in reinforcing a calm and relaxed mind, which in turn relaxes the body and helps restore the heart to a normal rhythm.

Deep breathing exercises allow the mind to focus only on the breath—where it begins, how long to inhale, how long to exhale, and where to feel the exhalation. This slows the mind and the bodily responses that are affected by an anxious mind. Autogenic training is also particularly useful for reducing and eliminating heart palpitations. The repetition of a series of specific phrases takes you through a systematic process of relaxing the entire body. Other techniques to aid in reducing stress and other emotional issues include biofeedback, psychotherapy, yoga, and meditation.

Therapeutic Massage

Swedish massage may be an excellent source of relaxation for both treating and preventing heart palpitations brought on by emotional issues. The rhythmic movements, along with gentle pressure, may loosen tense muscles, allowing a freer flow of blood throughout the body. During a Swedish massage, you will be encouraged to focus on your breathing, thereby reducing anxiety and returning the heart to a normal rhythm.

Lifestyle Recommendations

Keep a journal. Since it may be difficult to determine the underlying cause of heart palpitations, maintaining a daily journal may be useful. Record your intake of foods, beverages, and nutritional supplements; the duration and frequency of physical activity; and how you feel emotionally, mentally, and physically. Be sure to list specific times you exert yourself and any special circumstances. Also, record when you have heart palpitations. You may find that they are the result of a food intolerance, vigorous exercise, or emotional stress. If you are able to note a pattern, you may be able to make lifestyle changes that reduce or eliminate the palpitations. However, if the palpitations continue, you should consult with your doctor.

Quit smoking. The nicotine in cigarettes, which is a stimulant, may cause heart palpitations. Smoking also increases blood pressure and reduces the amount of oxygen to the heart.

Reduce or eliminate caffeine. Caffeine may be found in coffee, tea, chocolate, soft drinks, over-the-counter stimulants, pain medications, cold medications, and appetite suppressants. If you are consuming these products, they may be contributing to your heart palpitations. You may benefit from reducing your intake or eliminating them completely.

Reduce stress. Reduce the stress in your life and take measures to control the stresses you cannot eliminate. Consider meditating or some other way to calm yourself. Any form of meditation in which the mind is focused on a particular object, sound, visualization, breath, or activity is helpful in reversing the body's fight-or-flight response to stress. Yoga and tai chi are considered meditation in movement and help to relax muscles, quiet the mind, and create inner peace. You can also meditate while you are lying down or in a seated position. When you meditate while seated, be sure to sit properly—upright on a chair or the floor, with your back straight.

Hemorrhoids

Also known as piles, hemorrhoids are clusters of dilated veins in the anus. Located in the lowest section of the rectum and anus, hemorrhoids develop when repeated straining or pressure causes the veins in the rectum to enlarge.

There are two types of hemorrhoids, internal (inside the rectum) and external (around the anus). While internal hemorrhoids are usually not painful, passing stool may irritate them and cause them to bleed. Blood may appear on stool or toilet tissue, or in the toilet bowl. Sometimes, straining may push an internal hemorrhoid out through the anal opening. This is known as a prolapsed hemorrhoid. With a prolapsed hemorrhoid, you may have constant, dull, aching pain, as well as itching and bleeding. External hemorrhoids tend to be quite painful. The blood inside may collect and form a clot (thrombus), which may trigger severe pain and inflammation. When irritated, external hemorrhoids tend to itch and/or bleed.

Hemorrhoids are extremely common. By the age of 50, about half of all men and women have some evidence of this disorder.

A Quick Guide to Symptoms

☐ **Itching and burning**
☐ **Bleeding consisting of bright red blood**
☐ **Tenderness and swelling around the anus**
☐ **Painful bowel movements**
☐ **Lumps around the anus**

Causes and Risk Factors

Hemorrhoids are caused by a number of factors. These include the straining or pressure associated with constipation, diarrhea, and the expulsion of diarrhea stools, waiting too long to have a bowel movement, sitting too long on the toilet, frequent coughing or sneezing, heavy lifting, injury to the anus, some liver diseases, and sitting or standing for extended periods of time.

You may also inherit the tendency to develop hemorrhoids. Stress increases the risk of a hemorrhoid flare-up, as does the excess intake of alcohol. With age, the risk for hemorrhoids increases. And people who are obese have a greater risk.

Signs and Symptoms

While hemorrhoids may be symptom-free, they are often associated with a number of symptoms. These include itching, burning, bleeding of bright red blood, tenderness and swelling around the anus, painful bowel movements, and lumps around the anus that may be as large as a walnut.

Conventional Treatments
Dietary Modifications

Eating lots of high-fiber foods coupled with drinking a good deal of water helps to prevent constipation. Good sources of fiber are raw and cooked vegetables, such as cabbage and carrots, and whole-grain cereals with bran.

Medications

If you have mild to moderate pain, your doctor may prescribe a cream or ointment that contains witch hazel, zinc oxide, hydrocortisone, or petroleum jelly, and/or medicated suppositories that are placed inside the rectum.

Nonsurgical Procedures

Hemorrhoid banding or rubber band ligation. In these procedures, used to treat protruding internal hemorrhoids, the doctor places a tight band around the enlarged vein. The vein is then cut open, and the blood clot is removed. Within a few days, the vein heals and the scab falls off.

　　Other nonsurgical treatments. Your doctor may use freezing, electrical or laser heat, or infrared light to destroy a hemorrhoid. Or it may be shrunk by injecting a chemical around the vein (sclerotherapy).

Sitz Baths and Cold Packs

Try sitting in lukewarm water for about 15 minutes, two or three times a day. You may also want to place a cloth-covered ice pack on the anus for 10 minutes, four times a day.

Surgery

If you are in severe pain from hemorrhoids and none of the previously noted nonsurgical methods has provided sufficient relief, your doctor may recommend the surgical removal of the hemorrhoids (hemorrhoidectomy). Before the procedure begins, you will be given general or spinal anesthesia or the anus area will be injected with an anesthetic. In some instances, the procedure may require a 1- or 2-day hospitalization.

Complementary Treatments

Some of the most effective remedies and treatments for hemorrhoids are the ones that you may practice yourself. Dietary changes, exercise, and over-the-counter herbal supplements may not only relieve symptoms associated with hemorrhoids; they may also eliminate the condition.

Diet

Be sure to eat a diet that includes complex carbohydrates, fiber, and flavonoids. These foods may help strengthen the veins, promote regular bowel movements, and decrease the severity of irritating symptoms. Foods containing complex carbohydrates include beans, peas, vegetables, and whole grains. Flavonoids are the substances that give fruits and vegetables their color. Eat lots of fresh fruits and vegetables every day to obtain these substances to help decrease the swelling, inflammation, and bleeding associated with hemorrhoids.

　　It is important to increase high-fiber foods gradually. If you rapidly increase your intake of these foods, you may have uncomfortable symptoms such as diarrhea, gas, bloating, and cramping. High-fiber foods help to create stool that is soft, bulky, and easier to pass. Bran is a good source of fiber, but it has a tendency to bind with minerals such as calcium and zinc, which may result in deficiencies of these minerals. Limit or avoid foods that have little or no fiber, such as cheese, meat, and processed foods.

　　You should also increase your intake of fluids. Each day, try to consume about eight 8-ounce glasses of fluids—plain water is best—that do not contain caffeine or alcohol, substances that may promote dehydration.

Herbal Medicine

To help alleviate symptoms and speed healing, a number of herbs have been proven appropriate for internal use and for topical use as an ointment.

Butcher's broom. Butcher's broom tones the veins and reduces inflammation, helping to shrink hemorrhoids. In capsule form, the recommended daily dose is a standardized extract that provides 50 to 100 milligrams of ruscogenins (the active ingredient) per day. It may also be taken as a liquid extract, 1 teaspoon twice a day.

Horse chestnut. Horse chestnut has been found useful in reducing pain and alleviating the swelling associated with hemorrhoids. The recommended daily dose is 50 milligrams, three times a day, of 16 to 21 percent of standardized extract of aescin. It is also available in a tincture and as a topical cream. Be sure to avoid the leaves and nuts, which are toxic. If you suffer from liver or kidney problems, you should not use this herb.

St. John's wort. This herb is used as a topical ointment applied directly on hemorrhoids to reduce pain and inflammation.

Witch hazel. To ease discomfort and shrink hemorrhoids, witch hazel may be used in a sitz bath. Add 1 cup of distilled witch hazel to 6 inches of lukewarm bath water. Sit in the water for 15 minutes. Distilled witch hazel may be purchased over-the-counter at any pharmacy. For emergency use, a bottle of witch hazel may be kept in the refrigerator. Soak a cotton ball with cold witch hazel and dab directly on the external hemorrhoid. As witch hazel causes blood vessels to contract, this may be especially effective on bleeding hemorrhoids.

Homeopathy

Various over-the-counter homeopathic remedies may be useful depending upon the type of hemorrhoids you have and their symptoms. There are remedies to reduce inflammation, bleeding, and itching. They are readily available at natural and organic health food and grocery stores. Homeopathic practitioners will also take into account your constitution (emotional, physical, and psychological makeup) in addition to your symptoms when suggesting a remedy and dose.

Nutritional Supplements

Certain supplements can promote the healing process by strengthening the immune system and tissues.

- Vitamin C: 1,000 milligrams daily in divided doses of 500 milligrams. Helps shrink hemorrhoids and tone the veins.

- Vitamin E: 400 IU daily. Promotes healing.

- Zinc: 30 milligrams daily. Helps the recovery process.

Lifestyle Recommendations

Add additional fiber. To help regulate bowels and keep stools soft, it may be necessary to add additional fiber to your diet. Dissolve 1 tablespoon of psyllium seed powder in 8 ounces of water or juice; drink twice a day. A tablespoon of ground flaxseed may also be used.

Avoid dry, colored, or scented toilet paper. Dry toilet paper may cause further irritation. So, after a bowel movement, wipe with moist towelettes or wet toilet paper. A towelette that contains horse chestnut and/or witch hazel may relieve some symptoms and speed healing. Colored or scented toilet paper may increase irritation as well.

Avoid scratching. Scratching at inflamed hemorrhoids may actually irritate the walls of the veins and increase inflammation, thereby aggravating the condition.

Exercise. Participating in some form of regular exercise will help to keep the blood flowing in your veins, regulate bowel movements, and help to avoid constipation. Regular exercise reduces the pressure inside your colon, moves food along faster, and promotes the normal functioning of the bowels. One of the best exercises for constipation is a daily 20- to 30-minute walk. Regular exercise also helps maintain a healthy weight. Due to the excess pressure placed on the lower extremities, overweight individuals are more prone to hemorrhoids.

Preventive Measures

Exercise. Exercise may help to prevent constipation. Individuals who are constipated have higher risk for hemorrhoids.

Avoid long periods of sitting or standing. To help keep your blood flowing, periodically move around.

Dietary modifications. The same dietary modifications that are used to treat hemorrhoids may be used to prevent them—increase the fluid and fiber content of your diet.

Don't strain. Straining to pass a stool places increased pressure on the veins in the lower rectum. Straining due to lifting heavy objects has the same effect.

Limit the use of laxatives. Diarrhea may irritate the anus area.

Respond to your bowel. When you feel the urge to pass a bowel movement, don't delay. If you wait too long, the urge may pass and the stool will become drier and harder to pass.

Try an inflatable doughnut cushion. The cushion may be useful for hemorrhoid sufferers who are required to sit for long periods of time.

High Blood Pressure

Blood pressure is the amount of pressure that blood exerts against the arteries as it travels through the circulatory system. Three key organs are involved in the regulation of blood pressure: the heart, arteries, and kidneys. Your heart pumps the blood that flows throughout your body. If your heart must work harder to move the blood, it exerts more force on the arteries. As blood rushes through arteries, they expand and contract. If your arteries have narrowed or lost their elasticity, then your heart must use more force to propel your blood where it needs to go. Your kidneys regulate the amount of water-retaining sodium in your body. When excess salt leads to extra fluid in your body, your blood pressure may increase. Other factors such as stress can also affect your blood pressure.

In the United States today, high blood pressure is an extraordinarily common medical problem. It affects approximately 30 percent of adults. Every year, approximately 2 million additional cases are diagnosed.

If high blood pressure, which is also known as hypertension, is not treated, it has the potential to do serious harm to the body. High blood pressure has been linked to heart failure, kidney failure, damage to arteries, arteriosclerosis, aneurysm, coronary artery disease, left ventricular hypertrophy, eye problems, stroke, heart attack, and premature death. It is believed that high blood pressure contributes

Measuring Blood Pressure

The measurement of blood pressure involves two numbers. The first number is known as systolic pressure. This represents the amount of pressure in your arteries when the heart contracts and ejects blood into the aorta (the main blood vessel leading from the heart). The second number is the diastolic pressure, which indicates how much pressure remains in the arteries between heartbeats, when the heart is relaxed and filling with blood. The two numbers are written as if they are a fraction, with the systolic pressure on the top and the diastolic pressure on the bottom. The systolic number is higher than the diastolic one.

Ideal blood pressure for adults is 120/80 mm Hg or less ("mm Hg" refers to the number of millimeters that a column of mercury will reach in response to a given level of pressure). Though not necessarily ideal, a reading of up to 129/84 or less is considered normal. Systolic pressures between 130 and 139 mm Hg and diastolic pressures between 85 and 89 mm Hg are viewed as high-normal or borderline. When your blood pressure is higher than that, you may be diagnosed with high blood pressure.

Blood pressure readings tend to fluctuate throughout the day. They increase when your heart is working harder, such as during periods of physical exercise or during times that are particularly stressful. Your doctor will probably request a number of separate blood pressure readings before deciding whether you have high blood pressure. Try to take these around the same time each day.

to three-fourths of all strokes and heart attacks, and it causes about 30 percent of all cases of kidney failure. Every year, high blood pressure plays a direct or indirect role in more than 10 percent of the deaths in the United States. Nevertheless, many of those who have high blood pressure are unaware that they have this potentially life-threatening condition. Only about half of those who know that they have high blood pressure are receiving treatment, and only about 25 percent of people with high blood pressure have it under control.

In the vast majority of cases, high blood pressure develops slowly. Though it is rare, high blood pressure may also happen quickly, a condition known as malignant or accelerated hypertension. It occurs more often in people with uncontrolled high blood pressure or heart failure and requires emergency treatment.

There are two main forms of high blood pressure, essential and secondary. About 95 percent of adults with high blood pressure have the essential form, in which no single cause of the hypertension is identified. On the other hand, with secondary high blood pressure, there is a known underlying cause, such as a hormone abnormality or kidney disease. So, when the medical problems leading to secondary high blood pressure are managed, the blood pressure will often drop.

Causes and Risk Factors

As might be expected, some people are more vulnerable to high blood pressure than others. In the United States, African Americans who live in the Southeast have the highest incidence of all groups in the country. But all African Americans seem to have a higher risk for this disorder. They are almost twice as likely as whites to have high blood pressure. Although in traditional societies throughout the world, where people are leaner and more active, blood pressure tends to remain the same throughout life, in the United States, where older people have more body fat and are less active, the risk for developing hypertension increases with age. High blood pressure is relatively uncommon in people under 35. At the same time, more than half of people who are 65 or older have high blood pressure. Americans who are now

Medications as a Cause of Hypertension

If you are being evaluated for high blood pressure, be sure to tell your doctor about all the medications and supplements that you are taking. Some medications have the ability to cause high blood pressure; others will further raise existing elevated pressure. The following are groups of medications that may be of particular concern.

- ☐ **Monoamine oxidase inhibitor (MAOI) antidepressants**
- ☐ **Steroids**
- ☐ **Appetite suppressants**
- ☐ **Cold remedies and nasal decongestants**
- ☐ **Cyclosporine**
- ☐ **Oral contraceptives**

55 years of age or older have a 90 percent chance of developing high blood pressure during their lifetimes.

It is well known that high blood pressure runs in families. If either of your parents has or had high blood pressure, consider yourself to be at higher risk. Young and middle-age men have a higher risk than women.

The following factors also place people at higher risk.

- Obesity

- Excess alcohol consumption

- Smoking

- Sodium sensitivity (Each individual's blood pressure responds differently to the intake of sodium.)

- Lack of exercise

- High cholesterol

- Diabetes

- Emotional disorders, such as anxiety or depression

- Heart failure

It is important to note that the degree of risk that these factors add may be reduced through changes in behavior, diet, and medication.

One study looked at whether there is an association between sleep-disoriented breathing (apnea) and hypertension. Researchers followed more than 700 people with sleep-disoriented breathing for more than 4 years. Individuals with even a few periods of apnea had a 42 percent higher chance of having hypertension, compared with those without apnea. Those with 15 or more apnea events for every hour of sleep had three times the risk for hypertension compared with those without apnea.

Signs and Symptoms

Because high blood pressure rarely has any symptoms, it has frequently been called "the silent killer." Still, there are a few subtle symptoms such as nosebleeds, dizziness, ringing in the ears, blurred vision, and headaches. Then again, these symptoms are so common among the population at large that it may be hard to connect them to high blood pressure. Less than 1 percent of people with high blood pressure—usually those who are faced with the life-threatening malignant or accelerated hypertension—do have noticeable symptoms. These include nausea, loss of vision, headache, confusion, and drowsiness.

A Quick Guide to Symptoms

☐ **Often no symptoms are apparent**
☐ **Nosebleeds**
☐ **Dizziness**
☐ **Ringing in the ears**
☐ **Blurred vision**
☐ **Headaches**

Conventional Treatments

There are essentially two main ways to reduce blood pressure: lifestyle modifications and medications.

Lifestyle Modifications

Unless the situation requires immediate intervention, most doctors advise beginning with lifestyle modifications. These include eating a more healthful diet, losing weight, exercising regularly, reducing your intake of sodium, quitting smoking, limiting alcohol consumption, and developing better methods to deal with stress. Many people who make these lifestyle changes have been able to avoid taking medication or are able to take reduced doses of medication.

Medications

If lifestyle modifications do not sufficiently reduce blood pressure, the next step is likely to be some type of medication. There are many types of high blood pressure medication, which are also known as antihypertensives. You and your doctor may need to try a few before finding one that is suitable for you, and some people take a combination of drugs. The following are the most common categories.

ACE (angiotensin-converting enzyme) inhibitors. Angiotensin-converting enzyme (ACE) inhibitors prevent the body from producing a substance that causes the arteries to constrict. As a result, arteries remain wider, and blood may flow more freely. Though ACE inhibitors seem to have rela-

Self-Testing

Blood pressure is measured in an easy, painless manner with an instrument known as a sphygmomanometer. The sphygmomanometer has an inflatable cuff that wraps around your arm, an air pump, and a column of mercury (or a digital device that performs the same function). Some allow you to monitor your own blood pressure, and your doctor may ask you to purchase one so that you can take periodic readings at home. If you do buy one, be sure to select a sphygmomanometer that is easy to use. Consider an automatic version in which the results are digitally displayed.

To improve the accuracy of your tests, do not eat a big meal, drink caffeine or alcohol, or smoke for at least 30 minutes beforehand. These actions may raise your blood pressure and give a false reading.

tively few side effects, about 20 percent of the people who take them develop a dry cough. This is more likely to occur with women than men. Sometimes, the cough will become so annoying that a change in medication may be needed. Other potential side effects include reduced appetite, rash, and a changed sense of taste. ACE inhibitors are usually not advised for people with serious kidney problems.

Alpha-blockers. In addition to lessening the constriction of arteries, alpha-blockers mildly reduce the levels of total blood cholesterol as well as triglyceride levels. Since they also improve urine flow, men who have prostate problems may benefit from them.

Alpha-blockers are available in both short- and long-acting forms. They may have side effects. When an alpha-blocker is first prescribed, it may cause you to feel dizzy or even faint. Therefore, your doctor will probably start you on a very low dose, which should be taken at bedtime. As you adjust to the medication, the dose may be increased. Other potential side effects include weakness, a pounding heartbeat, nausea, and headache.

Angiotensin II receptor blockers. Angiotensin II receptor blockers are among the newest drugs being used to treat high blood pressure. They prevent arteries from constricting and the kidneys from retaining water and salt. About as effective as ACE inhibitors, they do not trigger an annoying cough. Though side effects are relatively rare, some people report pain in the back and legs, diarrhea, indigestion, insomnia, dizziness, and nasal congestion.

Beta-blockers. Although originally developed to treat coronary artery disease, beta-blockers are now commonly used to treat high blood pressure. Beta-blockers block the effects of the hormone norepinephrine and cause a dilation of blood vessels as well as a decrease in heart rate. Additionally, they slow the kidneys' release of renin, an enzyme that is integral to the production of angiotensin II, a hormone that narrows blood vessels, thus increasing blood pressure.

The two most common side effects of beta-blockers are fatigue and a diminished capac-ity for exercise. Other potential side effects include the loss of sex drive, erectile dysfunction, depression, sleep problems, small increases in the triglyceride level in the blood, a minor lowering of HDL levels, and cold hands. Because of the possibility of negative side effects, people with asthma, heart failure, peripheral vascular disease, insulin-dependent diabetes, chronic obstructive pulmonary disease, and Raynaud's disease may be advised not to take some or all beta-blockers.

Calcium-channel blockers. These medications relax arterial walls, and some also lower the heart rate. There are two main types of calcium-channel blockers, short-acting and long-acting. Short-acting calcium-channel blockers reduce blood pressure quickly, but they must be taken several times a day. Long-acting forms require a longer time to lower blood pressure, but the pressure remains lower for an extended period of time. Potential side effects from calcium-channel blockers include rapid heartbeat, constipation, rash, and swelling of the gums and the feet and/or lower legs.

If you are taking the calcium-channel blockers felodipine (Plendil), nifedipine (Nimotop), nisoldipine (Sular), diltiazem (Cardizem and others), or verapamil (Norvasc), consume grapefruit or grapefruit juice with enormous care. In fact, you may wish to avoid grapefruit products entirely. Grapefruit contains a substance that prevents an enzyme from breaking down calcium-channel blockers. As a result, they may accumulate in the blood. Blood levels may become too high and trigger side effects, such as angina, headaches, palpitations, and ankle swelling.

Centrally acting drugs. These medications stop the brain from sending messages to the nervous system to increase the heart rate and narrow blood vessels. As a result, the heart rate slows and blood flows more freely. Examples are methyldopa and clonidine (Catapres). Unfortunately, centrally acting drugs may have negative side effects such as extreme fatigue or drowsiness. In addition, they have been correlated with weight gain, impaired thinking, erectile dysfunction, dry mouth, headaches, and psychological problems such as depression. Also, when centrally acting drugs are discontinued, they may cause blood pressure to rise to dangerous levels. If you have been taking one and must stop, work with your doctor to find a method that is safe for you.

Diuretics. Diuretics are some of the most frequently prescribed medications for high blood pressure. Effective and inexpensive, they are often the first hypertension medication prescribed by doctors. Diuretics prompt the body to excrete water and salt. Thus, less fluid presses against artery and vein walls. But these drugs also remove potassium, so if you are on a diuretic, you may need to eat some potassium-rich foods such as nectarines, tangerines, watermelon, oranges or orange juice, bananas, mangoes, strawberries, apricots, and cherries.

Complementary Treatments

There are many complementary approaches for reducing blood pressure. Most may be used in conjunction with or even, in the case of diet, as part of conventional treatment.

Acupuncture

Acupuncture is very effective in treating hypertension. For best results, it is often combined with conventional medicine. Along with treatments, physical exercise will probably be encouraged. To locate an acupuncturist in your area, visit the Web site of the National Certification Commission for Acupuncture and Oriental Medicine (NCCAOM) at www.nccaom.org.

Aquatic Therapy

Aerobic exercise and relaxation techniques have been shown to lower blood pressure. Aquatic therapy is a gentle way to begin an aerobic exercise program and reduce stress. Water is an ideal environment to promote relaxation. The rhythmic movements and simple stretches help the mind and body to unwind and reduce stress.

Diet

Doctors who work with people who have hypertension often recommend the Dietary Approaches to Stop Hypertension (DASH) diet. In research studies, it has been proven to reduce blood pressure. The DASH diet is high in whole grains, fruits, and vegetables. In fact, it recommends seven or eight servings of grains each day and eight to 10 servings of fruits and vegetables; four or five servings of legumes, nuts, and seeds are also advised. Dairy products are limited to two or three servings a day, and these should be low-fat or fat-free. And there are no more than two servings each day of lean red meat, fish, or poultry without the skin.

The DASH diet advises no more than 2,400 milligrams of sodium per day, which is less than the 3,000 to 4,000 milligrams that many Americans consume. On a daily basis, your body actually needs only 500 milligrams of sodium. An important part of controlling sodium is limiting your salt intake (ordinary table salt is a form of sodium; it is 40 percent sodium and 60 percent chloride). The recommended maximum of 2,400 milligrams a day is about the amount contained in a single teaspoon of table salt. Some doctors suggest an even lower figure—about 1,500 milligrams of sodium per day. As you attempt to estimate your salt intake, remember that prepared foods, including restaurant foods, tend to contain higher amounts of salt than the food you make at home. Soy sauce generally has high amounts of salt, and there may even be salt in your antacid.

Since some recent studies have shown that sugar increases blood pressure in both animals and humans, it is also recommended that those with high blood pressure limit their intake of sugar. Be sure to check prepared foods for sugar content as well.

Reducing the Sodium in Your Diet

There are many simple, commonsense ways to reduce the amount of sodium in your diet.

☐ **Reduce your consumption of processed food and try to use as many fresh foods as possible. If you must use frozen or canned food, try to use those without added salt.**
☐ **Eat fresh meat, poultry, and fish rather than the canned or processed varieties, such as prepared cold cuts and hot dogs.**
☐ **Check ingredient labels whenever you purchase canned soups, packaged mixes, broths, and salad dressings. All of these tend to be high in salt.**
☐ **Prepare foods such as pasta and rice without adding salt to the water.**
☐ **Remove the saltshaker from the table.**
☐ **Don't add salt to cooked food.**
☐ **Limit your consumption of condiments such as ketchup and mustard.**
☐ **Watch your intake of olives and pickles. They may be high in salt.**

Herbal Medicine

Garlic. The use of garlic as a medicinal herb dates back thousands of years. Research has determined that ingesting 600 to 900 milligrams of garlic extract daily for a 4-week period significantly lowers blood pressure. While fresh garlic is the most effective, garlic supplements may also be useful. When taken fresh, garlic may be used liberally. If you can tolerate it, chew one clove daily. With garlic supplements, look for enteric-coated tablets or capsules with standardized allicin potential. To get up to 5,000 micrograms of allicin, take 400 to 500 milligrams of garlic, once or twice per day. Since garlic has anticoagulant properties, if you are taking prescription anticoagulant medication, check with your doctor before increasing your intake of garlic or beginning a garlic supplementation regimen. If you are planning to have surgery, you should inform your physician about your intake of garlic. It may be best to discontinue garlic for at least 2 weeks prior to surgery.

Ginkgo biloba. Ginkgo is an antioxidant that supports circulation. It is available in capsule form. The recommended daily dose is 120 milligrams twice a day of extract standardized to 24 percent of flavone glycosides and 6 percent terpene lactones. The flavone glycosides give ginkgo its antioxidant benefits, and terpene lactones increase circulation and have a protective effect on nerve cells. However, if you are taking prescription blood-thinning medication, be sure to consult your doctor before taking ginkgo supplements.

Grape seed extract. Grape seed extract contains flavonoids called procyanidolic oligomers or PCOs (also known as proanthocyanidins). Often referred to as PAC, grape seed extract is a valuable antioxidant that rids the body of damaging free radicals and has been shown to reduce blood pressure. The typical recommended dose is a 100-milligram capsule three times a day of extract standardized to contain 92 to 95 percent PCOs.

Green tea. Green tea contains high levels of substances called polyphenols, which have powerful antioxidant properties. It also helps to decrease cholesterol, lower blood pressure,

and prevent the clogging of arteries. Green tea may be taken as a tea or in capsules. Prepared tea bags are readily available in grocery and health food stores. You may also brew a tea from leaves. Steep 1 teaspoon of the leaves in 1 cup of boiling water for 2 to 3 minutes. Green tea can become bitter if steeped too long. Drinking 3 cups of tea per day may provide 240 to 320 milligrams of polyphenols. In capsule form, standardized extract of EGCG (a polyphenol) may provide 97 percent polyphenol content. This is the equivalent of drinking 4 cups of tea per day without the caffeine.

Hawthorn. Hawthorn works to decrease cholesterol and lower blood pressure. In addition, hawthorn helps to strengthen the heart muscles, improve circulation, and rid the body of unnecessary fluid and salt. Hawthorn is available in capsule or tincture form, standardized to 2.2 percent total bioflavonoid content. The recommended daily dose of hawthorn capsules varies widely, ranging from 100 to 300 milligrams two to three times per day. Be aware that higher doses may significantly lower blood pressure, which may, in turn, cause you to faint. In tincture, the recommended dose is 4 to 5 milliliters three times per day. It may take up to 2 months before you see the effects of this herb.

Hibiscus. Recent studies are showing that hibiscus tea may be as effective as captopril, a popular drug used to treat mild to moderate hypertension. It was also reported that results can be obtained quickly. Study participants had more than a 10 percent drop in both systolic (top number) and diastolic (bottom number) pressure in just 2 weeks. You should have your blood pressure monitored carefully to ensure that it does not drop too low, particularly if you are presently taking blood pressure–lowering medications.

Nutritional Supplements

Some nutritional supplements have a favorable effect on hypertension. If you are on prescription medication, check with your doctor before beginning a nutritional supplement regimen.

- Calcium: 1,500 milligrams daily in divided doses of 500 milligrams. Effective against high blood pressure.

- Coenzyme Q_{10}: 100 milligrams daily in divided doses of 50 milligrams. Lowers blood pressure.

- Magnesium: 750 milligrams daily in divided doses of 250 milligrams. Deficiency linked to high blood pressure.

- Omega-3 fatty acids: 1 tablespoon of flaxseed oil daily. Lowers blood pressure, triglyceride levels, and cholesterol.

Relaxation/Meditation

Many doctors recommend various relaxation/meditation techniques to help patients with high blood pressure reduce their stress. Results from a study sponsored by the National Institutes of Health (NIH) and published in 2007 showed that transcendental meditation lowered high blood pressure. Other clinical trials have found a combination of biofeedback, yoga, and meditation to be successful in reducing blood pressure. Also effective for the treatment of hypertension include the gentle movement therapies of qigong and tai chi.

When meditating, finding the right mix of elements is a subjective process. Your goal is to create a setting that allows you to sit or lie down comfortably. Some people like to listen to soft music, while others prefer a sound such as ocean waves or a low hum. Still others prefer complete quiet. You may want to light a candle to gaze at, which may help pull you away from your busy thoughts.

Next, focus on your breathing. Inhale through your nose as if smelling a rose; then exhale with enough force to blow out a candle. Continue as long as you wish. Such deep, cleansing breaths create an overall sense of relaxation and openness.

Lifestyle Recommendations

Begin exercising. One of the key elements in controlling high blood pressure is moderate exercise. Exercise strengthens your heart, which enables it to pump greater amounts of blood with less effort. If the heart does not need to work as hard, then there is less force placed on the arteries. Try to make time for at least 30 minutes of aerobic activity, such as walking or running, as often as possible. Exercising every day is ideal. However, before beginning any exercise routine, it is best to check with your doctor.

Drink concord grape juice. The polyphenols found in grape juice help lower blood pressure. Studies suggest this may be due to their relaxation effect on artery walls. If sugar is a problem, concord grape juice is available unsweetened.

Limit your caffeine consumption. The relationship between high blood pressure and caffeine consumption is still the topic of some debate. However, it is known that caffeine temporarily raises blood pressure, which can stay elevated for up to 2 hours.

Reduce alcohol consumption. If you consume alcohol, do so in moderation. Excessive alcohol intake raises blood pressure, but drinking smaller amounts does not appear to raise blood pressure. Moderate drinking is considered safe. For men, that is no more than two drinks per day; for women or small-framed men, that is no more than one drink per day. However, if you have been drinking larger amounts of alcohol, do not suddenly stop. It is safer to reduce slowly, as stopping suddenly could send your blood pressure soaring.

Other alcohol-related issues include the fact that, when mixed with alcohol, certain blood pressure medications may have undesirable side effects. For example, beta-blockers slow heart rate and relax blood vessels. So, if you drink alcohol around the same time you take a beta-blocker, you might feel light-headed. You may have a similar response if you mix alcohol and ACE inhibitors or calcium antagonists. Drinking some extra water may help to alleviate the symptoms. Since alcohol and central-acting agents are sedatives, mixing the two could make you feel depressed.

Stop smoking. If you smoke, stop. It has been estimated that about a third of the people with high blood pressure smoke. People who have high blood pressure and smoke are three to five times more likely to die from a heart attack or heart failure than people who do not smoke. And they die of a stroke more than twice as often as those with high blood pressure who do not smoke.

Preventive Measures

In the industrial world, the lifetime risk for hypertension exceeds 90 percent. Excessive weight, elevated blood fats, diabetes, insulin resistance, and aging are other risk factors associated with hypertension. Preventive measures are key to a more healthful life.

Avoid loneliness. Research has shown that being lonely can elevate your blood pressure by as much as 30 points. Make sure you take the time to stay connected socially, especially if you live alone.

Consider a vegetarian diet. Studies have shown that a vegetarian diet can significantly lower the risk of hypertension. Soy, a staple in vegetarian diets, has been shown to reduce blood pressure, LDL cholesterol, and triglycerides. A study published in the May 2007 issue of the *Archives of Internal Medicine* stated that participants who ate $1/2$ cup of soybeans each day for 8 weeks lowered their blood pressure and cholesterol levels.

Get moving. In addition to being useful for people who already have high blood pressure, exercise may prevent your blood pressure from becoming too high. Recent studies show exercise improves the nerve reflexes that control blood pressure and heart rate. Researchers noted that weakened nerve reflexes are a risk factor for sudden death after a heart attack. If you do not have hypertension and remain sufficiently active, you may never develop this disorder; studies show that men who are physically active can reduce their risk of developing hypertension up to 70 percent.

Lose excess weight. Excess weight is associated with high blood pressure. In fact, it is related to a number of chronic medical problems, including diabetes and stroke. If you are overweight, ask your doctor to determine if there is a medical reason, such as a thyroid imbalance. If no medical reason is found, you may wish to begin a weight-loss program.

Reduce stress. By itself, stress does not necessarily cause high blood pressure. Many people lead stressed lives, but their blood pressure remains normal. And there are people who are generally relaxed who have high blood pressure. Nevertheless, stress may, at least temporarily, raise your blood pressure. When you are stressed, your body releases hormones that narrow your blood vessels and increase your heart rate. If this happens frequently, it has the potential to damage your brain, kidneys, heart, eyes, and arteries. Try to reduce some of the stresses in your life. Develop some stress-coping mechanisms that work for you. You may wish to learn relaxation techniques such as deep breathing and meditation.

Use your senses to create a relaxing environment. By combining your senses of smell, sight, and hearing, you can create a therapeutic environment that is conducive to relaxation. Essential oils that may actually lower blood pressure are clary sage, lavender, lemon, marjoram, and ylang-ylang.

Try filling your bathtub with warm water and adding a few drops of the above oils. Then dim the lights, and light a blue or green candle, as both of these colors have a relaxing, calming effect on the body. Finally, play some relaxing music, lie back, and enjoy. When you are finished, wrap yourself in a blue or green towel, and climb into bed for a good night's sleep.

High Cholesterol

Cholesterol is a naturally occurring substance in the blood. Your body needs it to support nerve cells, produce hormones, and manufacture vitamin D on the skin's surface. The majority of the cholesterol in your blood is made by your liver from the carbohydrates, proteins, and fats that you consume. Large amounts of cholesterol are found in animal foods such as dairy products and red meats.

High cholesterol, or hypercholesterolemia, is a condition in which the level of cholesterol in your blood is too high. When this occurs, deposits of fat, called plaque, form inside the walls of the blood vessels. Over time, the blood vessels thicken and narrow, creating a medical problem known as atherosclerosis. This results in reduced bloodflow and increases your risk for heart disease and stroke. Heart disease is the most common killer of both men and women in the United States. Every year, about 1 million Americans have a heart attack and about 500,000 die from heart disease. High levels of cholesterol have also been linked with Alzheimer's disease.

High cholesterol is extremely common. About half of all Americans have it.

Causes and Risk Factors

A number of factors affect your cholesterol levels. Some you are unable to alter, such as your age and sex. As you age, your cholesterol levels tend to rise. In addition, genes play a role in cholesterol—high cholesterol runs in families.

But there are cholesterol-altering factors that you *can* control. If you eat a diet that is high in cholesterol and saturated fat, you

Two Types of Cholesterol

There are two primary components of cholesterol, low-density lipoprotein (LDL) and high-density lipoprotein (HDL). Both LDL and HDL carry cholesterol through your blood. LDLs leave fatty deposits on the vessel walls, thereby contributing to heart disease. On the other hand, HDLs clean artery walls and eliminate excess cholesterol from the blood, reducing the risk of heart disease. That is why LDL is often referred to as "bad" cholesterol and HDL is said to be "good" cholesterol. You should aim for higher levels of HDLs and lower levels of LDLs. Ideally, total cholesterol should be less than 200 milligrams/dL (milligrams of cholesterol per deciliter of blood), HDL should be 60 milligrams/dL or higher, and LDL should be less than 100 milligrams/dL. Some authorities use the ratio of total cholesterol to HDL cholesterol to more accurately predict individuals at greater risk for coronary heart disease. Though authorities vary on the ideal ratio, depending upon other risk factors such as tobacco use, age, and high blood pressure, men should strive for a ratio of less than 6.4.

increase your risk. People who are overweight or who have hypothyroidism, type 2 diabetes, or metabolic syndrome—a constellation of factors that includes high blood sugar, blood pressure, and triglycerides as well as excess abdominal fat—are also at greater risk.

Signs and Symptoms

Most often, high cholesterol is a silent disease. You will experience no symptoms until there is a dramatic event, such as leg pain while walking that is caused by the narrowed or blocked arteries in your legs or the chest pain of a heart attack.

Conventional Treatments

The goal of lowering your cholesterol is to reduce the risk for heart disease and stroke. Most likely, you will begin with therapeutic lifestyle changes (TLCs)—various forms of dietary modifications, physical activity, and weight management. If those fail to achieve the desired result, you will probably be advised to take medications.

A Quick Guide to Symptoms

☐ **Often, you will experience no symptoms**
☐ **First sign may be a dramatic event, such as chest or leg pain while walking or the chest pain of a heart attack**

Dietary Programs

A number of dietary programs might prove helpful for dealing with high cholesterol.

The DASH (Dietary Approaches to Stop Hypertension) diet. Doctors who treat high cholesterol often recommend the Dietary Approaches to Stop Hypertension (DASH) diet. In addition to reducing blood pressure, it has been shown to lower cholesterol. The DASH diet is high in grains, fruits, and vegetables. In fact, it recommends seven or eight servings of grains each day and eight to 10 servings of fruits and vegetables; four or five servings of legumes, nuts, and seeds are also advised. Dairy products are limited to two or three servings of low-fat or fat-free items a day. And there should be no more than two servings a day of lean meat, fish, or poultry (without the skin). Oily fish, such as salmon, is considered especially beneficial.

Mediterranean diet. The Mediterranean diet focuses on heart-healthy fiber and nutrients such as omega-3 fatty acids and antioxidants. Though it has a relatively high fat content of between 35 and 45 percent, the vast majority of the fat is monounsaturated and polyunsaturated. The diet includes olive oil, which improves insulin and blood glucose levels and reduces blood pressure, and canola oil, which is filled with omega-3 fatty acids. Avoid high-fat dairy and meat products, and rely on fish as the primary source of protein. The diet relies heavily on fresh fruits and vegetables and relatively high amounts of nuts, legumes, beans, and whole grains. Enjoy a daily glass or two of wine, and season food with garlic, onions, and herbs.

The Ornish program. If you're following the Ornish program (named after its creator, Dean Ornish, MD), you'll need to severely limit your intake of saturated fats. Only 10 percent of the diet may be obtained from even the healthier types of fat. At the same time, carbohydrates compose 75 percent of the diet. So, most of your meals will consist of lots of whole grains, legumes, and fresh fruits and vegetables. If you follow this diet, you will need to couple it with regular stress reduction techniques and at least 90 minutes of exercise three times each week. You will not be allowed to smoke. And you can't consume more than 2 ounces of alcohol each day.

The TLC diet. This diet focuses on eating low-saturated fat, low-cholesterol foods. If you elect to follow this diet, less than 7 percent of your calories can come from saturated fats. And you should eat no more than 200 milligrams of dietary cholesterol per day. This diet includes higher amounts of soluble fiber and foods that contain plant stanols or plant sterols (naturally occurring substances that are believed to reduce the absorption of cholesterol from the gut), such as cholesterol-lowering margarine and salad dressings.

Foods that are low in saturated fat include skinless poultry, whole grains, lean meats, fish, fat-free or 1 percent fat dairy products, fruits, and vegetables. Use liquid margarine or margarine that is in a tub. Since some margarines contain unhealthy trans fats, be sure to read the label. Restrict your intake of full-fat dairy products, organ meats, and egg yolks. Good sources of soluble fiber include

Self-Testing

There are a number of cholesterol self-tests sold in pharmacies, discount stores, and online sites. Some test only for total cholesterol, while others determine total cholesterol, HDL cholesterol, and LDL cholesterol. In order to use the kits, you must obtain a few drops of blood from your finger. All the supplies that you need are included, but be sure to read the instructions carefully. However, you should be aware that many doctors question the accuracy of these tests. If the test results indicate that your cholesterol is not within the normal range, schedule an appointment with your doctor.

oranges, pears, brussels sprouts, carrots, dried peas, beans, and oats.

Physical Activity

You need at least 30 minutes of physical activity almost every day. It has been determined that burning at least 250 calories a day raises HDL levels, thereby protecting against coronary artery disease. This may be accomplished by 45 minutes of walking or 25 minutes of running. Plus, resistance (weight) training reduces LDL levels.

Weight Management

If you are overweight, losing weight may help lower your LDL levels. This is particularly important if your triglycerides are high and your HDL level is low, and if you are a man with a waist measurement over 40 inches. When it comes to health, carrying most of your excess weight in your hips and thighs or lower body (pear shape) is considered better than carrying most of your excess weight in your waist (apple shape).

In general, 1 pound of fat equals about 3,500 calories, so you can lose approximately 1 pound a week if you reduce your intake of calories by about 500 calories each day.

Medications

If you are unable to achieve sufficient improvement in your cholesterol levels from diet and exercise, your doctor will likely recommend medications. It is important to realize that medications should be used in conjunction with lifestyle changes, not instead of them.

Bile-acid binding resins. Bile-acid binding resins attach to bile in the digestive tract and the bile is then excreted in the feces. With less bile in the body, the liver uses greater amounts of cholesterol to produce more bile. So, more cholesterol is removed from the bloodstream and LDL levels drop. Examples are cholestyramine (Questran, Questran Light), colestipol (Colestid), and colesevelam (Cholestagel, Welchol). With these medications, there are frequent reports of side effects such as heartburn, gas, constipation, and other gastrointestinal problems. Colesevelam, the newest bile-acid binding resin, seems to have the fewest number of side effects. Nevertheless, after 1 year, about 40 percent of people on these medications stop taking them.

Bile-acid binding resins may contribute to calcium loss as well as deficiencies of vitamins A, D, E, and K. There have been rare reports of liver toxicity. Do not take bile-acid binding resins at the same time that you take digoxin (Lanoxin), warfarin, beta-blocker drugs, or any of a number of medicines used to treat hypoglycemia. Take these medications at least 1 hour before or 4 to 6 hours after taking your bile-acid binding resin.

Nicotinic acid. If your HDL is very low, your doctor may recommend nicotinic acid, the active component found in niacin (vitamin B_3). Examples are Niacor, Nicolar, and Slo-Niacin; there is also an extended-release form called Niaspan. When used in high doses, nicotinic acid raises HDL more than any other anticholesterol medication and also lowers both LDL and triglycerides. However, many find the side effects too uncomfortable. These include flushing of the face and neck, itching, headache, blurred vision, gastrointestinal problems, dry skin, darkening of the skin, and dizziness. Because of the side effects, after 1 year, about 40 percent of those who start nicotinic acid stop taking it.

About 3 to 5 percent of those taking nicotinic acid develop liver abnormalities. Fortunately, these disappear when the medication is stopped. If you have a chronic liver problem, you should not take any form of this medication. Since nicotinic acid elevates uric acid, if you have gout, you should not take it.

Statins. The statins—such as lovastatin (Mevacor), pravastatin (Pravachol), simvastatin (Zocor), fluvastatin (Lescol), and atorvastatin (Lipitor)—work directly in the liver to block a substance needed for the production of cholesterol. These are the most effective drugs for treating high cholesterol. While especially useful for lowering LDL, the statins also raise HDL and reduce triglycerides. There is evidence that they reduce inflammation in the arteries and help curtail blood clotting. Statins are generally considered the first choice for most people with high cholesterol and are particularly helpful for those who have type 2 diabetes.

A study published in the *New England Journal of Medicine* reported that intensive therapy with statin drugs not only lowered levels of LDL cholesterol, but also lowered a substance known as C-reactive protein. This is helpful because in people with coronary artery disease, the progression of the disease is apparently slowed by reducing both LDL cholesterol and C-reactive protein.

Statin drugs tend to be well tolerated. Nevertheless, reported side effects include gastrointestinal discomfort, skin rashes, headaches, muscle aches, sexual dysfunction, drowsiness, dizziness, nausea, constipation, and peripheral neuropathy (numbness or tingling in the hands or feet). Since statins may affect the liver, liver function tests should be given periodically. Statins should be taken with caution by anyone with liver problems, and they may interact with other cholesterol-lowering medications. If you are taking a statin medication, do not consume grapefruit juice or sour oranges, found in marmalades, as these may increase the potency of your medication.

Complementary Treatments

Complementary medicine treats high cholesterol in much the same way as conventional medicine, including dietary and lifestyle changes.

Tips for Taking Nicotinic Acid

There are ways to reduce the side effects of nicotinic acid. The following are a few suggestions.

☐ **Avoid hot drinks.**
☐ **Start with lower doses and slowly work up to the dose recommended by your doctor.**
☐ **Try taking a low-dose aspirin about 30 minutes before taking nicotinic acid. This seems to prevent flushing.**
☐ **Try the extended-release form.**

Diet

Beans and legumes contain pectin, a water-soluble fiber that helps move cholesterol out of the body. Eat one serving of beans ($1^1/_2$ cups) each day. Especially good choices are soybeans, lima beans, kidney beans, navy beans, pinto beans, black-eyed peas, and lentils.

Fruits also contain pectin and should be eaten regularly. Carrots, cabbage, broccoli, and onions have pectin in the form of calcium pectate, which helps remove cholesterol. Starting your day with half a grapefruit and eating two raw carrots at lunch is an ideal way to begin lowering your cholesterol.

Recent research has shown that certain nuts and seeds contain high levels of phytosterols, a group of chemicals found in plants that are known to reduce blood cholesterol levels. Nuts with the highest levels of phytosterols are pistachios, sunflower seeds, pumpkin seeds, pine nuts, almonds, macadamia nuts, and black walnuts.

A compound found in skim milk may actually inhibit cholesterol production in the liver.

It's a good idea to curtail large amounts of red meat. However, moderate amounts of lean red meat, with all visible fat removed, may be included in the diet.

Herbal Medicine

Garlic. Garlic has the ability to reduce cholesterol. Fresh garlic is the most effective, but garlic supplements may also be useful. However, some deodorized garlic supplements do not lower cholesterol. Look for enteric-coated tablets or capsules with standardized allicin potential. Take 400 to 500 milligrams, once or twice per day, to provide up to 5,000 micrograms of allicin. Since garlic has anticoagulant properties, if you are taking prescription anticoagulant medication, check with your doctor before increasing your intake of garlic or beginning a garlic supplementation regimen. If you are planning to have surgery, you should inform your physician about your intake of garlic. It may be best to discontinue garlic for at least 2 weeks prior to surgery.

Green tea. Green tea contains high levels of substances called polyphenols, which have powerful antioxidant properties. Green tea also helps to decrease cholesterol, lower blood pressure, and prevent the clogging of arteries. The tea may be taken as a beverage or in capsules. Prepared tea bags are readily available in grocery and health food stores. You may also brew a tea from leaves. Steep 1 teaspoon of the leaves in 1 cup of boiling water for 2 to 3 minutes. Green tea can become bitter if steeped too long. Drinking 3 cups of tea per day may provide 240 to 320 milligrams of polyphenols. In capsule form, standardized extract of EGCG (a polyphenol) may provide 97 percent polyphenol content. This is the equivalent of drinking 4 cups of tea per day without the caffeine.

Hawthorn. Hawthorn works to decrease cholesterol and lower blood pressure. In addition, hawthorn helps to strengthen the heart muscles, improve circulation, and rid the body of unnecessary fluid and salt. Hawthorn is available in capsule or tincture form, standardized to 2.2 percent total bioflavonoid content. The recommended daily dose of hawthorn capsules varies widely, ranging from 100 to 300 milligrams, two or three times per day. Be aware that higher doses may significantly lower blood pressure, which may, in turn, cause you to faint. In tincture, the recommended dose is 4 to 5 milliliters, three times per day. It may take up to 2 months before you see the effects of this herb.

Nutritional Supplements

The following supplements help lower total cholesterol and raise HDL cholesterol.

- Vitamin C: 1,000 milligrams daily in divided doses of 500 milligrams. Prevents plaque buildup in arteries. Improves HDL cholesterol, decreases LDL and triglycerides.

- Vitamin E: 400 IU daily. Works with vitamin C in preventing plaque buildup and raising HDL.

- Calcium: 1,500 milligrams daily in divided doses of 500 milligrams. Lowers total cholesterol.

- Magnesium: 750 milligrams daily in

divided doses of 250 milligrams. Works with absorption of calcium.

- Niacin: 100 milligrams daily. Lowers total cholesterol.

Lifestyle Recommendations

Add psyllium powder to your diet. Studies have shown that adding psyllium powder to your diet helps lower cholesterol. Psyllium powder is derived from the husks of the seeds.

Drink concord grape juice. The polyphenols found in grape juice help lower LDL cholesterol. If sugar is a problem for you, concord grape juice is available unsweetened.

Red wine, another grape product, has similar benefits. A number of studies have found that drinking one or two glasses of red wine each day improves cholesterol.

Stop smoking and stay away from smokers. Cigarette smoking lowers HDL levels. When you stop smoking, your HDL levels will naturally rise. However, secondhand smoke also lowers HDL levels, so you don't want to spend too much time around smokers. In addition, smoking as few as 20 cigarettes a week may increase your total cholesterol level.

Preventive Measures

Begin exercising. Becoming physically active is as close as you can get to having a magic solution for preventing high cholesterol. A regular exercise program not only raises HDL levels, it also helps decrease total blood cholesterol, blood pressure, body fat, and risk of heart disease and diabetes, and helps you maintain a healthy weight. Begin a regular exercise program before you are diagnosed with high cholesterol; include both weight-bearing and resistance exercises. Try to do some form of aerobic exercise for at least 30 minutes five times a week.

Change your diet. Reduce your consumption of saturated fats and eat lots of fresh fruits and vegetables, whole grains, and fish and poultry. Add more soluble fiber to your diet. Foods high in soluble fiber include oat bran, oatmeal, beans, peas, rice bran, barley, citrus fruits, strawberries, barley, prunes, and apples. Eat more fish, especially fish that are high in omega-3 fatty acids, such as salmon, mackerel, and herring. Eat more soy products, which contain isoflavones, substances that regulate cholesterol. Soy has been shown to reduce LDL cholesterol and triglycerides. A study published in the May 2007 issue of the *Archives of Internal Medicine* stated that participants who ate $\frac{1}{2}$ cup of soybeans each day for 8 weeks lowered their LDL cholesterol level by as much as 11 percent. If you make these modifications, you may avoid the disorder completely.

Drink tea. The catechins (flavonoid phytochemical compounds) found in green, oolong, and black tea may help keep cholesterol in the normal range. Because of how it's processed, green tea has the most catechins; oolong has the second highest. Black tea has the least because its fermentation process makes the catechins less potent. While regular tea drinking may be beneficial, it must be combined with other dietary recommendations.

Reduce stress. Studies have shown that transcendental meditation can help to significantly reduce total cholesterol levels.

Indigestion

Indigestion is that uncomfortable or burning feeling in your upper abdomen. Also known as dyspepsia, this condition often appears with other medical problems such as belching, abdominal bloating, nausea, and, on occasion, vomiting. Bending over or lying down tends to make the pain worse.

Indigestion is quite common. Though some believe that the figure is higher, it has been suggested that about one in four people experience indigestion each year.

Causes and Risk Factors

Indigestion is frequently the result of certain behaviors, such as eating too much, eating too quickly, and eating high-fat foods. Other causes of indigestion include eating while dealing with a stressful situation, living a stressful life, excess consumption of alcohol, fatigue, and taking medications that tend to upset the stomach (such as anti-inflammatory drugs).

Indigestion may also be caused by a medical problem, such as a gastric or duodenal ulcer or gastroesophageal reflux disease (GERD). A gastric ulcer is an open sore on the inside lining of the stomach, and a duodenal ulcer is a similar sore on the lining of the beginning portion of the small intestine. There is a good chance that the ulcer was caused by the bacterium *Helicobacter pylori*. In GERD, the acid from the stomach backs up into the esophagus, the tube that connects the mouth to the stomach. When people with celiac disease, an autoimmune disorder, ingest foods that contain gluten (wheat, oats, barley, or rye), they may have significant indigestion. On rare occasions, indigestion is triggered by stomach cancer.

Sometimes, there is no apparent cause for indigestion. In such cases, the condition is known as functional or nonulcer indigestion. People with this form of indigestion may have a problem with the motility or muscular squeezing action of the stomach, which leads to a delayed emptying of the stomach.

Indigestion tends to occur more often as you age. If you are overweight or if you smoke, you are also at increased risk.

A Quick Guide to Symptoms

☐ **Gnawing and burning sensation in the upper middle part of abdomen**
☐ **Burping**
☐ **Nausea**
☐ **Stomach feels bloated and excessively full**

Signs and Symptoms

With indigestion, there is a gnawing and burning sensation in the upper middle part of your abdomen. You may burp and feel nauseated. Your stomach may feel bloated or excessively full.

Conventional Treatments
Lifestyle Changes

Treatment for indigestion normally begins with several lifestyle changes. These include eating smaller meals, sitting or standing after you eat, limiting fatty foods, avoiding foods and drinks that tend to be more problematic (such as citrus fruits and chocolate), losing weight, and avoiding or limiting alcohol. You may also be advised to stop smoking and make time for relaxation.

Since some medications may contribute to indigestion, your doctor will probably want to review all your medications. Some medications that are known for causing indigestion include nonsteroidal anti-inflammatory drugs (NSAIDs), such as aspirin, ibuprofen, and naproxen.

Medications

If you have not achieved sufficient relief from lifestyle changes and changes in medication, your doctor may suggest a medication.

Acid blockers. Acid blockers (also called H-2 blockers) reduce the secretion of stomach acid. Some acid blockers are available over-the-counter, while others are sold only by prescription. Well-known examples of these drugs are cimetidine (Tagamet HB) and famotidine (Pepcid AC). On occasion, these medications may have side effects such as dry mouth, dizziness, drowsiness, and bowel changes. Be sure to ask your doctor if they might interfere with other medications you are taking.

Antacids. Over-the-counter antacids, which neutralize gastric acid, may relieve your symptoms. Common examples are Tums and Rolaids. However, when antacids are consumed

> **Since indigestion may be a sign** of a more serious illness, if you have symptoms such as weight loss, appetite loss, black tarry stools, blood in vomit, recurrent vomiting, and severe pain in the upper abdomen, see your doctor.

frequently, they may trigger constipation or diarrhea. Also, some antacids may interfere with the effectiveness of other medications, particularly those prescribed for kidney and heart disease. Antacids that contain magnesium may cause a buildup of magnesium in the body, which may contribute to kidney disease, especially in people who have diabetes. And consuming too much calcium, which can also

Indigestion and Heart Attacks

It is well known that as people age, they may confuse a bout of indigestion with a heart attack. Many people have rushed to hospital emergency departments believing that they are having a heart attack, only to be diagnosed with indigestion. But it is also true that some people who are having a heart attack misinterpret their symptoms as indigestion and delay going to the hospital. If you experience intense pain in the center of the chest, and if it spreads to one or both arms and the lower jaw, you may be having a heart attack. You need to seek emergency medical care.

be found in antacids, may place you at risk for kidney stones. Antacids are also known to interfere with the absorption of some medications such as ciprofloxacin (Cipro), tetracycline, and propranolol (Inderal). To prevent these interactions, take these medications either 1 hour before or 3 hours after the antacid.

Antibiotics. If you have a history of peptic ulcer disease, active gastric ulcer, or an active duodenal ulcer with evidence of *H. pylori*, your doctor will probably want to eradicate the infection. Curing *H. pylori* is usually associated with a higher rate of ulcer healing and a reduction in complications and recurrences. There are at least four different treatment regimens for *H. pylori* infection that range in duration from 10 to 14 days. Typically, a proton-pump inhibitor (see below) or acid blocker is used in combination with two antibiotics and the possible addition of an antacid. Some of the recommended antibiotics include amoxicillin, metronidazole, clarithromycin, and tetracycline.

Prokinetics. If your doctor believes that your indigestion is caused by the motility or muscular squeezing action of your stomach, he or she may prescribe a medication to control this action. These are known as prokinetic drugs. They may help GERD by counteracting some of the physical abnormalities that may be present. Drugs such as metoclopramide (Reglan) may increase the pressure of the lower esophageal sphincter, improve emptying of the stomach, and encourage the normal digestive muscular contractions.

Proton-pump inhibitors. Proton-pump inhibitors are a newer class of drugs that block the final stage of acid production. Omeprazole (Prilosec) and lansoprazole (Prevacid) are examples. Potential side effects include headache, diarrhea, and abdominal pain.

Itopride. In one study done in Germany, researchers gave people with a type of indigestion known as functional dyspepsia three different strengths of itopride as well as a placebo. They randomly assigned individuals with dyspepsia to one of three drug treatments or placebo for a period of 8 weeks. Although the symptoms of dyspepsia improved in all groups, including the placebo treatment group, itopride produced superior symptom relief in those taking the medication. Itopride is currently unavailable in the United States.

Surgery

Unless your indigestion is caused by certain specific types of GERD or stomach cancer, your doctor is unlikely to consider surgery as a treatment option for this medical problem.

Complementary Treatments

Complementary medicine aims to find the underlying cause of indigestion and ultimately make appropriate nutritional and lifestyle changes in order to reduce it.

Diet

Individual constitutions are so specific and symptoms of indigestion so subjective that it is hard to pinpoint and recommend general dietary advice. Some people have trouble digesting wheat or lactose (found in dairy products). To determine if you have a food intolerance, you might wish to list everything you eat in a food journal. Keeping track of what you eat, when you eat, how you feel when you eat (such as stressed, relaxed, or rushed), and how you feel after you eat may help find trigger foods that are causing indigestion. You can then begin the process of eliminating specific foods that you feel are causing your problem. Do you feel better when you don't eat them? You may be able to reintroduce these foods after certain changes are made, such as eating in a relaxed environment, eating slowly, or chewing your food completely.

Herbal Medicine

Herbs may be helpful either in relieving specific symptoms of indigestion or as a general tonic. You can use herbs for indigestion either individually or in combination. Herbs known as carminatives help to expel gas and prevent it from forming in the intestines. Antispasmodic herbs aid in preventing involuntary muscle cramps. And herbs known as stomachics stimulate digestion and tone the stomach.

Chamomile and peppermint. Chamomile is an antispasmodic and stomachic. It also fosters relaxation and reduces stress, which is a trigger for indigestion. Peppermint is a stomachic and carminative and is extremely useful for indigestion that is caused by overeating. It reduces acidity in the stomach and accelerates the stomach's emptying process by more than 40 percent. These two herbs are popular teas and may be taken to relieve indigestion. Both chamomile and peppermint are available as a dried herb or in prepared tea bags. When using the dried herb, pour 1 cup of hot water over 1 tablespoon of the herb, and steep for 10 minutes. When using the tea bags, follow the directions on the package. Peppermint tea may be taken throughout the day, but save chamomile for the evening, because it is especially good for relaxing before bedtime.

Fennel. Fennel seeds have a calming effect on the digestive system, and chewing them after a meal may eliminate indigestion. For quick relief, carry some fennel seeds in a tin to chew at any time on the road or at work.

Goldenseal. By increasing the flow of gastric juices, goldenseal promotes good digestion. To create a powerful treatment to relieve bloating or gas, add a few drops of goldenseal tincture to a cup of chamomile or peppermint tea. Goldenseal's antiseptic properties have been shown to be very effective against intestinal bacteria. However, if you suffer from high blood pressure, goldenseal should be used sparingly.

Slippery elm. The inner bark of the slippery elm tree (*Ulmus rubra*) contains mucilage that helps protect the throat and digestive tract. It also soothes irritated mucous membranes and neutralizes the excess stomach acid that may lead to indigestion. Prepare a tea from 1 tablespoon of the dried herb or 1 tablespoon of liquid extract poured over a cup of hot water. Drink 1 to 3 cups daily.

Homeopathy

Homeopathy may provide excellent results for treating the various symptoms associated with indigestion. The remedies are specific to the type and severity of symptoms. Natural health food stores carry remedies for milder conditions, while a homeopathic practitioner may prescribe stronger remedies.

Hydrotherapy

A moist heating pad or hot water bottle placed over the abdomen after meals may relieve symptoms of indigestion.

Nutritional Supplements

Digestive enzymes, available in a wide variety of over-the-counter preparations, may be helpful in battling indigestion. Lactase, for example, is a digestive enzyme necessary to break down the milk-sugar lactose found in dairy products. Some people who produce inadequate amounts of this enzyme take a lactase enzyme such as Lactaid prior to eating dairy products. There are other specific enzymes that are made in the body to digest protein, fats, and carbohydrates. Bromelain and papain, two enzymes that digest protein, are found in pineapple and papaya. Some products have a combination of enzymes to break down fats, protein, and carbohydrates. Take these products as directed on the label.

Relaxation/Meditation

To relieve stress, which directly affects the digestive process, practice relaxation, meditation, or deep breathing techniques. To work efficiently, the digestive system needs a large supply of blood. When the body is in a state of stress, it redirects the blood and uses it in other areas, such as the muscles, heart, and lungs, for the "fight-or-flight" response. This disturbs the digestive process, causing problems such as indigestion. A regular routine of meditation, deep breathing, tai chi, or yoga may reduce stress. Biofeedback may help you target why and how stress is affecting you and ways to reduce it.

Preventive Measures

Avoid swallowing air. To avoid excessive bloating or belching, do not chew with your mouth open, talk while eating, or chew gum.

Don't exercise or lie down after eating. Exercise after eating diverts blood away from your stomach, hindering digestion. Schedule your exercise either before eating or at least 30 minutes after eating. It is fine to relax after eating, but don't lie down flat for 2 to 3 hours. It may be useful to raise the head of your bed by 3 inches—this small change in elevation may prevent acid reflux.

Don't rush your meals. Eating quickly increases your risk for indigestion. Take time to eat and chew your food properly.

Don't smoke. People who smoke increase their risk for indigestion since smoking can irritate the stomach lining.

Watch what you eat. Reduce your intake of acidic foods, spicy foods, fatty foods, carbonated beverages, and caffeine. These have all been correlated with indigestion. Caffeine, in particular, increases gastric secretions and irritates intestinal muscles.

Influenza

Also known as the flu, influenza is a contagious illness caused by the influenza virus. Most often passed from person to person in respiratory droplets of coughs and sneezes, the flu may also be spread when a person touches respiratory droplets on another person or object and then touches his or her mouth or nose. While some people infected with the flu virus do not experience symptoms, most symptoms tend to begin 1 to 4 days after infection. So, you may begin spreading the flu a day before you actually feel symptoms and continue spreading the flu for another 3 to 5 days. Most people recover within a week or two, although older people may take longer.

Every year, millions of people in the United States become sick with influenza. It has been estimated that between 5 and 20 percent of the population become ill with this disease. About 200,000 people who catch influenza require hospitalization, and 36,000 die from it.

There are two types of influenza virus, A and B. Type A causes the most severe influenza epidemics. Type B also causes epidemics, but they are milder than type A. Cases of influenza generally appear in the late fall, winter, and early spring.

Causes and Risk Factors

Influenza comes on suddenly and attacks the respiratory tract—nose, throat, and lungs.

Though anyone may become ill with the flu, very young people, people with chronic medical problems, and those over the age of 65 are most at risk for complications, such as pneumonia, bronchitis, postinfectious cough, and sinus and ear infections. Complications often occur after you are feeling better.

Signs and Symptoms

The symptoms of influenza include fever at 101°F or above, headache, tiredness, dry cough, sore throat, nasal congestion, chills, and body aches. Symptoms of flu-related complications are high fever, shaking chills, chest pains with each breath, and coughing that produces thick, yellow-greenish-colored mucus.

Conventional Treatments

For fever and muscle aches, your doctor will probably recommend aspirin, acetaminophen,

A Quick Guide to Symptoms

- ☐ Fever at 101°F or above
- ☐ Headache
- ☐ Tiredness
- ☐ Dry cough
- ☐ Sore throat
- ☐ Nasal congestion
- ☐ Chills
- ☐ Body aches

Precautions with Antiviral Medications

If you have a chronic lung disease such as asthma, you need to share that information with your doctor. And you need to use zanamivir (Relenza) with care. It may cause bronchospasm. After using zanamivir, you may have trouble breathing. Be sure to have a fast-acting reliever bronchodilator on hand.

or ibuprofen. Be sure to rest and drink plenty of liquids. To treat your congestion, cough, and nasal discharge, try an over-the-counter decongestant and antihistamine.

Antibiotics

If you have an influenza-related complication such as pneumonia or a sinus or ear infection, your doctor may prescribe antibiotics. Antibiotics are used to treat infections caused by bacteria. Since the flu is a viral infection, antibiotics are not routinely used to treat it.

Antiviral Medications

Your doctor may suggest taking antiviral drugs, taken within the first 2 days of becoming ill. The adamantanes include amantadine (Symmetrel) and rimantadine (Flumadine). The newer medications are the neuraminidase inhibitors zanamivir (Relenza) and oseltamivir (Tamiflu). Amantadine and rimantadine are older medications that treat only type A influenza and are associated with several toxic side effects. Oseltamivir and zanamivir are useful for both types A and B influenza. These medications may reduce the symptoms, shorten the duration of the illness, and make you less contagious to others. Only oseltamivir has been found to reduce some of the complications that require antibiotics. Neuraminidase inhibitors are also useful for helping to prevent infection with the flu virus. Trials of long-term prophylactic use of zanamivir and oseltamivir in healthy adults, adolescents, and the elderly have shown reductions in the incidence of influenza. So, you may ask your doctor for a prescription if the flu is prevalent in your community or workplace or if a family member has the flu. Potential side effects include stomach upset, insomnia, and nervousness.

Complementary Treatments

Complementary medicine is extremely beneficial in helping to relieve the symptoms associated with the flu. By supporting and strengthening the immune system, the body is better able to fight the flu virus.

Diet

Eat light, easily digestible foods such as vegetable soups, broth, salads, and rice. Consume liberal amounts of garlic and onion, which have antiviral and immune-boosting properties.

Drink plenty of liquids. Make sure you get a good eight to ten 8-ounce glasses of fluids daily. Laboratory studies have shown that the tannins contained in grape juice may kill viruses. In addition, grape juice is rich in vitamin C, which may help boost the immune system. Other good choices include any juice high in vitamin C, such as orange juice, cranberry juice, and grapefruit juice, as long as the acidity does not bother the gastrointestinal tract. However, you should avoid juices containing high amounts of added sugar. Stay away from caffeine and alcohol as these can contribute to dehydration. Alcohol also robs the body of vitamin C.

Herbal Medicine

Astragalus. Astragalus root has been shown to increase the production of white blood cells, which help fight invading viruses. Because it helps strengthen the body against disease, astragalus should be taken at the first onset of symptoms. Take one 500-milligram capsule, four times a day, until symptoms abate, and then reduce dosage to one capsule, twice a day, for 1 week. Products should contain standardized extract of the root with 0.5 percent glucosides and 70 percent polysaccharides.

Echinacea. Echinacea also stimulates the immune system and increases white blood cell production and should be taken at the onset of symptoms. A study using 900 milligrams of *Echinacea purpurea* daily showed that, in 3 days, there was a significant decrease in body aches, headache, cough, and lethargy. For best results, echinacea should be used for 1 to 2 weeks at a time. When echinacea is used for an extended period of time, the body tends to build up a tolerance, making it less effective. The recommended daily dose to decrease flu symptoms is 500 milligrams of standardized

extract per day containing at least 3.5 percent echinacosides, the active ingredient. If taken in liquid extract form, 1 teaspoon, three times a day, is the recommended dose. Echinacea tincture is often combined with goldenseal, a very effective herb for preventing the flu as well as a treatment at the onset of flu symptoms. Goldenseal contains berberine, which helps to activate white blood cells to destroy the flu virus.

Elderberry. Elderberry flowers contain properties that help stop the flu virus from infesting cells of the respiratory tract. The most effective treatment using elderberry is a patented drug called Sambucol. Clinical trials have shown that 90 percent of people with flu who took Sambucol recovered after 3 days. In 24 hours, 20 percent showed considerable relief from muscular aches and fever, and after 48 hours, 73 percent reported feeling better. The recommended dose is 4 tablespoons, three times a day, for 3 days.

Garlic. Garlic stimulates the immune system and is also effective in preventing respiratory complications such as bronchitis. Garlic cloves may be eaten raw, cooked in food, or taken as a capsule or tincture. Garlic is available in enteric-coated tablets or capsules to prevent stomach upset. The recommended daily dose is 500 milligrams, twice a day. Or take 2 to 4 milliliters of garlic tincture three times daily. If you have a choice, select fresh garlic over supplements. The supplements contain concentrated extracts, which may increase the risk of excessive bleeding.

Other herbs. Combine the herbs coltsfoot, mullein, peppermint, and wild cherry bark in equal amounts and brew a tea to assist in releasing mucus and eliminating phlegm. Fill a saucepan with water and add equal amounts of the herbs. For each cup of water, use a table-

Because the viral material in flu vaccines is grown in eggs, if you are allergic to eggs, you should not have a shot. You should also avoid a shot if you have a history of Guillain-Barré syndrome.

spoon of each herb. Bring the mixture to a boil, turn off the stove, and let the mixture steep for at least 1 hour. Drink the tea throughout the day. Due to their antiviral properties, other teas helpful in relieving the flu are forsythia, honeysuckle, and lemon balm.

Homeopathy

Oscillococcinum (Oscillo) is a homeopathic remedy, manufactured by Boiron, that speeds up the recovery process from the flu virus. The active ingredient in Oscillo is Anas barbariae hepatis et cordis extractum 200CK. Inactive ingredients are sucrose and lactose. Following the directions on the package, take Oscillo at the first sign of flu symptoms. Homeopathic remedies often make symptoms more severe for the first day or two, but recovery from the virus is much quicker.

Nutritional Supplements

Since zinc boosts the immune system, it has widely been used at the first sign of flu symptoms. When taken immediately, zinc can help

the body recover from influenza quicker. The recommended dose for influenza is a zinc gluconate lozenge every 2 hours as needed.

High doses of vitamin C taken at the onset of symptoms or right after exposure to someone with the flu can help shorten the duration of your illness. Take 1,000 milligrams (divided doses of 500 mg each) of vitamin C daily.

Lifestyle Recommendations

Eat chocolate. Theobromine, a chemical found in chocolate, has been found to be more effective at calming persistent coughs than codeine.

Get vaccinated. The best way to prevent becoming ill with influenza is to obtain a flu shot between early October and mid-November each year. Ideally, you want to be vaccinated 6 to 8 weeks before the flu season begins. Since the actual virus changes from year to year, you need a new shot every year. Some people (fewer than one-third) who get a flu shot will have some soreness around the site of the injection. In rare instances, there may be aches, pains, and fever.

In 2003, the FDA approved FluMist, an influenza vaccine that is administered nasally. It is approved only for healthy people between the ages of 5 and 49. Do not take FluMist if you meet any of the following specifications.

• You have a metabolic disorder such as diabetes or kidney dysfunction.

• You have a lung condition, such as asthma, or a heart condition.

- You have an immunodeficiency disease or are on immunosuppressive treatment.

- You have had Guillain-Barré syndrome.

- You have a history of being allergic or very sensitive to eggs or any part of FluMist.

Minimize exposure. During flu season, avoid crowds and crowded spaces, because the flu virus spreads easily. In fact, individuals can spread the virus even before they are symptomatic. To help prevent the spread of the virus, always sneeze into a tissue. If you live with someone suffering from the flu, do not share items that can easily spread the virus, such as towels, clothing, blankets, cups, dishes, and utensils.

Pay attention to your diet. During the flu season, it is especially important to pay attention to what you eat. Avoid fried foods and refined sugars, as these foods may place an added burden on your immune system.

Reduce stress. Avoid overexertion and don't get run down. Both physical and emotional stress may impair your immune system, making you more susceptible to the flu.

Relieve coughing. A tablespoon of warm honey with a sprinkling of cinnamon is effective in clearing the sinuses and relieving chronic coughs. Take 1 tablespoon a day to relieve flu symptoms. Gingerroot has been used for centuries as a natural cough suppressant. To help control a cough, chew a small, dime-size piece of raw gingerroot. It lubricates the throat by stimulating the salivary glands.

Preventive Measures

Quit smoking. According to the Centers for Disease Control and Prevention, research shows an increase in influenza in smokers as compared to nonsmokers. There is a higher mortality rate for smokers from the flu as compared to nonsmokers. Smoking suppresses the immune function, causing more upper and lower respiratory tract infections.

Take supplements. In addition to a daily multivitamin/mineral supplement, it is important to begin boosting your immune system in the fall months to ward off any impending influenza outbreak. Take additional vitamin C (1,000 milligrams daily), as well as echinacea, goldenseal, and astragalus as recommended in the herbal medicine section. Take them for 1 to 2 weeks, and then discontinue for 1 to 2 weeks. Repeat this on-again, off-again schedule until the flu season is over. This program will help stimulate your immune system, but it will avoid building up a tolerance to these supplements.

Wash your hands. Wash your hands thoroughly with soap and water for a minimum of 20 seconds several times throughout the day. To help reduce your chance of infection, avoid touching your eyes, nose, and mouth, as these are open passageways for germs to enter the body.

Insomnia

If you have insomnia, you are obtaining inadequate or poor-quality sleep. And it may occur in a few different ways. You may have difficulty falling asleep, or you may have a problem staying asleep, or you may awaken too early in the morning and be unable to go back to sleep. As a result of your disrupted sleep, you are tired during the day.

Almost everyone has occasional problems with sleep. Some types of insomnia, such as insomnia from jet lag or the noise of a thunderstorm, are relatively brief. Insomnia that lasts from a few days to a few weeks is termed transient. When the bouts with insomnia happen from time to time, they are called intermittent. Insomnia that continues for a month or longer is considered chronic. People with chronic insomnia spend a good deal of time worrying about whether or not they will be able to get the sleep they need, and that only adds to the insomnia problem.

Insomnia is very common. Every year, about one in three adults is affected, and approximately 10 to 20 percent of these cases are severe. Insomnia also takes a physical toll on the body. It is believed to increase the risk of heart failure, stroke, high blood pressure, coronary artery disease, obesity, and diabetes.

Causes and Risk Factors

Older adults are at greater risk for insomnia. They are more sensitive to noise, and they awaken more easily. As people age, they are more likely to have trouble falling into the deeper stages of sleep, and there is a good chance they will have a medical problem or be on a medication that may disturb sleep. It is often said that the need for sleep decreases with age. That is not true. Rather, as we grow older, we tend to lose the ability to sleep as well as we did when we were younger.

Insomnia may also be caused by a number of other factors. Transient and intermittent insomnia tend to be the result of stress, extreme temperatures, environmental noise, time changes, and the side effects of medication, particularly drugs containing caffeine.

Chronic insomnia is more multifaceted and may have a number of contributing factors. A frequent cause of chronic insomnia is depression. Other causes are heart failure, asthma, anxiety, hyperthyroidism, kidney disease, arthritis, restless legs syndrome, sleep apnea, Parkinson's disease, and narcolepsy.

Some people clearly have a genetic tendency. About 35 percent of people dealing

A Quick Guide to Symptoms

☐ An inability to fall asleep
☐ Awaken frequently during the night and have trouble returning to sleep
☐ Awaken too early in the morning and find yourself unable to fall back to sleep

with chronic insomnia have family history.

Still, behavioral factors play a role in chronic insomnia, including chronic stress and misuse of caffeine or alcohol. Cigarette smoking before bedtime or napping in the afternoon or evening may also be sources of chronic insomnia. Additionally, humans are designed to work during the day and sleep at night. People who do nighttime shift work or work in a position that requires frequent shift changes may be plagued by insomnia.

Signs and Symptoms

Insomnia is characterized by three main symptoms. You may have an inability to fall asleep, you may awaken frequently during the night and have trouble returning to sleep, or you may awaken too early in the morning and find yourself unable to fall back to sleep. The next day you are tired. In fact, you are so tired that you may be irritable and have difficulty concentrating on your work.

Conventional Treatments

Transient insomnia and intermittent insomnia are normally not treated. However, if they impact daily activity, your doctor may prescribe short-acting sleeping pills.

There are several methods for treating chronic insomnia. Your doctor will probably begin by looking for any medical or psychological causes. Sometimes, when these are addressed, the insomnia stops. For example, if your insomnia is caused by depression, then treating the depression may end the insomnia. Similarly, if your insomnia is a result of anxiety, treating the anxiety may improve your sleep. Also, your doctor will attempt to determine if any of your behaviors, such as smoking at bedtime or drinking alcohol, may be contributing to the situation.

Behavioral Techniques

Stimulus control. Treating chronic insomnia may require a reinterpretation of how you view your bed. Don't use your bed for anything other than sleeping or sex. Go to bed only when you are very tired, and try to think comforting thoughts. If you find that you are unable to sleep in 15 to 20 minutes, get out of bed and do not return until you are very sleepy. It is best to establish set times for going to bed and awakening. Also, do not nap during the day. Avoid nighttime activities that could produce anxiety, such as bringing work home or watching television programs that you might find disturbing. Another suggestion is listening to audiotapes of soothing sounds or music that facilitate deep breathing, which promotes relaxation.

Progressive muscle relaxation. Spend about 10 minutes a day practicing the following form of relaxation.

• Concentrate on a specific muscle group in your body, such as the muscles in your left foot.

- As you inhale, tense the muscle group for about 8 seconds.

- Quickly release the muscle group and let it stay limp for about 15 seconds.

- Repeat the sequence.

- Then, go on to other muscle groups in your body. Typically, you should go from the bottom portion of your body to the top.

Sleep restriction therapy. While dealing with insomnia, some people spend many hours in bed trying to sleep. They may be helped by a program that limits how much time they are allowed to be in bed. As their sleeping pattern improves, they will be permitted additional time.

Sleep restriction therapy begins by keeping a sleep diary for 2 weeks. Divide the amount of time that you sleep by the time in bed—the answer is your sleep efficiency number. So, if you spend 8 hours in bed, but you sleep only 5 hours, then your sleep efficiency number is 62.5 percent. Your goal should be to take actions that will increase your number to 85 to 90 percent.

Begin by going to bed 15 minutes later than usual. Until an 85 percent sleep efficiency is reached, decrease the amount of time in bed by 15 minutes every week. However, do not reduce the time in bed to fewer than 5 hours. When a 90 percent efficiency is reached, start increasing the time in bed by 15 minutes every week.

Medications

In order to break your pattern of chronic insomnia, your doctor may prescribe a short course of low-dose benzodiazepine sleeping pills. While you are taking these pills, your doctor may wish to monitor you carefully, and possibly lower the dose slowly. When certain sleeping medications are suddenly stopped, they may trigger a few nights of insomnia and produce side effects such as nausea, nightmares, dizziness, and headaches. These medications should never be mixed with alcohol.

While the older forms of sleeping pills, such as barbiturates, were known to be quite dangerous and had the potential to cause death when taken in high doses, the more recent medications are significantly safer. They have fewer side effects and are less likely to be addictive. Zaleplon (Sonata) is

Sleep Apnea

In sleep apnea, breathing periodically stops throughout the night. Episodes may last for as long as a minute and occur hundreds of times during the night. By morning, people with sleep apnea are tired and confused. Usually, sleep apnea is caused by partial blockage of the upper airway. Obesity aggravates the condition, and men are far more at risk for sleep apnea than women. People with this condition may be advised to lose weight. They may also be told to wear an apparatus known as a CPAP (continuous positive airway pressure) every night, which provides an air splint to the upper airway, thereby keeping the airway open. Though it is not comfortable, for many with sleep apnea it is a solution. Sleep apnea is a risk factor for cardiovascular disease.

useful for individuals who have difficulty falling asleep. An intermediate-acting medication, eszopiclone (Lunesta), helps those who have trouble staying asleep. Studies have generally supported the efficacy of these medications, including improvement in the time needed to fall asleep, decrease in awakenings, and improvement in sleep quality and total sleep time. But there may be side effects, such as dizziness, drowsiness, and problems with coordination. Anyone on sleep medications should be carefully monitored by a doctor. Sleeping pills should always be viewed as short-term solutions. They should never be used for a prolonged period of time.

Complementary Treatments

Complementary therapies assist in finding the underlying cause of insomnia and provide lifestyle changes and behavioral approaches that can promote better sleeping habits.

Acupuncture

Studies show that acupuncture and acupressure are very successful for the treatment of insomnia. They both increase production of serotonin, a relaxing hormone; promote relaxation; enhance sleep quality; and decrease awakening during the night. To locate an acupuncturist in your area, visit the Web site of the National Certification Commission for Acupuncture and Oriental Medicine (NCCAOM) at www.nccaom.org.

To find a practitioner trained in acupressure, visit the following Web site: www.aobta.org (American Organization for Bodywork Therapies of Asia) and www.ncbtmb.org (National Certification Board for Therapeutic Massage and Bodywork).

Ayurveda

Ayurvedic medicine treats insomnia by restoring balance to the *vata* dosha (according to Ayurvedic constitutional type). Maintaining a regular nightly routine is also important. A successful treatment routine includes massaging the scalp and soles of the feet with sesame oil. It is also useful to rub the areas around the forehead and eyes with a paste made of nutmeg and *ghee* (a cooked, clarified butter with all the moisture removed). Other ways to relax the *vata* dosha include a warm bath followed by a warm glass of milk containing the Ayurvedic herb Amrit Kalash, relaxing music, and comforting reading.

Diet

Eating a well-balanced diet that limits the amount of sugar, caffeine, and processed foods helps to reduce insomnia. Calcium, magnesium, and vitamins B_6 and B_{12} are all useful nutrients for their ability to calm the nervous system. Foods high in calcium and magnesium are milk and milk products (select low-fat or skim); tofu; shrimp; almonds; green leafy vegetables, such as spinach, kale, or broccoli; black beans; and potatoes. Meat, fish, and eggs are foods that naturally contain B_{12}. Vitamin B_{12} is also often added to breakfast cereal. Poultry and fish are the best natural sources for B_6.

About an hour before bedtime, consume some foods containing the amino acid tryptophan. In the brain, tryptophan converts into serotonin, which helps foster sleep. Since milk contains tryptophan, consider drinking a small glass. Other tryptophan-containing foods are cheese, bananas, and turkey.

Herbal Medicine

A number of herbs may help relieve anxiety, calm an overactive mind, and induce sleep and improve the quality of sleep.

Chamomile, hops, and vervain. These are relaxing teas to drink before bedtime. They are readily available in prepared tea bags. People who suffer from depression should not take hops. When taken for a prolonged period of time, hops may disrupt the menstrual cycle.

Passionflower and valerian root. Passionflower and valerian root calm the central nervous system, relieving anxiety and insomnia. They are available in prepared tea bags, tincture, and as dried herbs. For passionflower, look for products containing no less than 0.8 percent total flavonoids. As a tincture, take 1 to 4 milliliters in the evening to increase sleepiness. When using the dried herb, pour 1 cup of boiling water over 1 teaspoon of the dried herb, and steep for 10 to 15 minutes; drink before bedtime. When taking valerian root, look for products containing 0.8 percent valeric/valerenic acid. Since valerian may have a bitter taste and strong odor, you may prefer to take it in capsule form.

Take 400 to 450 milligrams an hour before bedtime. Passionflower and valerian are often rotated, using one for 2 weeks and then switching to the other. If you are taking other sleep-inducing products, before beginning a regimen of either passionflower or valerian, check with your doctor.

If there is any chance that you are pregnant, do not take passionflower.

Homeopathy

Various over-the-counter remedies for insomnia are readily available at natural and organic health food and grocery stores. *Coffea* is an effective homeopathic remedy for an overactive mind that will not shut down at night. *Nux vomica* is used for anxiety and is best taken at night. Take *Muriaticum acidum* for irritability and restlessness.

Melatonin

The supplement melatonin, a natural hormone produced at night by the pineal gland in the brain, is commonly used for insomnia. There have been different reports on its effectiveness, however. There is some indication that, under certain circumstances, people fall asleep faster on melatonin, but it does not appear to affect total sleep or feelings of fatigue during the day. Melatonin has some reported adverse side effects, such as nightmares, drowsiness, severe headaches, depression, low sperm count, and blood vessel constriction. If you decide to use melatonin, the typical recommended dose is 1 to 3 milligrams, 1 to 2 hours before bedtime. Start with a lower dose and increase as needed. Melatonin takes up to 2 weeks to affect a sleep pattern.

Nutritional Supplements

Nutritional supplements can help reduce stress, relax muscles, and have a calming effect.

- B-complex vitamins: Take as directed on the label. Effective for nervous system function and reducing stress.

- Calcium: 1,500 milligrams daily in divided doses of 500 milligrams. Natural sedating effects. Take with magnesium after meals and take the last dose 45 minutes before bedtime.

- Magnesium: 750 milligrams daily in divided doses of 250 milligrams. Helps relax muscles.

Therapeutic Massage

By relieving muscular tension, calming the nervous system, and improving circulation, therapeutic massage relaxes the body and the mind. So that you will experience these effects closer to bedtime, it is best to schedule massage appointments in the late afternoon or early evening.

Lifestyle Recommendations

Try a soak before turning in. Taking a shower or bath before bedtime is generally helpful in inducing restful sleep.

Begin exercising. Exercise is known to help with insomnia. Experts especially recommend brisk walks, runs, or bike rides late in the afternoon. They believe that afternoon exercise helps deepen sleep. Exercise raises body temperature. About 6 hours later, when the temperature falls, sleep will come more easily. So, people who exercise require less time to fall asleep. But avoid exercising at or right before your bedtime. Exercising 2 to 3 hours before bedtime may increase the chances of insomnia.

Practice deep breathing. Deep breathing can provide sound relaxation and improve your ability to fall asleep. While lying flat on your back, place both hands on your abdomen. Slowly inhale through your nose, pushing your abdomen up as if blowing up a balloon. Then, exhale slowly through your mouth, and feel your abdomen deflate. Practice this breathing process as often as possible.

Preventive Measures

Avoid fruit juice and high-sugar snacks before bedtime. High or low fluctuations in blood sugar levels can disrupt your sleep.

Control bedroom light and noise. Bright lights and loud noises disrupt sleep. If bright lights are streaming into your bedroom, you may wish to purchase light-blocking shades or lined drapes. You may even wish to try an eye mask. Excess outside noise that intrudes on the bedroom may be reduced with heavy curtains or drapes or by installing double-pane windows. Wearing earplugs and running a fan to create soothing white noise are other options.

Eat moderately at dinner. Eating a heavy meal for dinner tends to disturb sleep. On the other hand, a small bedtime snack is generally fine.

Establish a relaxing routine. Set up a prebedtime relaxing routine. Consider relaxation exercises or soaking in warm or hot water about $1\frac{1}{2}$ to 2 hours before bedtime. Don't take a hot bath too close to bedtime as it increases alertness. Consider reading or meditation before going to bed.

Keep a comfortable bedroom temperature. Although there is some disagreement among researchers, it is usually believed that the bedroom should be slightly cool. So, turn the thermostat down in the winter and consider an air conditioner, fan, or dehumidifier for the summer.

Make lists. Before going to bed, write down all the things that you accomplished throughout the day. Next, make a "to do" list of those items that you did not get a chance to complete and include any other items that popped up in your day. This helps to empty your mind by seeing your accomplishments and by knowing that you are ready for the following day. You can rest easy and not stay awake thinking about all the things you have to do or didn't do.

Limit alcohol consumption. While alcohol consumption directly before bed will calm you and help you fall asleep, drinking alcohol at bedtime increases the amount of times you awaken at night.

Limit caffeine consumption. Caffeine is contained in a number of foods, including chocolate, cola drinks, teas, and regular coffee. While some people dealing with insomnia may be able to consume foods that contain caffeine early in the day, others may need to eliminate all caffeine from their diets. Certainly, if you have insomnia, you may wish to avoid any caffeine-containing foods for at least 6 hours before bedtime. It may be better not to consume any caffeine-containing foods after lunch.

Limit evening fluid intake. If you drink a good deal of fluid during the evening hours, you may awaken to use the bathroom. After using the bathroom, you may then have difficulty falling back to sleep.

Stop smoking. Cigarettes contain nicotine, which is a stimulant. Smoking before bedtime increases the risk of insomnia. As you sleep, you experience nicotine withdrawal and the need for nicotine may awaken you. People who smoke are also known to have more nightmares.

When you first stop smoking, you increase your risk of insomnia. But that risk will soon fade, and you will reap the benefits of not smoking.

Kidney Stones

Kidney stones, also known as nephrolithiasis or urinary calculi, are hard masses of crystals that develop inside the kidneys. The most common types of stones are composed of calcium oxalate or calcium phosphate. A less common stone, called a struvite, contains magnesium ammonium phosphate. Uric acid stones are even less common, and cystine stones are rare.

If the crystals remain tiny, and they do in 70 to 90 percent of cases, they may pass through the urinary tract without being noticed. Problems may occur when a stone irritates the lining of the kidney or leaves the kidney and enters one of the two ureters that connect the kidneys to the bladder. The stone may become lodged in a ureter and prevent urine from flowing freely. The part of the ureter that is behind the blockage may dilate. As time passes, there may be injury to the kidney.

The kidneys filter a wide variety of substances, including calcium, oxalate, uric acid, and cystine. All four of these substances have a tendency to form crystals. Fortunately, when everything is working normally, citrate and magnesium, which are also in the kidneys, prevent crystal formation. Sometimes, however, the balance is upset. If your kidneys contain too much calcium, oxalate, uric acid, or cystine, or if they have too little citrate and magnesium, crystals may form. Crystal formation may also take place when the urine is too concentrated or is too acidic or alkaline. The key element in the development of kidney stones is supersaturation. That is, salts in the kidney become so concentrated that they are unable to dissolve, and they precipitate out and form crystals.

In the United States, more than 1 million cases of kidney stones are reported every year. During an average lifetime, an American has a 10 percent chance of developing a kidney stone. They are most common during the midlife years, and they occur three times more often in men than in women. Though it is not known why, over the past 20 years, the incidence has been rising.

Causes and Risk Factors

It is not always clear what triggers the imbalance that results in kidney stones. Family history is known to play an important role in the development of kidney stones. In those who are susceptible, diet may well play a role. And certain medical conditions have been associated with this disorder, including urinary tract infections, obesity, high blood pressure, gout, chronic diarrhea, kidney problems such as cystic kidney diseases, and metabolic problems such as hyperparathyroidism.

People who have chronic inflammation of the bowel or who have had an intestinal bypass operation or ostomy surgery are more likely to form calcium oxalate stones. Those who take the protease inhibitor indinavir, which is used to treat HIV and AIDS, are at higher risk for kidney stones. Other causes are high levels of uric acid in the urine, excess

A Quick Guide to Symptoms

- ☐ Excruciating pain (renal colic)
- ☐ Nausea and vomiting
- ☐ Pain in the genitals
- ☐ Blood in the urine
- ☐ A burning sensation and the need to urinate often
- ☐ Fever and chills

intake of vitamin D, and a urinary tract blockage. Some diuretics and calcium-based antacids add to the amount of calcium in the urine, thereby increasing the chance that you will have kidney stones. People who are confined to bed tend to reabsorb more calcium and are therefore at a greater risk.

White males have the highest risk for kidney stones. White people have a greater risk than African Americans. Being overweight also increases the possibility of kidney stones. Once you have had a kidney stone, you are more likely to have another. If you are not treated for your first bout with kidney stones, you have an 80 percent chance of having another episode within 10 years.

Signs and Symptoms

The most common first symptom of a kidney stone is excruciating pain, which may be referred to as renal colic by your doctor. At first, the sharp, cramping pain tends to be in the back and side—in the area of a kidney or

the lower abdomen. There may also be nausea and vomiting. As time passes, the pain may spread to the groin. You may feel pain in the genitals, particularly the testicles.

There may be blood in the urine, which may be cloudy and foul-smelling. When the stone approaches the bladder, you may have a burning sensation and feel the need to urinate often. You may also have a fever and chills, usually indicating an infection and a medical emergency. If you are experiencing these symptoms, you need to contact your doctor immediately or visit an urgent care clinic or the emergency room of a hospital.

Conventional Treatments

In about 85 percent of individuals, kidney stones are sufficiently small—less than the width of a pencil eraser—that they are able to pass during normal urination. If there is no infection, watchful waiting is a perfectly acceptable option. To help the stone pass, you should drink 2 to 3 quarts of water each day. Your doctor will give you a collection kit that contains a filter for collecting the stone.

Medication

During the acute attack, while waiting for the stone to pass, you will be given painkilling medications such as nonsteroidal anti-inflammatory drugs (NSAIDs). In some instances, you may be given opioids such as meperidine (Demerol). If there is an infection, you may be admitted to the hospital, where you will receive intravenous antibiotics. Even if you are not admitted, if you have an infection, your doctor will prescribe an antibiotic.

A number of medications can help prevent the formation of calcium and uric acid stones. The diuretic hydrochlorothiazide reduces the amount of calcium that is excreted. Allopurinol lowers the amount of uric acid production. Potassium citrate attaches itself to calcium, allowing the calcium to be removed safely from the body. Sodium cellulose phosphate may be given to those with a condition known as absorptive hypercalciuria. This medication binds to calcium in the intestines, thereby preventing it from getting into the urine. Cystine stone formation may be treated with penicillamine or tiopronin, which facilitates the body's breakdown of cystine.

If you have struvite stones that can't be removed, your doctor may prescribe aetohydroamic acid (AHA), which is used in conjunction with antibiotic medications.

Some studies have attempted to determine if treatment with medications, including calcium-channel blockers or alpha-blockers, helps with the passage of the stones. Pooled results of a number of experimental trials suggest that, under certain conditions, these medications may be useful. Since this option may enable you to avoid surgery, you may wish to discuss medications with your clinician.

Surgery

Extracorporeal shock wave lithotripsy (ESWL).

In this most common surgical procedure, shock waves are used to break the stones into small crystals that can be passed in the urine.

The procedure is best for stones that are less than 1 centimeter in size. Usually, you will first be given some form of anesthesia, then

> **The degree of pain** that you feel from a kidney stone is not necessarily a function of the size of the stone. A small stone with sharp edges may cause more pain than a larger stone that is smooth.

either placed on a soft cushion or partially submerged in water. An ultrasound device generates shock waves that travel through your body and hit the stones. Though you won't feel the shock waves, they create a great deal of noise. To protect your hearing, you will be asked to wear earplugs or headphones.

Assessing the Stone

After your kidney stone attack, your doctor may want additional blood and urine tests. The blood tests help determine the levels of blood urea nitrogen, creatinine, calcium, phosphate, and uric acid in your blood. The urine test is used to detect the specific chemical and biological factors that play a role in the stone formation. You will probably be asked to collect your urine for 24 hours. The urine will be evaluated for levels of acidity, calcium, uric acid, oxalate, citrate, and creatinine. This information is used to establish the cause of the stone.

When collecting your 24-hour urine, be sure to discard the first urine of the first day and to include the first urine of the second day. This allows for accurate counting for the entire 24-hour period.

As the shattered stones pass through the urinary tract, you may have some discomfort. It may take months for all the stones to pass. To aid the passage, your doctor may insert a stent or small tube through the bladder into the ureter. You may resume your regular schedule in a few days.

The most common complication of ESWL is blood in the urine, which may last for a few days. To reduce your risk, for 7 to 10 days before the procedure, you may be advised to stop taking aspirin or other NSAIDs. You may also have some bruising or minor discomfort in your back or abdomen. If the stone did not completely fragment, you may need another treatment. Success rates vary from 50 to 90 percent.

Percutaneous nephrolithotomy. If the stone is larger than 3 centimeters, or the ESWL was not successful, or there is evidence that your stone is blocking the flow of urine, damaging the kidney, or causing a urinary tract infection, your doctor may advise a percutaneous nephrolithotomy. In this procedure, your doctor makes a small incision in the back. Then, after a "tunnel" to the kidney is created, the stone is removed with an instrument known as a nephroscope. Sometimes, the stone must first be broken into smaller pieces.

Success rates with this surgery tend to be quite high—about 98 percent for stones in the kidney and 88 percent for stones in the ureters. About 3 percent of those who have this surgery have complications, which include scarring, blood loss, imbalances in the fluid used to irrigate the tunnel, collapsed lung, and injuries to the operative area.

Ureteroscopic stone removal. If your stone is stuck in the mid to low area of one of the ureters, your doctor may suggest a ureteroscopy. In this procedure, your doctor passes a ureteroscope, a small fiber-optic instrument, through the urethra and bladder into the ureter. After the stone is located, it will be held and removed by tiny forceps. Larger stones are generally shattered with an ultrasound. To help the ureter heal, a stent or small tube may be left in for a few days.

Treating Underlying Disorders

If the underlying cause of the kidney stones is determined, it is important that it be treated. Effective treatment of the underlying cause should significantly reduce the chances of another attack. For example, people with hyperparathyroidism have high amounts of calcium. As a result, they are at higher risk for kidney stones. Hyperparathyroidism is often caused by a tumor in one of the four parathyroid glands in the neck. When the tumor is removed, the condition is resolved.

Complementary Treatments

Complementary medicine treatments may be beneficial for pain relief of kidney stones. Herbs and dietary changes are useful in preventing further occurrences of kidney stones. Conventional medicine is the best course of action for this condition, especially when the stones are large and require immediate attention. Complementary medicine treatments should be used in conjunction with conventional medicine.

Diet

Diet plays a key role in the treatment and prevention of kidney stones, but before you make any changes in your diet, it is important to find out what type of stones you have. You may need to limit or eliminate foods containing calcium, salt, oxalate, protein, and potassium. While diet restrictions may vary, it is generally recommended that anyone with kidney stones avoid foods high in animal protein, fried foods, sugar, and processed foods.

Naturopathy

Since diet plays a key role in the treatment of kidney stones, visiting a naturopathic physician will be beneficial. A naturopath can also assist in nutritional supplement recommendations, if needed, along with other health and lifestyle changes to eliminate future stone attacks. To find a naturopathic practitioner in your area, contact the American Association of Naturopathic Physicians at www.naturopathic.org.

Nutritional Counseling

Contact a registered dietitian to help clear up any confusion associated with the type of stones you have and the foods to avoid. He or she will help you create a diet to reduce the incidence of future attacks.

Nutritional Supplements

A combination of nutritional supplements may be beneficial in preventing calcium kidney stones.

- B-complex vitamins: Take as directed on the label. B vitamins work best when taken together. B_6 in particular helps prevent crystallization and the reformation of calcium kidney stones. Take with magnesium.
- Magnesium: 500 milligrams daily. Take with B-complex vitamins. Do not take magnesium if you have kidney disease.

Lifestyle Recommendations

Apply heat. To provide relief while passing a kidney stone, apply moist heat to the lower back or soak in a hot tub.

Be careful of high-protein diets. Though it is not well understood, it is known that the incidence of kidney stones is associated with the amount of protein in the diet. Groups with higher intakes of dietary protein tend to have elevated rates of kidney stones. Since protein may aid stone production by increasing acidity of urine or facilitating the excretion of uric acid, phosphorus, and/or calcium, be careful with the amount of protein you consume.

Drink lemon juice. Fresh lemon juice may help reduce the pain of kidney stones and prevent future stone formation. For pain relief, add the juice of half a lemon to an 8-ounce glass of warm water. Drink a glass every hour. For the prevention of future stones, start your day with this same combination. Once a day is sufficient for prevention.

Preventive Measures

Avoid grapefruit juice. A number of studies have found that grapefruit juice increases the risk of kidney stones.

Use care when taking vitamin C. Because

most stones will not form in acidic urine, increasing your intake of vitamin C may be useful. However, if you've been told that you have too much urinary oxalate, a condition known as hyperoxaluria, you should avoid taking vitamin C supplements. Vitamin C, also known as ascorbic acid, may convert to oxalates.

Drink lots of fluid. If you have already had a bout with kidney stones or if you have been told that you are at increased risk, you should drink at least 10 to 14 glasses of fluid each day. Of that, at least half should be water. If you have a tendency for cystine stones, you need to drink more than a gallon of fluids each day. If your urine is dark or yellow rather than watery, you are not drinking enough fluids. Remember, during the warmer months or if you live in a warm climate, you should drink even more. You goal is to drink a sufficient amount of fluids to produce at least 2 quarts of urine every day.

Water helps dilute the urine and pushes out concentrations of harmful chemicals. If you are prone to uric acid stones or calcium oxalate stones, you should avoid cranberry juice and any other products containing cranberries, as recent studies have shown that cranberry juice can actually raise the risk for these types of kidney stones. The study did show, however, that cranberry juice lowered the risk for brushite stones, which are rare. Orange juice may help prevent stone formation.

Exercise. Regular exercise may remove excess calcium from the blood and transport it to the bones, where it is better utilized. The lack of regular exercise may increase the level of calcium in the blood, which may lead to kidney stones. Get at least 40 minutes of exercise daily.

Limit soft drinks. Many soft drinks contain phosphoric acid, which increases your risk for kidney stones.

Lose weight. If you are carrying around excess weight, try to lose it. But drop the pounds slowly, as losing weight too quickly increases the risk for kidney stones.

Reduce your sugar intake. Consuming sugar promotes the release of insulin by the pancreas, which, in turn, causes calcium to be released into the urine.

Restrict your sodium intake. Salt increases the amount of calcium in the urine and may aid in the formation of kidney stones.

Take care with calcium supplementation. Although research has found that the dietary intake of calcium appears to be protective against calcium oxalate stones, calcium supplements may raise your risk for other types of kidney stones. Supplementation up to 1,200 milligrams per day is considered safe. Do not exceed 2,000 milligrams per day, as that level of supplementation is clearly associated with increased risk. If you are at risk for kidney stones, you should discuss calcium supplementation with your doctor.

Try to relax. People who are stressed tend to have more kidney stones than those who are less stressed. Find a way to incorporate relaxation techniques into your life.

Macular Degeneration

When your vision is impaired, as it is with age-related macular degeneration (AMD or ARMD), objects may appear unclear. You may have difficulty with everyday functions such as driving and reading. Faces of other people may become blurred, and you may be unable to differentiate one person from another. You may have a hard time determining the colors and fine points of items that appear within the center of your field of vision. And what you do see will tend to be in black and white, rather than in color. Fortunately, the peripheral vision of those dealing with AMD is normally spared.

The macula is a light-sensitive layer of tissues located in the back of the eye at the center of the retina. When light, which enters the eye via the cornea and lens, focuses on the macula, it is transformed into nerve signals. These nerve signals are, in turn, transmitted to the brain. This process enables you to see central vision (what is straight ahead) in sharp, fine details, and allows you to distinguish different colors.

Macular degeneration is a relatively common disease. Approximately 1.6 million Americans have the advanced form of the disease, which threatens vision. Another 6 million Americans are considered at risk for developing advanced macular degeneration in at least one eye. Macular degeneration is believed to be the leading cause of legal blindness in US residents over the age of 55.

There are two types of AMD, dry AMD (atrophic) and wet AMD (exudative). Approximately 90 percent of those affected by this illness have dry AMD. While the cause is not known, in dry AMD the light-sensitive cells in the macula stop working. As time passes, central vision is lost. Dry AMD typically begins by affecting one eye, but it may ultimately affect both eyes.

Wet AMD is the rapidly advancing form of this illness. Ninety percent of those who experience severe AMD-related vision loss have wet AMD. In wet AMD, new, fragile blood vessels behind the retina grow toward the macula, and, in the process, they leak blood and fluid. This damages the macula, which may cause a relatively swift loss of central vision. On occasion, people with dry AMD may also develop wet AMD.

Causes and Risk Factors

The risk of AMD increases with age. Those in their fifties have about a 2 percent risk of developing AMD, but that figure jumps to 30 percent in people over the age of 75. In addition to age, there are other risk factors. There is strong evidence of an association between

A Quick Guide to Symptoms

- ☐ Mildly blurred vision
- ☐ Colors are harder to distinguish
- ☐ Blurred spot at the center of vision
- ☐ Straight lines that look wavy (wet AMD)
- ☐ Rapid loss of central vision (wet AMD)

smoking and AMD. Smoking reduces macular pigment up to 50 percent. The risk of AMD is about 2 to 4 times greater in smokers than nonsmokers. In smokers who have a certain genetic predisposition, the risk for AMD may be 34 times greater compared with nonsmokers without the genetic predisposition.

Some studies have found that women and whites are more likely to have AMD. Family history seems to play a role, as does elevated cholesterol, arteriosclerosis, high blood pressure, and smoking. Similarly, fair skin, light-colored eyes, extreme farsightedness, and prolonged exposure to sunlight add to the risk.

Using the Amsler Grid

If you are diagnosed with dry AMD, you should check your eyes daily with an Amsler grid, which is a grid with a pattern that looks like a checkerboard. In a small number of cases, dry AMD progresses to wet AMD, and you want to determine if that could be happening to you. The test allows you to see whether the disease is stable or progressing.

The Amsler grid has a black dot in the center. Be sure to place your grid in a convenient location, such as on the refrigerator. Stand 12 to 15 inches away from it. Cover your right eye when you look at the black dot with your left eye, and cover your left eye when you look at the black dot with your right eye. Keep a log, and record how the grid looks. One day, you may note that the straight lines in the pattern appear wavy, or they may simply be changed (appear blurry or distorted or discolored), or part of the grid may have disappeared.

If any of these events seems to be happening, make copies of the grid and use a new copy each day, and date it. Indicate the exact changes and their location on the grid. These symptoms may be a sign of wet AMD. If they occur, you need to visit your eye care professional quickly. Bring copies of the grid to your appointment. A picture of an Amsler grid is available on the Internet at www.nei.nih.gov/health/maculardegen/armd_facts.asp.

Signs and Symptoms

Neither form of macular degeneration triggers pain. The most frequent symptom of dry AMD is mildly blurred vision. For example, someone might notice that more light is needed for reading. Facial features and colors may appear harder to distinguish. Central vision colors will be difficult to determine, and objects will tend to be black or white. As the disease progresses, there may be a blurred spot at the center of vision. This spot may gradually grow larger and darker, thereby reducing still more of the central vision. When dry AMD occurs in only one eye, people usually do not notice any changes in their vision because they are still able to see fine details with the other eye. Often, dry AMD is first detected during a routine eye exam. Most people realize that there is a problem only when dry AMD affects both eyes.

Straight lines that look wavy are a frequent first symptom of wet AMD. This indicator is caused by newly formed blood vessels that are leaking fluid under the macula. Another symptom of wet AMD is a rapid loss of central vision, and there may also be a blind spot.

If you are experiencing any of these symptoms, you should immediately contact an eye care professional, such as an ophthalmologist or optometrist. Describe your symptoms on the phone, and underscore your need to be evaluated quickly.

If you suspect that you may have AMD, you should seek emergency assistance from an eye care professional.

Conventional Treatments for Wet AMD

Thanks to the use of laser surgery, new types of medications, and combinations of lasers and light-sensitive drugs, people with wet AMD are retaining more of their sight.

Antiangiogenesis Drugs

It is well understood that cancer tumors obtain some of their blood supply by growing new blood vessels. A certain group of medications, known as antiangiogenesis drugs, is used to stop the growth of these vessels. In recent years, researchers have been examining whether they would be similarly useful for treating the vessels formed in wet AMD. They inject the antiangiogenesis drugs directly into the eye. The goal is to inhibit substances, such as the vascular endothelial growth factor (VEGF), that facilitate the growth of these new vessels. Another possibility is using the antiangiogenic steroid triamcinolone acetonide, not to destroy the blood vessels but to limit the amount of leaking fluid. Though still in the experimental stage, these drugs are showing enormous promise.

Laser Surgery

When laser surgery is appropriate, it involves a visit to a highly trained ophthalmologist. The physician will dilate your pupil and apply drops to numb the eye. It may also be necessary to numb the area behind the eye. During the laser treatment, the physician will aim a high-energy beam of light directly at the leaking blood vessels. You may see flashes of light. Do not defer or delay this treatment. It should be done as soon as possible, before the blood vessels have harmed the fovea (the central part of the macula).

Following treatment, you will be able to return home, but, since you will be unable to drive, prearrange a ride. Because the eye remains dilated for several hours, you should also wear sunglasses. Your vision will be blurry for most of the day, and there may be some localized pain, which should respond well to pain medication.

It is important to realize that laser surgery treats wet AMD, but it is not a cure. New vessels will probably develop, and they may require additional laser surgery. You will need relatively frequent evaluations by your physician.

An FDA-approved laser treatment uses photodynamic therapy (PDT). A drug in the form of a green dye, known as verteporfin or Visudyne, is injected into a vein in the arm. It takes about 10 to 20 minutes for the dye to make its way to the eye, where it tends to enter abnormal vessels. A physician then focuses a low-power laser beam on the back of the eye, which activates the drug to attack the abnormal vessels. The retina is spared. Obviously, the procedure requires extraordinary precision and, for now at least, is expensive. While the progression of the disease stops in about two-thirds of the people who have the surgery, only 10 percent witness an improvement in their vision. Further, photodynamic therapy works for only a somewhat brief period of time, so individuals may need to be retreated every few months.

Laser surgery comes with a degree of risk, though when carried out by a highly skilled practitioner, that likelihood should be minimal. While very small, there is the possibility that the laser beam will be aimed incorrectly. When that occurs, healthy retinal tissue may be destroyed. Further, bleeding and scar tissue may form on the retina. Also, the area that received the laser beam has an increased chance of a loss of vision.

Radiation

Researchers are studying a form of radiation known as proton-beam therapy to determine if it may be useful for wet AMD. Proton particles are directed precisely at the abnormal vessels and lesions. Although the abnormal vessels and lesions may be destroyed, the healthy cells appear to sustain little damage. Researchers believe that radiation may prove to be quite effective, particularly in the early stages of this disease.

Surgery

Some researchers are attempting to preserve central vision by removing abnormal blood vessels (submacular surgery). And surgeons are investigating retinal translocation in which part of the retina is detached and moved away from the problematic new blood vessels. This may improve vision. However, it is very risky. People having this surgery may run the risk of losing all vision.

Conventional Treatments for Dry AMD

Currently, there are no conventional treatments for dry AMD. So, what should you do if you are diagnosed with this disease? See an eye care professional at least once a year. Obtain an Amsler grid and, as previously noted, test your eyes every day. Then, you will be able to notice any sudden changes from dry AMD to wet AMD.

Complementary Treatments

A treatment plan will vary from person to person, since each individual has a unique constitution, as well as characteristic lifelong habits. However, there are basic lifestyle guidelines that aid in the treatment of AMD.

Diet

Many studies indicate that certain nutrients—carotenoids, specific vitamins, and essential fatty acids—are beneficial to treating AMD. Some of these nutrients concentrate in the part of the retina where macular degeneration strikes. Others work to strengthen capillaries carrying blood to the eye muscles. These powerful nutrients can be found in common foods, so increasing your intake of these foods may aid in reducing the effects of macular degeneration.

Lutein and zeaxanthin are antioxidants in the carotenoid family. They concentrate in the part of the retina where macular degeneration occurs and protect the delicate cells of the macula from the damaging effects of ultraviolet light. People with AMD have been found to have lower levels of these substances in their bodies. Good sources of lutein and zeaxanthin include green, leafy vegetables, such as spinach, kale, and collard greens.

Anthocyanosides are compounds with antioxidant properties found in blueberries, cherries, raspberries, red or purple grapes, and plums. The European species of blueberry, the bilberry, has the highest level of anthocyanosides. Anthocyanosides help improve capillary circulation, which is very important in the retina.

Avoid foods high in hydrogenated fats, such as solid shortening, margarine, and deep-fried foods. Many processed snack foods, such as cookies and cakes, are high in fat. In fact, try to stay away from as much processed food as you can. These foods contribute to elevated cholesterol, arteriosclerosis, and high blood pressure, all risk factors in macular degeneration. A diet with lots of whole grains, vegetables, fruits, and cold-water fish, such as bluefish, cod, herring, mackerel, salmon, and tuna, is healthier. New studies have found that a diet high in omega-3 fatty acids may reduce the risk of advanced age-related macular degeneration.

Herbal Medicine

Ginkgo biloba. Ginkgo, which has been shown to improve memory and enhance concentration, is also beneficial for macular degeneration. Since ginkgo contains a variety of bioflavonoids, it acts as an antioxidant, increases the oxygen supply to the eyes, and assists in improving circulation and reducing oxidative damage. The recommended daily dose is 120 milligrams twice a day of extract standardized to 24 percent of flavone glycosides and 6 percent terpene lactones. The flavone glycosides give ginkgo its antioxidant benefits, and terpene lactones increase circulation and have a protective effect on nerve cells. Ginkgo should not be used if you are presently taking a blood-thinning medication.

Proanthocyanidin bioflavonoids. Often referred to as PAC or grape seed extract, this antioxidant may suppress the progression of macular degeneration by allowing macular tissue to adjust to oxygen fluctuations. It also reduces sensitivity to glare and sunlight. The typical recommended dose is 150 to 250 milligrams per day.

Nutritional Supplements

Antioxidant nutrients protect against the damage of free radical cells. Some of these nutrients concentrate in the retina, and deficiency can lead to macular degeneration.

- Vitamin C: 2,000 milligrams daily in divided doses of 1,000 milligrams. Protects against oxidative damage from sunlight, thereby decreasing the symptoms of macular degeneration. Do not take with selenium.

• Vitamin E: 400 IU daily. Antioxidant that neutralizes free radicals. Take with selenium.

• Bilberry extract: 100 milligrams of extract three times a day. Improves capillary circulation, which is very important to the retina.

• Copper: 2 milligrams daily. Long-term use of zinc may interfere with copper absorption and supplementation may be necessary.

• Lutein: 10 milligrams daily. Protects cells of the macula from the damaging effects of ultraviolet light.

• Selenium: 200 micrograms daily. Antioxidant that neutralizes free radicals.

• Zeaxanthin: 0.6 milligram daily. Protects cells of the macula from the damaging effects of ultraviolet light.

• Zinc: 50 milligrams daily. Essential since zinc concentrates in the retina. Prevents AMD, prevents vision loss in those with AMD, and reduces symptoms of AMD.

Lifestyle Recommendations

Discuss related medications with your doctor. Elevated cholesterol levels increase the risk for AMD, so it's a good idea to have your cholesterol level checked. If it is high, revamp your diet and discuss with your doctor whether you are a candidate for a cholesterol-lowering drug. Similarly, high blood pressure has been correlated with higher risks for AMD. If your blood pressure tends to be high, you may wish to discuss medications with your physician.

Drink a glass of red wine. Red wine contains bioflavonoids such as quercetin, rutin, and resveratrol, which have antioxidant activity to prevent oxidative damage. This can help slow the progression of macular degeneration. It may also play a role in prevention.

Exercise. Exercising increases the delivery of nutrients to the eyes and facilitates the removal of waste products. In addition, maintaining a regular exercise program helps reduce many of the risk factors associated with macular degeneration. The most important exercise for eye health is aerobic—consider walking, running, or swimming on a regular basis.

Try microcurrent stimulation. In this procedure, a TENS (transcutaneous electrical nerve stimulation) unit is used to apply electrical stimulation to key nerves around the eyes. For the treatment of wet and dry macular degeneration, electrodes are placed on the skin over the nerve areas and a low-voltage electrical pulse is then applied. Supporters of this noninvasive procedure contend that it improves bloodflow to the macula, and there are patients who indicate that it has increased visual acuity and color perception.

Preventive Measures

Get your vitamin D. Getting 10 to 15 minutes of direct sunlight several times a week can ensure that your body absorbs sufficient vitamin D. New findings show that individuals with higher levels of vitamin D may reduce the risk of developing early-stage age-related macular degeneration by 40 percent. Remember to use sunscreen if you spend longer than the recommended 10 to 15 minutes in the sun. If you are unable to spend time in the sun, you can get vitamin D in your diet through eggs and fish such as cod, mackerel, sardines, salmon, and tuna. It is also available in supplement form. Take 400 IU daily or at least three times a week.

Stop smoking. The direct correlation between macular degeneration and smoking is well documented. It appears that smokers are $2^1/_2$ times more likely than nonsmokers to develop AMD. While the average age that a nonsmoker will become ill with AMD is 71, the average age that a smoker will develop AMD is 64.

Wear a hat and sunglasses. Most eye professionals believe that ongoing exposure to sunlight increases the risk of AMD. It is a good idea to wear a protective hat and sunglasses that block out 100 percent of ultraviolet (UVA and UVB) rays and filter out at least 85 percent of blue-violet sun rays. Some contend that brown to yellow lenses are better alternatives. Be aware that there are medications that make the skin and eyes even more sensitive to light. Ask your doctor if any of your medications has this potential. If you are taking such a medicine, you need to be extra vigilant with sun protection.

Male Menopause

Often referred to as andropause, male menopause consists of the physical and psychological changes men experience at midlife. As men age, their testes and adrenal gland produce less of the male hormone testosterone—a condition known as hypogonadism. While these changes may appear anytime between the ages of 30 and 70, they tend to occur when a man is in his forties and fifties. About 13 percent of men between the ages of 40 and 60 have lower than normal testosterone levels. An average 70-year-old man has 25 to 50 percent less testosterone than he had at the age of 20.

While the very existence of male menopause is controversial, those who believe that it is a real disorder also contend that it is somewhat common. It has been estimated that as many as 5 million men over the age of 40 in the United States have this condition.

With male menopause (also known as low testosterone syndrome, and climacteric), there is a decrease in the production of testosterone in the testicles, although this is more variable than the estrogen deficiency seen in women who have undergone menopause. Lower levels of testosterone may induce loss of muscle mass, weakness, and osteoporosis. The osteoporosis that is caused by andropause may result in higher risk of fracture. However, this usually occurs about 10 years later than it does in women.

The changes associated with male menopause may be divided into two main categories, urinary/sexual changes and more generalized physical and psychological changes. For example, a man with a lower level of testosterone may have a reduced interest in sexual relations and may have mood swings. But low levels of testosterone are not believed to have any effect on fertility.

Theoretically, all men at midlife are at risk for male menopause. Evidently, however, not all men experience the symptoms linked to this disorder.

A Quick Guide to Symptoms

- ☐ **Increases in fat, decreases in muscle and bone mass**
- ☐ **Decrease in strength and endurance**
- ☐ **Irritability and mood swings**
- ☐ **Difficulty concentrating**
- ☐ **Hot flashes**
- ☐ **Sleep problems**
- ☐ **Lack of energy**
- ☐ **Depression**
- ☐ **Erectile dysfunction**
- ☐ **Problems with urination**

Signs and Symptoms

Common symptoms of male menopause include increases in fat, decreases in muscle and bone mass, decreased beard growth, decrease in strength and endurance, irritability, difficulty concentrating, hot flashes, sleep problems, lack of energy, decline in performance at work, depression, erectile dysfunction, mood swings, and problems with urination.

Conventional Treatments

If you have low levels of testosterone and your doctor believes this requires treatment, then you may be given a prescription for testosterone replacement therapy (TRT). This is available as injections, patches, or a rub-on gel. Men who receive TRT must be closely monitored for prostate cancer. Though there is no evidence that TRT causes prostate cancer, it may potentially accelerate the growth of any existing prostate cancer. Men who have been diagnosed with prostate cancer should not take TRT, and men taking TRT must be carefully watched. In addition, there is some evidence that TRT may increase bad cholesterol and decrease good cholesterol. Plus, TRT may potentially harm the liver, stimulate benign growth of the prostate, and aggravate sleep apnea.

Complementary Treatments

Whether andropause is part of the normal aging process or a condition unto itself, complementary medicine offers numerous options to relieve and eliminate symptoms associated with male menopause.

Acupuncture

Due to its ability to produce a more controlled, higher level of continuous stimulus, using electro-acupuncture for the treatment of erectile dysfunction has shown positive effects, according to numerous studies. In electro-acupuncture, needles are inserted at specific points on the body. After insertion, an electric current is passed through the needles.

There is a saliva self-test that evaluates levels of testosterone, but it is generally viewed as somewhat unreliable. If you are at midlife, are experiencing the previously noted symptoms, and believe that you may be going through andropause, you should visit your doctor.

Diet

Maintain a healthy weight by eating lots of whole grains, fruits, and vegetables. In addition to assisting with weight maintenance, eating foods high in nutrients keeps the body properly nourished. These foods help keep the vascular system healthy, thereby maintaining proper bloodflow to the penis, which is necessary for erections. Try to include a minimum of five servings of vegetables, four servings of fruit, and six servings of whole grains each day.

Eliminate foods that are high in fat and sugar. They not only have an adverse effect on weight, but they rob the body of essential nutrients and interfere with their absorption. Also, stay away from foods and supplements that contain caffeine. While caffeine is a stimulant, it relaxes muscles and may interfere with normal function of the genital area. Avoid alcohol, which robs the body of zinc. Studies have shown that zinc deficiency may lead to prostate problems. Zinc is found in pumpkin and sunflower seeds, so try to include these in your diet.

Exercise

Regular, moderate exercise is beneficial both for relieving the symptoms of male menopause and for slowing the male aging process.

Regular exercise lowers your risk for diabetes, heart disease, and osteoporosis. It also increases the release of endorphins, brain chemicals that help regulate body temperature and decrease stress, mood swings, and depression.

Without exercise, bones diminish in size and strength. At any age, bones may be rebuilt with weight-bearing activity, such as walking. Weight-bearing exercise also helps normalize the flow of sugar from the blood into muscle tissue, where it may be properly metabolized, reducing the risk of diabetes. Exercise improves muscle mass, strength, and gait, while facilitating flexibility, balance, and coordination.

Regular exercise slows the loss of dopamine, a neurotransmitter that prevents shaking and stiffness. Dopamine also supports our ability to react, thereby reducing the risk of falling.

You should create an exercise routine that includes an overall body program. It should incorporate weight-bearing exercises, strength training for the arms and legs, and postural training to support the back. Any exercise is better than none, but try to exercise at least 40 minutes per day. Since they increase flexibility and strength, yard work and gardening are considered exercise. Simply walking a minimum of 20 minutes, three times a week, may enhance bloodflow.

Herbal Medicine

A number of herbs can help balance the hormones and are considered precursors to progesterone and testosterone.

Asian ginseng. Asian ginseng helps maintain an erection and is known to improve male potency. The recommended daily dose is 100 to 200 milligrams, standardized to 4 to 7 percent ginsenosides. However, do not use ginseng if you have high blood pressure, heart disorders, or hypoglycemia.

Damiana. Damiana may be more effective when combined with other, similar-acting herbs such as sarsaparilla. To make a tea, place 1 gram of dried leaves in 1 cup of water and steep for 10 minutes. Drink 2 to 3 cups per day. Damiana is also available in tincture and capsule form. Take 2 to 3 milliliters of the tincture, two or three times per day. In capsules, take 400 milligrams, twice a day.

Ginkgo biloba. Ginkgo has been shown to increase overall circulation as well as bloodflow to the penis. It is available in capsule form. The recommended daily dose is 120 milligrams, twice a day, of extract standardized to 24 percent flavone glycosides and 6 percent terpene lactones. The flavone glycosides give ginkgo its antioxidant benefits, and terpene lactones increase circulation and have a protective effect on nerve cells. However, if you are taking a prescription blood-thinning medication, be sure to consult your doctor before taking ginkgo supplements.

Maca. Maca is a perennial crop from Peru that has been used for centuries. It is grown at elevations of 12,000 feet and higher, is in the same family as turnips and radishes, and is a highly nutritious food. It has an overall nutritive effect that improves physical vitality, endurance, and stamina. Maca is also known for the treatment of male menopause because of its ability to increase sexual desire and performance. It is available in capsule form. The recommended daily dose is 550 milligrams twice a day.

Sarsaparilla. Sarsaparilla has long been regarded as a restorative for the male reproductive organs. It has been used for centuries in Central and South America for the treatment of impotency and as a general tonic for physical weakness. Take 1 cup of dried root tea 2 or 3 times daily. Sarsaparilla is available as packaged tea in natural health food or organic grocery stores. The powdered root is also available in capsules containing 1 to 2 grams of the root powder. In tincture form, take 2 to 3 milliliters of plant extract twice each day.

Hypnosis

Hypnosis has been successful for treating psychological symptoms of male menopause, particularly erectile dysfunction.

To learn more about hypnosis and to locate a qualified practitioner in your area, visit the Web site of the American Society of Clinical Hypnosis at www.asch.net. Schedule an introductory visit to determine his or her experience in treating your condition as well as your comfort level with this person.

Nutritional Supplements

Supplements can increase energy, reduce stress, and help restore normal sexual function.

- Multivitamin/mineral: Take as directed on the label. Ensures proper nutrient level for overall health and vitality.

- B-complex vitamins: Take as directed on the label. Reduce stress.

- L-arginine: 1,000 to 2,000 milligrams daily. Necessary for production of nitric oxide, which is needed to obtain a normal erection.

- Omega-3 fatty acid, like flaxseed oil or fish oil: 1 tablespoon of flaxseed oil daily or 4,000 milligrams daily of fish oil capsules. Beneficial for heart health and mood swings.

- Zinc: 30 milligrams daily. Necessary for normal sexual function in males.

Lifestyle Recommendations

Most men with sexual issues do not consult their physician. Consider bringing up the topic at the next office visit.

Improve your lifestyle. Find time to exercise more. Eat a healthier low-fat, high-fiber diet. Reduce your intake of caffeine and alcohol. Get the sleep that you require.

Lower your cholesterol. Studies have shown that high levels of cholesterol increase your risk for erectile dysfunction.

Reduce stress. Since stress speeds the aging process, find ways to relax, unwind, and reduce your stress. Every day, try to find at least 10 minutes to close your eyes, empty your mind, and breathe deeply.

Stop smoking. Men who smoke are at greater risk for erectile dysfunction than those who don't.

Memory Loss

Having problems remembering places, people, objects, or events? There are two main types of memory loss. Short-term memory loss is forgetfulness of a recent event. Were you just introduced to somebody? Have you already forgotten that person's name? That is short-term memory loss. Long-term memory loss is forgetfulness of something that took place a long time ago. There are three forms of long-term memory loss. Semantic memory involves recalling knowledge, such as an event of historical significance. Procedural memory relates to remembering how to do something, such as driving a car. Episodic memory concerns how you recollect everyday events, such as where you placed your keys. Aging is most likely to affect episodic memory.

There is also a profound form of memory loss known as amnesia, in which there is the partial or total loss of recall. Amnesia may be temporary or permanent.

As people reach midlife, some degree of memory loss is quite common. Fortunately, for most people, the degree of memory loss is mild. The vast majority of people do not develop a serious impairment that interferes with their daily lives.

A Quick Guide to Symptoms

- ☐ **Forgetting everyday things such as where you put your keys**
- ☐ **Trouble immediately recalling the names of friends**
- ☐ **Failing to recall your own home address or other familiar locations (dementia)**
- ☐ **Neglect of personal hygiene and not remembering to eat (dementia)**
- ☐ **Impairment in thinking, judgment, and the ability to perform everyday tasks (Alzheimer's disease)**

Causes and Risk Factors

Though a certain amount of memory loss tends to occur with the aging process, memory loss may have other causes, including dementia, in which there are severe problems with memory and thinking. The two most common types of dementia are Alzheimer's disease, in which large numbers of brain cells die, and multi-infarct dementia, in which a series of small strokes or changes in the blood supply cause the death of brain tissue. Multi-infarct dementia is believed to be associated with high blood pressure.

Other causes of memory loss are thyroid disease, head injury, chronic alcohol abuse, use of hallucinogens, menopause, barbiturates, combinations of certain medications, vitamin B_{12} or B_3 (niacin) deficiency, strokes, seizures, infections, depression, atherosclerosis (hardening of the arteries), Parkinson's disease, Pick's disease, electroconvulsive therapy (ECT), and surgery in the temporal lobe of the brain.

Memory loss associated with a progressive illness such as dementia will tend to worsen. Over time, this kind of memory loss interferes with more and more of the activities of daily living.

Your risk for memory problems increases as you age. The simple act of aging places you at risk.

Signs and Symptoms

If you have memory loss, you forget things. Maybe you walk out of the grocery store without the item you most wanted to purchase. Or perhaps you fail to remember what you intended to retrieve when you entered your bedroom. You may have trouble immediately recalling the names of friends. You should realize that forgetfulness is ubiquitous. Everyone experiences some degree of memory loss, but, as you age, certain symptoms of memory loss tend to become more common. For example, it is more likely that you will have trouble learning new material. And you may require longer periods of time to remember already learned information, such as names.

If you have memory loss from a medical problem, you will probably have symptoms of that particular condition. Thus, if you have memory loss from hypothyroidism (low thyroid function), you may experience other symptoms such as fatigue; weight gain; brain fog; feeling cold; intolerance to cold; loss of hair; dry, scaly, itchy skin and scalp; leg cramps; and depression. Or if you have memory loss from depression, you may have a number of additional symptoms, such as depressed mood, agitation, irritability, sleep disturbances, a diminished energy level, reduced self-esteem, slowed movement, and thoughts of death or suicide.

While the early stages of memory loss from a serious progressive illness such as dementia may appear similar to other forms of memory loss, as the disease process continues, the symptoms become more troublesome. During the early stages, you may forget where you placed your keys. As dementia progresses, you may not be able to recall how to use your keys. Similarly, during the early stages, you may forget a phone number. As the disease worsens, you may forget how to use a phone.

It is not uncommon for people with dementia to fail to recall their own home address or other familiar locations. They may neglect personal hygiene and not remember to eat. Eventually, they fail to recognize family and friends. Alzheimer's disease tends to begin slowly, but as the disease continues, there is impairment in thinking, judgment, and the ability to perform everyday tasks. Multi-infarct dementia symptoms typically appear fairly quickly. People with this condition generally improve after a single stroke, and, if more strokes occur, become ill again. The symptoms of both Alzheimer's and multi-infarct dementia may appear together in the same person.

Conventional Treatments

Most mild cases of age-related memory loss are not treated. However, to improve your memory, you may wish to use a number of coping mechanisms.

- Whenever possible, follow a routine. Keep lists of the things you need to do. Record

While there are a number of informal memory tests available on the Internet, you will probably be aware if you have been experiencing trouble with your memory. You may wish to keep a diary of your memory loss to record the dates and times of your memory losses. What were you doing? Had you taken a certain medication or combination of medications?

future events on your calendar, and check the calendar often.

• When driving around your town, use landmarks to help you remember places.

• Always store certain items, such as keys, in the same place.

• When you meet new people, repeat their names or even write them down.

If your doctor determines that your memory loss has been caused by a medical disorder, then the underlying cause should be addressed. Thus, if you are found to have hypothyroidism, you will be told to take medication upon awakening every day. If you are found to be depressed, your doctor will likely prescribe medication and advise you to see a therapist. In both instances, when the primary medical problem is corrected, the degree of memory loss should lessen.

Medications

A few medications are helpful for those in the early and middle stages of Alzheimer's disease. By increasing the amount of acetylcholine in the body, they improve memory and delay the worsening of symptoms. These medications include tacrine (Cognex), donepezil (Aricept), rivastigmine (Exelon), and galantamine (Reminyl). Potential side effects include nausea, insomnia, vomiting, diarrhea, fatigue, muscle cramps, and liver damage. To monitor for possible liver damage, periodic liver function tests are ordered. People with multi-infarct dementia need to prevent future strokes by controlling their blood pressure, cholesterol, and diabetes. Since behavior problems are often seen in people with dementia, doctors may prescribe medications for agitation, anxiety, depression, and sleeping problems.

Complementary Treatments

Nutritional and lifestyle changes are often recommended to treat memory loss.

Diet

The old saying "You are what you eat" may easily be connected to memory loss. Your brain can function only as well as you feed it. So, it is extremely important to maintain a diet that is high in nutrient-rich foods and to avoid fried foods, hydrogenated fats, and processed foods containing artificial colors and other chemicals. Be sure to include lots of fresh fruits and vegetables and whole grains in your daily diet. Try to include a minimum of five servings of vegetables, four servings of fruit, and six servings of whole grains each day. Vitamin C and beta-carotene, found in many fruits and vegetables, have been shown to improve memory performance. Antioxidants, which are also found in fruits, vegetables, and soy products, may slow memory loss. Preliminary research has shown that monounsaturated fats, such as olive oil, may protect against memory loss and age-related cognitive decline (ARCD).

Herbal Medicine

A number of studies have shown that the antioxidant herb *Ginkgo biloba* improves mental clarity and memory, in addition to overall circulation to the brain. The typical recommended dose is 120 milligrams, twice daily, of extract standardized to 24 percent flavone glycosides and 6 percent terpene lactones. The flavone glycosides give ginkgo its antioxidant benefits, while terpene lactones increase circulation and have a protective effect on nerve cells. If you are also taking prescription blood-thinning medications, be sure to check with a doctor before using ginkgo supplements.

Melatonin

Melatonin, a hormone secreted by the pineal gland in the brain, has been shown to be useful for improving sleep, mood, and memory. As we age, our production of melatonin decreases. Since sleep and mood may affect our ability to remember and to maintain mental clarity, melatonin may be valuable. Take one 1-milligram tablet 30 minutes before going to bed if you have trouble falling asleep. You may need to increase the dose if you are having trouble staying asleep. Generally, 3 milligrams is the highest dose recommended. To ensure proper dosing and to prevent interactions with any other prescription or mood-enhancing medications, check with your doctor before supplementing with melatonin.

Nutritional Supplements

Nutritional deficiencies may lead to various forms of memory loss.

- Multivitamin/mineral: Take as directed on the label. Should include copper, zinc, calcium, and magnesium to help the brain retain memory.

- B-complex vitamins: Take as directed on the label. Essential in preventing and reversing memory loss. B_3 improves circulation to the brain while deficiency may produce dementia, B_1 can decrease effects of senility, and B_6 aids in long-term memory.

- Vitamin B_{12}: Injections. Deficiency may impair mental ability. Injections of B_{12} show improvement in memory.

- Vitamin C: 2,000 milligrams daily in divided doses of 1,000 milligrams. Antioxidant effects help reduce memory loss.

- Vitamin E: 400 IU daily. Antioxidant effects help reduce memory loss.

- Acetyl-L-carnitine: 1,000 milligrams daily in divided doses of 500 milligrams. Improves memory. Take with meals.

- Selenium: 400 micrograms daily, in divided doses of 200 micrograms. May protect the body against toxic effects of mercury.

Psychotherapy

Consider some form of psychotherapy. Internal pressures may lead to an increase in anxiety, anger, depression, and other dysfunctional behavior. When these pressures are addressed, the mind is able to concentrate more clearly and focus better.

Lifestyle Recommendations

Drink plenty of water. If your body lacks sufficient water, you may become dehydrated, feel tired, and have more trouble concentrating. Drink at least eight 8-ounce glasses a day.

Exercise. If you do not already exercise, begin a program of regular exercise. It will improve the flow of blood to your brain. Your exercise program should include some form of aerobic activity (brisk walking, bicycling, or swimming) at least 5 days a week, strength training (weight lifting) at least two or three times per week, and stretching every day.

Learn relaxation techniques. If you are nervous or anxious, you will have a harder time concentrating. Anxiety has been linked to poor memory performance. Studies show that individuals with chronic stress, anxiety, or anger throughout life have a greater chance of cognitive decline in later years. Find ways to reduce your stress.

Make associations. When trying to remember something, begin by thinking of associations. Gradually, the pieces may lead you to what you have forgotten. For example, when attempting to remember the name of a book, you may recall first that it was a mystery. Then, you might realize that it was a hardcover book, and you read it at the beach. Soon, you may be able to think of aspects of the story, even the author's name. Eventually, your mind will be refreshed and activate your memory to remember the title.

Rewrite notes. When trying to remember something, write it down. Then, within 5 hours, rewrite your notes. This will help to ensure that your brain files the information.

Preventive Measures

Avoid alcohol and recreational drugs. These may contribute to memory loss.

Get sufficient sleep. When you don't obtain adequate amounts of sleep, your mind feels foggy, and it is more difficult to concentrate, which contributes to memory loss.

Read labels. Some prescription medications, and even some over-the-counter medications such as antihistamines, may contribute to forgetfulness. Check the side effects of your medications or ask your doctor to determine if these may be contributing to your memory loss.

Stay intellectually challenged. Keep stimulating your mind.

- Enroll in a course at your local community college.
- Learn to play a new instrument.
- Join a study group.
- Attend political and cultural events.
- Do crossword puzzles or play Scrabble.
- Pick up a new hobby.
- Create an interesting part-time business.
- Volunteer.

Metabolic Syndrome

With metabolic syndrome, also known as insulin resistance syndrome, your fat, muscle, and liver cells are unable to respond appropriately to the hormone insulin. As a result, your pancreas keeps making high amounts of insulin. Metabolic syndrome also involves excess body fat, especially around the waist, abnormal blood lipid levels, and borderline or elevated blood pressure.

If your body is unable to regulate blood sugar levels, as is the case in about 25 percent of those affected by insulin resistance, you may develop type 2 diabetes. Type 2 diabetes is associated with a number of serious medical problems, such as heart disease, blindness, and kidney disease. In most instances, however, you will not develop type 2 diabetes. Instead, your body will simply keep producing increasing amounts of insulin, a condition known as hyperinsulinemia. Your glucose levels remain high, but within normal limits. Still, the high levels make you more vulnerable to a host of other medical problems, such as heart disease, stroke, and high blood pressure.

According to the National Cholesterol Education Program, if you have any three of the following medical problems, you probably have metabolic syndrome: blood pressure of at least 130 (systolic) or at least 85 (diastolic), fasting blood sugar of at least 110 (or greater than 140 at 2 hours into the glucose tolerance test), fasting triglycerides of at least 150, fasting HDL ("good") cholesterol of less than 40, or abdominal obesity. Abdominal obesity is defined as a waist size of greater than 40 inches in males and 35 inches in females.

Some believe that metabolic syndrome is responsible for as many as 50 percent of all heart attacks. Even when there is no evidence of diabetes or cardiovascular disease, men with metabolic syndrome are at increased risk for cardiovascular disease and mortality from any cause. In addition, since the presence of metabolic syndrome is a significant predictor for type 2 diabetes and cardiovascular disease, it may help identify those at high risk for these disorders.

Research has also linked insulin resistance to the formation of more dense LDL (bad) cholesterol, high levels of fat in the blood after eating, slow clearance of fat from the blood, a decreased ability to break up blood clots, and high blood levels of uric acid.

Metabolic syndrome is very common. The prevalence is around 6.7 percent for individuals between the ages of 20 and 29 to around 43.5 percent for people between the ages of 60 and 69. Mexican Americans have the highest prevalence. African American women have a

A Quick Guide to Symptoms

- ☐ Weight gain, especially around the waist
- ☐ Frequent cravings for sweets, breads, and other simple carbohydrates
- ☐ Fatigue, particularly after meals

57 percent higher prevalence than African American men, and Mexican American women have 26 percent higher prevalence than Mexican American men. According to 2000 census data, about 47 million US residents have metabolic syndrome.

Causes and Risk Factors

While the exact cause of metabolic syndrome is unknown, it is quite apparent that family history plays a strong role. You are at increased risk if your family members tend to have type 2 diabetes, high blood pressure, or cardiovascular disease, or if you have a history of glucose intolerance, gestational diabetes, high blood pressure, elevated triglycerides and low HDL cholesterol, or cardiovascular disease. Also, risk increases after the age of 40.

Nonwhites are at higher risk than whites. People with European ancestry have lower risks than those with non-European ancestry. Polynesian Islanders and Native Americans have an extremely high risk. But lifestyle factors appear to be equally important. Lack of physical exercise, obesity, a diet high in carbohydrates, and cigarette smoking all contribute to this disorder.

Signs and Symptoms

People with metabolic syndrome tend to gain weight, especially around the waist, have frequent cravings for sweets, breads, and other simple carbohydrates, and complain of fatigue, particularly after meals.

Conventional Treatments

Since insulin resistance grows worse as the pounds increase, treatment for metabolic syndrome generally begins with a weight loss program that includes exercise. To keep the glucose under control, your body has been producing more insulin. As your weight drops, your insulin resistance will improve. In many instances, weight loss and exercise are the only treatments needed.

Medications

When weight loss and exercise are unable to control metabolic syndrome, your doctor may prescribe medications to treat the problems associated with the disorder. Thus, if your lipids are high, you will probably be given a lipid-lowering medication, and if you have high blood pressure, you will probably be given a blood pressure–lowering prescription. On occasion, a medication for diabetes, such as metformin, may be prescribed for someone with metabolic syndrome.

Complementary Treatments

The focus of complementary medicine is on examining lifestyle habits that may lead to conditions resulting in the metabolic syndrome. This includes a sedentary lifestyle and a diet high in nutrient-poor foods. Because the metabolic syndrome is a cluster of symptoms that are related, eliminating some of these may work toward improving the others.

Diet

Diet plays an important role in preventing and reversing metabolic syndrome. It is important to understand what foods to avoid and why you should avoid them. Simple carbohydrates such as breads, pasta, bagels, white flour, white rice, sweets, and other foods made with sugar and other concentrated sweeteners impair your ability to control blood sugar. These foods increase the risk for type 2 diabetes, increase triglycerides, and lower HDL. Complex carbohydrates such as whole grains, corn, and potatoes may also raise blood sugar levels. If you already have metabolic syndrome, these foods should be eliminated until your blood pressure, blood fats, and weight are normalized. Nonstarchy vegetables, such as salad greens, asparagus, green beans, spinach, and broccoli, may be eaten freely. They raise the blood sugar only minimally and are filled with other nutrients and fiber.

Protein stimulates the production of a hormone called glucagon that opposes insulin. Because it helps to burn stored fat and prevents the urge to overeat carbohydrates, protein is useful when consumed in small amounts throughout the day. Good sources of protein are fish, poultry, and high-protein dairy foods such as eggs, cottage cheese, and tofu. However, beans, which also contain protein, are not good for individuals with metabolic syndrome, as they may raise blood sugar and insulin levels.

Omega-3 fatty acids lower blood pressure, reduce the risk of heart attack and stroke, and may help with weight gain—all issues associated with metabolic syndrome. Good sources of omega-3's are cold-water fish such as salmon, tuna, herring, and mackerel. In fact, eating cold-water fish once a week may reduce the risk of heart attack. Extra-virgin olive oil, grape seed oil, flaxseed oil, hempseed oil, and walnut oil should replace vegetable oils when cooking and preparing foods.

Fried foods, margarine, and any other foods that contain partially hydrogenated oils should be eliminated from the diet, as should sweetened fruit drinks, sodas, and alcohol.

Herbal Medicine

As it helps maintain normal liver function, milk thistle is extremely beneficial for preventing or reversing metabolic syndrome. The liver plays a role in maintaining blood sugar. Milk thistle is available in capsule form. The typical recommended daily dose is 300 milligrams per day. Look for capsules containing 80 percent silymarin.

Nutritional Supplements

Nutritional supplements play a role in proper insulin function.

- Vitamin C: 1,000 milligrams daily in divided doses of 500 milligrams. Helps normalize blood sugar and insulin function.

- Vitamin E: 400 IU daily. Helps normalize blood sugar and insulin function.

- Alpha-lipoic acid: 200 milligrams daily in divided doses of 100 milligrams. Helps normalize blood sugar and insulin function. Increases the potency of vitamins C and E.

- Calcium: 1,500 milligrams daily in divided doses of 500 milligrams. May improve insulin sensitivity in those with high blood pressure.

- Chromium picolinate: 200 micrograms daily. Deficiency disturbs normal insulin function. Necessary for preventing or reversing metabolic syndrome.

- Coenzyme Q$_{10}$: 200 milligrams daily. May reduce glucose and insulin blood levels.

- Glucomannan (bulk-forming dietary fiber derived from konjac root): dosage to be determined by your health-care provider. Drink at least 8 ounces of water with each dose. Stabilizes blood sugar in insulin-resistant individuals, reduces triglycerides and LDL cholesterol, and raises HDL cholesterol. Do not take if you have any esophageal disorder.

- L-carnitine: 1,000 milligrams daily in divided doses of 500 milligrams. May reduce glucose and insulin blood levels.

- Magnesium: 750 milligrams daily in divided doses of 250 milligrams. Deficiency disturbs normal insulin function. Necessary for preventing or reversing metabolic syndrome.

- Omega-3 fatty acids: 1 tablespoon of flaxseed oil daily. Lowers blood pressure and reduces risk of heart attack and stroke.

- Zinc: 30 milligrams daily. Deficiency disturbs normal insulin function. Necessary for preventing or reversing metabolic syndrome.

Lifestyle Recommendations

While obesity and physical inactivity do not cause metabolic syndrome, they do make the condition worse. Losing weight will help lower your insulin levels. Even a loss of only 10 to 15 pounds may significantly reduce insulin levels. And a loss of weight will make the body more insulin sensitive, so that less insulin is required for the same task of moving sugar from the bloodstream into various tissues.

Exercise will lower insulin and blood triglyceride levels while also raising HDL cholesterol. In the beginning, especially if you have been sedentary, you may be able to exercise for only 5 to 10 minutes. Try to build up to a minimum of 30 minutes of aerobic exercise at least three or four times each week. In people with insulin resistance, the combination of aerobic activity with strength training works best. In addition to the previously mentioned benefits, regular exercise also reduces stress, lowers blood pressure, and strengthens the heart and blood vessels. Of course, before beginning an exercise program, you should check with your doctor.

Preventive Measures

Reduce stress. Studies have shown that stress may lead to decreased insulin sensitivity. Meditation, biofeedback, and relaxation techniques such as deep breathing are all good ways to reduce stress.

Stop smoking. Researchers have determined that smokers are more insulin resistant and have higher insulin levels than nonsmokers. Smokers also have higher levels of blood triglycerides and lower HDL cholesterol levels. By smoking, you increase your probability of developing metabolic syndrome. Secondhand smoke and nicotine patches have the same effect as smoking.

Watch salt intake. Salt should be used in moderation, whether you currently have metabolic syndrome or are trying to prevent it.

Muscle Cramps

During a cramp, a muscle involuntarily and painfully contracts. Muscles are bundles of fibers that produce movement by contracting and expanding. Muscle cramps, which are also called muscle spasms, may occur in part of a muscle group, over an entire muscle group, or in several muscle groups.

The most likely muscles to cramp are those that span two joints, such as the calves (gastrocnemius), the back of the thighs (hamstrings), and the front of the thighs (quadriceps). However, you may experience muscle cramps in other parts of the body, such as the arms, abdomen, hands, feet, and along the rib cage. If you spend a good deal of time writing with a pen or pencil, you may even have muscle cramps in your thumb and first two fingers.

Muscle cramps may vary in intensity, ranging from a slight tic to severe pain. A badly cramped muscle may feel quite hard to the touch. It may appear distorted under your skin. And you may see it twitching. A muscle cramp may last a few seconds or more than 15 minutes, and it may recur.

Muscle cramps are extremely common. At some point, just about everyone has experienced them.

Causes and Risk Factors

Though the exact cause of muscle cramps is unknown, some contend that muscles that have not received adequate stretching or muscles that are fatigued are at increased risk for cramps. Other factors that may be associated with muscle cramps include exercising or working in intense heat, dehydration, and the depletion of salt and minerals known as electrolytes, such as calcium, magnesium, and potassium.

Muscle cramps and pain may also be associated with the use of statin drugs to lower cholesterol. Some studies report 1 to 5 percent incidence of these symptoms in statin users. In order to prevent muscle pain and cramps, you should use the lowest dosage of statin needed to lower cholesterol, and report any muscle pain immediately to your doctor.

Because of the normal muscle loss that comes with aging, we are at increased risk for muscle cramps as we age. Aging places us at particular risk for cramps that occur at night while we are sleeping. Inactivity only exacerbates the risk for muscle cramps. On the other hand, endurance athletes, such as those who run marathons, also have a greater risk for muscle cramps.

Muscle Cramps May Signal a Serious Illness

While most muscle cramps are benign, sometimes they indicate a more serious condition. Some of the medical problems that may cause muscle cramps include narrowing of the spinal canal (stenosis), thyroid disease, chronic infections, cirrhosis of the liver, hardening of the arteries, spinal nerve irritation or compression (radiculopathy), and amyotrophic lateral sclerosis (ALS or Lou Gehrig's disease).

Signs and Symptoms

With muscle cramps, the most significant symptom is pain. You may also be able to feel the cramped muscle and to see it twitching under the skin.

Conventional Treatments

Muscle cramps may be treated in a number of ways. Begin by relaxing the cramped muscle and gently massaging the area. Then, slowly stretch the muscle.

If you have muscle cramps that repeatedly disturb your sleep, your doctor may prescribe diazepam (Valium). It relaxes muscles and decreases stiffness. Other muscle relaxants include verapamil (Calan, Isoptin, Verelan), chloroquine (Aralen), and hydroxychloroquine (Plaquenil).

Complementary Treatments

Diet

Many nutrients play an important role in preventing muscle cramps. As a nutritional deficiency may be the cause of your muscle cramps, don't overlook the following nutrients.

• Bioflavonoids: found in many fruits and vegetables

• Potassium: found in bananas, oranges, broccoli, dates, and raisins

• Magnesium: found in whole grains, beans, almonds, and brewer's yeast

• Calcium: found in dairy foods, tofu, figs, green leafy vegetables, and salmon

Iron and vitamin E are also helpful in preventing cramps. Iron may be found in brewer's yeast as well as in fortified cereals and dried fruit. Vitamin E is found in wheat germ, soybeans, whole grains, green leafy vegetables, and vegetable oils.

Exercise

Both the lack of exercise and excessive exercising may cause muscle cramps. Whether you have been exercising too little or too much, if you have been experiencing muscle cramps, start over with moderate, limited exercises. Gradually, over time, increase your routine. Don't use stretching as your warmup. Begin with a slow jog or walk to warm the body and supply oxygen and nutrients to the muscles, then stretch. Remember that the cooldown period is just as important as the warmup. After you cool down, end with some final stretches.

Homeopathy

Nux vomica 9C and *Cuprum metallicum* 9C are two homeopathic treatments commonly used for muscle cramps. Alternate three pellets of each, three times per day. Another homeopathic treatment, arnica, is available as an ointment. Apply it to the affected area as directed. In order to obtain the best treatment for your particular muscle cramps, you may consider consulting with a homeopath, who will be able to individualize your treatment plan. To find a practitioner trained in homeopathy, visit the Web site of the National Center for Homeopathy at www.homeopathic.org.

Hydrotherapy

Alternating hot and cold compresses may bring relief to a muscle cramp. Wring out a washcloth soaked in hot water and apply it to the affected area for 2 minutes. Place the washcloth back in the hot water and wring out a washcloth soaked in cold water with ice. Place this over the affected area for 40 seconds. End by placing the hot cloth on the muscle again for 2 more minutes.

Nutritional Supplements

Certain supplements help improve circulation and prevent muscle cramps.

- Vitamin C: 2,000 milligrams daily in divided doses of 1,000 milligrams. Improves circulation.
- Vitamin E: 400 IU daily. Deficiency may cause muscle cramping in the legs.
- Calcium: 1,500 milligrams daily in divided doses of 500 milligrams. Works well with magnesium in preventing muscle cramps.
- Magnesium: 750 milligrams daily in divided doses of 250 milligrams. Prevents muscle cramps, promotes good night's sleep.

Therapeutic Massage

Regular massage therapy has been shown to relax muscles and increase circulation, providing oxygen and nutrients to tired, overworked muscles. For centuries, massage has been used as a preventive measure against muscular cramping as well as a therapeutic treatment to release muscle cramps.

Stretches for Your Muscles

Consider beginning and ending your exercise routine with the following stretches. These can also be practiced before going to bed. Hold each stretch for 30 to 45 seconds and repeat each one two or three times. Do not bounce when stretching. Bouncing activates the reflex that actually tightens the muscles. Also, the excess bouncing may cause muscles to rip.

☐ Calf muscle stretch: Stand 2½ to 3 feet from a wall. Lean forward and place your hands on the wall. Keeping your heels down, gradually move your hands up the wall as high as you can. Lean in toward the wall and hold the position for 45 seconds.

☐ Hamstring muscle stretch: Sit with one leg folded with the foot against the side of the other leg, which should be straight out with the foot upright. Lean forward and touch the foot of the straightened leg or come as close to touching the foot as you can without straining. Change leg positions and repeat.

☐ Quadriceps muscle stretch: While you are standing, bend your leg up behind you and hold the top of the foot with the opposite hand; pull the foot toward the buttocks. (Use your other hand on the wall or a chair to maintain your balance.) Repeat with the opposite leg.

Lifestyle Recommendations

Consider a medication change. If you are on a diuretic medication, check with your doctor. Often, because of dehydration from the diuretic, an adjustment in the dose will relieve muscle cramps.

Try tonic water. Quinine, found in tonic water, has been used for years as a remedy for muscle cramps.

Visit a physical therapist or personal trainer. Physical therapists and personal trainers are able to design special exercises to reduce your bouts with muscle cramps. By completing these exercises regularly, you may see considerable improvement in your condition.

When you exercise, drink extra fluid. If you can, about 2 hours before you begin physical activity or exercising, begin drinking fluid—at least 2 cups. For every 15 to 20 minutes of physical activity or exercise, try to drink another cup or more of fluid. Drink another cup of fluid upon completion of exercise.

Preventive Measures

Avoid overheating. Muscle cramps are one of the first signs of heat stroke. If you are exposed to warm temperatures for a prolonged period of time, the best prevention is to drink plenty of fluids, especially sports drinks with electrolytes.

Get your vitamin D. Getting 10 to 15 minutes of direct sunlight several times a week can ensure that your body absorbs sufficient vitamin D. Vitamin D is essential for absorption of calcium, which helps to prevent muscle cramps. Remember to use sunscreen if you spend longer than the recommended 10 to 15 minutes in the sun. If you are unable to spend time in the sun, you can get vitamin D in your diet through eggs and fish such as cod, mackerel, sardines, salmon, and tuna. It is also available in supplement form. Take 400 IU daily or at least three times a week.

Improve your posture. If you spend hours each day hunched before a computer, you increase your risk for neck and leg cramps due to a shortening of the muscles and poor circulation.

Loosen your bed covers. To reduce your risk for muscle cramps while you sleep, loosen your covers at the foot of the bed to prevent your feet from pointing down.

Participate in aquatic exercise. Regular exercise in water will stretch, lengthen, and strengthen your muscles, making them less likely to cramp.

Practice deep breathing. To help avoid side stitches (rib cage muscle spasms), practice slow, deep breathing exercises regularly.

Remain hydrated. To help avoid muscle cramps, drink six to eight glasses of water or other fluids every day.

Stretch regularly. Throughout the day, periodically stretch your muscles.

Nail Fungus

It's unsightly, it's aggravating, and it's persistent. Nail fungus, also known as onychomycosis or ringworm of the nail, is a parasitic infection in the nails of the fingers or toes. Most often, a nail fungal infection involves a group of fungi called dermatophytes, which include *Trichophyton rubrum* and *Trichophyton mentagrophytes*. They thrive on keratin, the protein in the nail. But a nail fungus may also thrive on yeasts (*Candida albicans* or *Candida parapsilosis*), mold, or even the acrylic nail bonding agent methyl methacrylate, which may be used by discount salons instead of the safer ethyl methacrylate. Toenails are more likely to be affected than fingernails. The big toes and little toes have the highest risk, probably because they are exposed to the most friction from shoes.

Nail fungus is a relatively common problem. Though many people are unaware of the condition, it has been estimated that 12 million Americans have this disorder. Men are twice as likely as women to have a nail fungus, and the incidence appears to increase with age.

Causes and Risk Factors

A nail fungal infection usually occurs when a nail is damaged or exposed over an extended period of time to a warm, moist environment. People who spend a good deal of time working with water, such as dishwashers and cleaning personnel, are at increased risk. Those with diabetes or HIV are also at greater risk, as are those who tend to perspire a lot from their feet and/or have a history of athlete's foot. Other factors that add to the risk include poor circulation and hot, humid weather.

> **Fungi** are simple parasitic plant organisms. Since they lack chlorophyll, they do not need sunlight to grow.

Signs and Symptoms

A nail fungus usually begins with a small separation between the end of the nail and the skin under the nail (the nail bed). With time, a yellow material forms in this separation, and the nail becomes thick and yellow or brown. There may be white spots on the nail, and foul-smelling debris under the nail. Unless the area becomes infected or is so thick that it presses against the inside of your shoes, there should be little or no pain. But when a nail is infected, there may be a good deal of pain, and you may find it uncomfortable to walk or stand. However, in time, the nail separates, and you are left with a moderately destroyed yellow nail that may fall off. Even if the nail falls off, the new nail will grow in with the fungus.

Conventional Treatments

Unfortunately, without treatment, nail fungus persists. So, unless you are content to watch your nails deteriorate, see a doctor. Your treatment may begin with your doctor attempting

A Quick Guide to Symptoms

☐ Separation between the end of the nail and the skin under the nail
☐ Nail becomes thick and yellow or brown
☐ White spots on the nail
☐ Foul-smelling debris under the nail

to remove as much of the affected nail as possible. This may involve trimming the nail with clippers, filing it down, or dissolving it with a paste that contains urea and bifonazole.

If the affected area is relatively small, your doctor may prescribe a medicated nail polish that contains ciclopirox (Loprox). This should be applied to the nail daily until the fungus is completely gone. This treatment is more effective than placebo and appears to be safe. It may be useful for people who are unable to take oral antifungal drugs. Studies are needed to demonstrate how long the nail will remain free of the fungus.

Medications

Since nail fungus often involves a wider area or more than one nail, your doctor may prescribe an antifungal drug that is taken orally for several months, which is necessary because nails grow slowly. Terbinafine (Lamisil) and itraconazole (Sporanox) are each taken for up to 3 months and may be up to 70 percent effective. Griseofulvin (Fulvicin, Grisactin) is taken for 6 months and is up to 40 percent effective. The use of griseofulvin has been superseded by terbinafine and itraconazole.

These medications have potential side effects such as nausea, rash, vomiting, stomach upset, and headaches. Less common side effects are blood disorders and liver damage. Because of possible liver problems, itraconazole should not be used by people taking simvastatin, lovastatin, triazolam, or cisapride. Before beginning treatment, your doctor will test your liver enzymes, and again during the course of your treatment.

As an alternative, your doctor may recommend fluconazole (Diflucan). The recommended dose is one 150-milligram tablet a week for 26 weeks. While this drug's efficacy of 48 percent may not be as high as for the other medications, it has fewer side effects, and with only one pill per week, it is easier to take.

It should be noted that for all of these medications, the rate of relapse—where the fungus reappears—is high.

Surgery

If the nail fungus does not respond to treatment and is causing you pain, you may need permanent removal of the infected nail.

Complementary Treatments
Herbal Medicine

Chamomile, echinacea, goldenseal, rosemary, sage, and thyme. Chamomile, echinacea, and goldenseal have antiseptic properties. As a bonus, echinacea boosts the immune system, helping to fight off infections. Additional herbs that have antifungal properties are rosemary, sage, and thyme. Look for topical creams containing these herbs and use according to the directions on the label.

Garlic. Eating garlic has been shown to be effective against fungus.

Grapefruit seed extract. Provides antibacterial and antifungal protection while boosting the immune system. Grapefruit seed extract is available in capsule and tincture form. Take a 100-milligram capsule daily or add 10 drops of extract three times a day to a small glass of water.

Tea tree oil. A number of reliable studies have shown that tea tree oil may kill fungus and bacteria and is effective in treating fungal infection of the nails, even those that are resistant to some antibiotics. As it is toxic when swallowed, tea tree oil is always used topically and never taken internally. If used near the eyes, nose, and mouth, it could potentially cause burning. The oil is safe to use full strength on the nail, but it should be diluted when applied to the skin. In fact, it is best to use small amounts and to test for any sensitivity that may cause a rash or itching.

Lifestyle Recommendations

Drink plenty of fluids. Cracking nails may be a sign of fluid deficiency. Be sure to drink lots of fluids throughout the day to help prevent cracks where fungi can grow.

Preventive Measures

Get treatment for athlete's foot. If you have athlete's foot, be certain it is treated adequately. The fungus causing athlete's foot can cause a toenail infection, which is much more difficult to eradicate.

Care for your nails. Keep your nails short, dry, and clean. After bathing or showering, dry your toes and the area between your toes.

Change your socks. If your feet tend to swell or sweat, change your socks several times each day.

Don't pick at your nails. If you pick at the skin near the nail, you can create an entry point for fungi.

Use foot powder. A good-quality foot talcum (not cornstarch) will absorb excess perspiration.

Wear shoes, sandals, or flip-flops. Walking around a public pool, locker room, or shower without shoes places you at high risk for fungal infection. Also, wear comfortable shoes that have room for your feet to breathe.

Obesity

Obesity is extremely common: About one in three Americans is considered to be obese, and among those between the ages of 50 and 60, that figure may be twice as high. Obesity in America appears to be growing among people of all ages and ethnic groups.

People who are obese are seriously overweight. In addition, they have an abnormally high proportion of body fat, often defined as a body mass index (BMI) of 30 or higher. If you are obese, you have a far greater risk for a host of other medical problems. These include high blood pressure (hypertension), type 2 diabetes, abnormal blood fats, coronary artery disease, stroke, osteoarthritis, sleep apnea and other sleep disorders, emotional problems, binge eating, gout, gallbladder disease, heart attack, gum disease, non-Hodgkin's lymphoma, multiple myeloma, and cancer (of the esophagus, colon, rectum, liver, gallbladder, pancreas, prostate, and kidney). Since obesity takes a toll on the muscles and bones, people who are obese are more likely to have hernias, low back pain, and problems with arthritic conditions. It has been estimated that about 300,000 lives in the United States could be saved each year if people maintained a healthy weight.

Causes and Risk Factors

In general, obesity is caused by consuming far more calories than you are able to burn in your everyday life. Since calories that are not needed for energy are stored as fat, if you consistently eat excess amounts of food, you will gain weight. Eventually, you become obese. After the age of 25, there is a tendency to gain about a pound a year. Since muscle and bone mass decrease with age, the actual gain in fat per year is closer to 1½ pounds. By midlife, many Americans weigh at least 30 pounds more than they did in their twenties.

Your risk for obesity increases if you regularly consume high-fat foods as well as sugary soft drinks, candy, and desserts. Some people eat to fill a psychological void, an unhealthy eating pattern that can lead to weight gain.

Genes, which help to determine the amount and location of body fat, also play a role. Ex-smokers have higher rates of obesity, as do people who work the late shift (between 4:00 p.m. and 8:00 a.m.).

Leading an inactive life also raises your risk. Since men have more calorie-burning muscle than women, women are at greater risk for obesity. As we age, our metabolism slows and we tend to have less muscle. Both of these factors raise the risk for obesity. Weight gain in men tends to plateau around age 50.

A small number of medications may also cause weight gain. These include corticosteroids, some antipsychotic agents, and tricyclic antidepressants. And it is believed that less than 2 percent of obesity may be traced to a medical problem, such as a slow thyroid (hypothyroidism) or imbalanced hormones.

Signs and Symptoms

If you are obese, there is a good chance that you know it. You may have some of the symptoms of weight-related medical problems. For example, excess weight may have resulted in elevated blood pressure or type 2 diabetes.

Conventional Treatments
Behavior Modification Therapy

With behavior modification, you change your daily patterns associated with eating. Begin by keeping a diary of everything you eat. Record when you eat and what you are doing while you eat. How long does each meal take? What is your emotional state? Then, review your diary with a therapist. If you always eat while watching TV, you may be advised to try eating in another room or to simply turn off the TV. Check with your local hospital for programs to treat obesity. You may want to enroll in a behavior modification program led by a psychologist.

Diet

Most weight loss begins with some form of calorie restriction. Normally, you need to reduce your daily caloric intake by 500 to 1,000 calories, and allow no more than 30 percent of your total calories to be from fat. Eliminate as much saturated fat as possible. Severely restrictive diets of less than 1,100

A Quick Guide to Symptoms

- [ ] **Significantly overweight**
- [ ] **Body mass index (BMI) of 30 or higher**
- [ ] **Symptoms of weight-related medical problems such as high blood pressure**

calories per day are typically not a good idea. You should never embark on such a program without proper medical monitoring.

Many people advise those who wish to lose weight to replace higher-fat foods with lower-fat, higher-fiber alternatives. While 1 gram of fat has nine calories, 1 gram of carbohydrates or protein has only four calories. Moreover, dietary fat converts more easily than carbohydrates and proteins to body fat.

Fat substitutes have become popular additions to many foods. A number of these have been used for decades and are considered safe. These include carrageenan (made from seaweed), guar gum, gum arabic, and the cellulose gel Avicel. Olestra, a more recently created fat substitute, leaves some people with cramps and diarrhea, and there is concern that it may deplete the body of some vitamins. If you plan to eat foods containing olestra on a regular basis, you should discuss vitamin supplementation with your doctor or nutritionist.

Insoluble fiber is especially useful for weight loss. It is found in whole grains, seeds, wheat bran, fruit, and vegetable peels. Pectin, a soluble fiber found in apples, provides a

Self-Testing

Since a body mass index (BMI) of 30 or higher is an indicator of obesity, begin by determining your BMI. Multiply your weight in pounds by 703, then divide it by your height in inches squared. For example, if you are 5'10" (70 inches) tall and weigh 200 pounds, 200 multiplied by 703 equals 140,600; then 140,600 divided by 70 squared (4,900) is 28.69, rounded off to a BMI of 29. (To square a number, you simply multiply it by itself; 4 squared is 4 times 4, which equals 16.) You can also calculate your BMI on the Internet at www. nhlbisupport.com/bmi/.

Another frequent self-test involves measuring your waist. A man whose waist is larger than 40 inches may be obese. You may also want to determine the distribution of body fat around the abdomen and hips. To do this, divide your waist size by your hip size. Lower ratios are preferable—the risk of heart disease increases when a man's ratio is above 1.0. Discuss your results with your doctor.

sense of fullness, so you may potentially eat less.

Although consuming sugar does not appear to be a key factor in the development of obesity, you should limit your sugar intake. In some instances, you may wish to use a sugar substitute, such as aspartame (Nutra-Sweet, Equal), acesulfame K (Sweet One), or sucralose (Splenda).

High-protein diets have been around for decades and periodically reemerge in a variety of formats. Though they may lead to quick weight loss, one by-product of this diet is the release of ketones, which may cause bad breath, nausea, and lightheadedness. To ensure that you are a good candidate for a high-protein diet, you should check with your doctor.

Exercise

A key element of any weight loss program is exercise. If you are obese, before starting an exercise program, you should visit your doctor. Generally, you will be advised to work up to about 45 to 60 minutes of daily aerobic exercise, such as walking, dancing, or hiking. But you may need to begin with only 5 to 10 minutes per day. Don't forget to include resistance or strength training at least two or three times each week. But you should realize that exercise alone tends to lead to only minimal weight loss—although it may result in greater total body fat loss compared to a restricted calorie intake without the exercise component.

Medications

Due to issues surrounding efficacy, potential abuse, and possible side effects, the role of medication in weight loss programs is frequently questioned. Still, there are a number of over-the-counter natural and prescriptive medications used for weight loss. Collectively, these are known as anorexiants. Acutrim and Dexatrim are over-the-counter medications that contain phenylpropanolamine. While these suppress the appetite, when taken in doses of 75 milligrams or higher in the immediate-release form, they may cause high blood pressure or stroke.

A number of over-the-counter weight loss products contain ephedrine, a component in adrenaline. Ephedrine may trigger high blood pressure, rapid heartbeat, insomnia, heart rate irregularities, nervousness, tremors, strokes, psychosis, seizures, and death. Pseudoephedrine, which is found in many antihistamines and is sometimes used by dieters, may have similar side effects. Benzocaine is a local anesthetic that is sold as a gum; when chewed, it numbs the mouth and alters taste, which may make food seem less appetizing.

The appetite suppressant phentermine was previously prescribed in conjunction with fenfluramine ("fen-phen"), which was found to have some serious side effects and is no longer available. Potential side effects of phentermine include dizziness, drowsiness, and lightheadedness. This drug should not be mixed with certain medications, and it may alter the way some medications react in your body. Be sure to tell your doctor about every medicine you are taking. Also, this drug should be used for no more than a few months.

Sibutramine (Meridia) improves mood and energy levels while it increases metabolism and the feeling of fullness. Obese people do lose weight on this prescription medication, but when the medication is stopped, the weight may return. Frequent side effects include constipation, insomnia, and dry mouth. There are also reports of increases in blood pressure and heart rates. It should not be taken by people who have high blood pressure or a history of stroke or arrhythmias. Other people who should avoid sibutramine are those taking a decongestant, a monoamine oxidase inhibitor (MAOI), or a selective serotonin reuptake inhibitor (SSRI), or those using a bronchodilator.

Orlistat (Xenical) is a prescription medication that reduces the body's absorption of fat. After 1 year of use, expect to achieve a 5 to 10 percent drop in weight. But there may be gastrointestinal side effects, and orlistat may interfere with the absorption of the fat-soluble vitamins A, D, E, and K and other nutrients. Adhering to a low-fat diet tends to lessen the side effects.

In one study, researchers attempted to determine if topiramate (Topamax), an anti-seizure medication, would help obese patients with type 2 diabetes lose weight. For 40 weeks, people in the study were divided into three treatment groups. The first group received a placebo, the second group received 96 milligrams of topiramate each day, and the third group received 192 milligrams of topiramate each day. At the end of the study, the placebo group averaged a 2.5 percent weight loss, the low topiramate group averaged a 6.6 percent weight loss, and the high topiramate group averaged a 9.1 percent weight loss. Still, it is important to note that the FDA has not approved topiramate for weight loss management.

Surgery

Surgery is generally reserved for those who are dangerously obese. Typically, your BMI should be more than 40, and you should be at least 180 percent more than your ideal weight. There are two main types of surgery. Both should be considered only after more conservative weight loss efforts have failed. In a study published in the *New England Journal of Medicine*, surgery for severe obesity was associated with weight loss over the long term and a decreased overall mortality compared to those individuals who did not have surgery.

Gastric bypass. In this procedure, most of the stomach is blocked off. In a Roux-en-Y gastric bypass, a small stomach pouch is created and connected to the small intestine. Potential complications include obstruction, problems with the staple line, and overexpansion of the pouch. In about 10 to 20 percent of cases, these complications result in additional surgery. Weight loss occurs because the stomach is much smaller. In addition, the connection to the small intestine may cause some malabsorption of calories; only a portion of consumed calories are actually absorbed.

Normally, within about 2 years of the procedure, you will lose about two-thirds of your excess weight, and your weight-related health problems should improve. The most common side effect is vomiting. Another frequent problem is "dumping syndrome," which occurs when food moves too quickly through the intestine. It may cause weakness, nausea, and faintness, especially after eating sweets. You may develop anemia and require supplements of folic acid and vitamin B_{12}. In addi-

tion, the surgery increases your risk for bone loss and osteoporosis.

The lap-band. In this procedure, which is also known as laparoscopic gastric banding, tiny incisions are made in the abdomen. A surgeon then uses special laparoscopic instruments to place a silicone band around the upper portion of the stomach. This limits the amount of food that you are able to eat and leaves a feeling of fullness. Attached to the band is a small balloonlike reservoir that contains saline, which may be added to tighten the band or removed to loosen it. Weight loss tends to be significant. But there are potential complications, including infection, bleeding, and slippage or rupture of the band. In rare instances, there may be blood clots, pneumonia, or perforation of the stomach. If the band needs to be removed, the intestinal tract returns to normal.

Weight Loss Programs

There are many commercial weight loss programs. Some provide a good deal of personal attention, while others emphasize group support. Most programs have prepared foods that you can purchase. Examples of these commercial programs are Jenny Craig, Nutri-System, and Weight Watchers.

There are two well-known nonprofit sources for weight loss support as well. TOPS Club Inc. (Take Off Pounds Sensibly) consists of weekly group meetings, confidential weigh-ins, talks by various professionals from the community, and support from other members and volunteers. Before beginning the program, you are encouraged to see your doctor. If you believe that you are a compulsive overeater or one who is recovering from this problem, you may wish to consider Overeaters Anonymous (OA), which is based on the same 12-step program used by Alcoholics Anonymous.

Complementary Treatments

Acupuncture

Auricular (ear) acupuncture may be useful in regulating your appetite. To locate an acupuncturist in your area, visit the Web site of the National Certification Commission for Acupuncture and Oriental Medicine (NCCAOM) at www.nccaom.org.

Ayurveda

An Ayurvedic medicine practitioner may help you eliminate foods that are not appropriate for your body's constitution. These foods may be contributing to your weight gain. There is no professional organization that offers membership to Ayurvedic practitioners. However, the Ayurvedic Institute may provide the names of appropriate professionals in your area. The Institute may be contacted through its Web site: www.ayurveda.com.

Diet

Start by eating a healthy diet that includes lots of fresh fruits, vegetables, and whole grains. Try to include a minimum of five servings of vegetables, four servings of fruit, and six servings of whole grains each day.

Eliminate from your diet foods high in fat, such as fried foods and fatty meats, as well as highly processed foods, fast foods, and foods high in sugar. In addition to increasing weight, these may contribute to many other health problems, including high cholesterol and high blood pressure. Also, it has been shown that eating foods such as white rice, white flour products, and potatoes may increase your hunger after they are consumed, thereby encouraging the intake of more food. Try substituting with brown rice, bran, whole grains, and cereals.

Studies have shown that sensitivity to certain foods may lead to overeating, causing obesity. To assist in eliminating certain foods from your diet, it may be useful to consult with a nutritionist or doctor who specializes in food intolerances.

Herbal Medicine

Cayenne pepper. Studies have shown that 10 grams of cayenne pepper consumed with meals may increase the metabolism of dietary fats and reduce appetite. Capsaicin, a main component of cayenne peppers, may also suppress the appetite. A study found that individuals eating a meal containing capsaicin reduced food intake by 200 calories.

Hoodia. Hoodia, a plant indigenous to the Kalahari Desert in South Africa, has been getting widespread attention as an appetite suppressant for its ability to fool the brain into thinking the stomach is full. It has been used for centuries by South African Bushmen. It took 30 years of researching the plant by the South African national laboratory to find the appetite-suppressing ingredient. Once the ingredient was found, the laboratory applied for a patent and licensed it to a company called Phytopharm, which is working to farm enough Hoodia in South Africa to make products such as shakes and bars containing the plant. For now, these products are not available in the United States, as clinical trials of Phytopharm's patented ingredient are ongoing. Many products currently on the market claim to contain Hoodia, but their quality is questionable.

Naturopathy

Naturopathy is a system of holistic therapy that relies on natural remedies, such as homeopathy, hydrotherapy, diet, herbs, massage, acupuncture, and exercise. A naturopath may investigate your lifestyle and potential food intolerances and recommend an appropriate diet and exercise program for your obesity. Contact the American Association of Naturopathic Physicians at www.naturopathic.org to find a naturopathic practitioner in your area.

Nutritional Counseling

What we should eat and what we do eat are rarely the same. Many factors, from lifestyle and time constraints to culturally learned eating habits, determine our diets. Nutritionists offer education on numerous subjects, including facts about nutrition, eating patterns, and vitamins/minerals while also providing motivational support. Nutritionists will help individuals design specific diets that provide both variety and proper nutrition.

Nutritional Supplements

Nutritional supplements are beneficial for fat burning and providing additional nutrients when on a low-calorie diet.

- Multivitamin/mineral: Take as directed on the label. Can help make up for any nutritional shortfalls on a low-calorie diet.

- Chromium: 150 micrograms daily. Trace mineral that metabolizes carbohydrates and fats.

- L-carnitine: 500 milligrams daily. Amino acid that helps burn fat and lowers the fat level in the blood.

Psychotherapy

Since it can aid in the resolution of emotional problems that may be causing you to overeat, psychotherapy may be useful for obesity. Psychotherapy focuses on the healing of the mind and the emotions. It provides a good listener and comfortable, safe surroundings, giving the individual an opportunity to identify conflicts, release emotions, and find useful coping strategies.

Lifestyle Recommendations

Beware of natural weight loss products. Natural weight loss products come in a variety of forms. Some are teas that contain laxatives such as rhubarb root, aloe, buckthorn, senna, cascara, and castor oil. These may result in gastrointestinal distress. Neither chitosan, a dietary fiber made from shellfish, nor garcinia (mangosteen), a tropical fruit that contains hydroxycitric acid, has been proven to result in weight loss.

Don't get discouraged. When you have a great deal of weight to lose, it is easy to become disheartened, especially when the pounds drop slowly. Maintain your routine of healthy eating and other therapies. You will ultimately be rewarded. Remember, it took a long time to become obese, so now you need time to lose the weight.

Don't starve yourself. Maintaining a high metabolism should be the ultimate goal in losing weight. By eating several smaller meals throughout the day along with daily exercise, you can increase your metabolism. By doing this, your body becomes accustomed to burning energy through exercise and using food properly. Food is used as energy, and what is not used is stored for later use. Many individuals starve themselves thinking it is the fastest way to lose unwanted pounds. What they don't realize is that they end up slowing down their metabolism because the body panics and takes whatever food

is eaten and immediately stores it as fat.

Forgive your setbacks. Adhering to your new routine will not be easy, and you may have an occasional setback. Learn to forgive yourself.

Keep a food diary. Record when and what you are eating. Also, keep a record of your exercise activities. This will help ensure that you are following a reasonable program.

Preventive Measures

Consume smaller portions. Americans tend to eat far too much. Reduce the amount of food that you eat at each meal. When eating in a restaurant, consume half of the meal and take the rest home. You will be less likely to gain weight. Avoid all-you-can-eat buffets.

Eat a healthier diet. Eat lots of fruits and vegetables as well as low-fat, protein-rich foods such as fish and skinned chicken. Eat far fewer higher-fat foods such as red meat, and eliminate your consumption of processed foods, saturated fats, and refined sugar.

Start to exercise. If you want to prevent obesity, it is important to exercise. Try to find time for at least 30 minutes of daily aerobic exercise. And don't forget to add some form of resistance or weight-bearing exercise several times a week.

Osteoarthritis

Osteoarthritis causes pain, swelling, and loss of motion in joints. It's easy to understand the symptoms when you understand what's taking place inside the joints: With osteoarthritis there is a deterioration of the cartilage that cushions the ends of the bones in the joints. As this occurs, the smooth surface of the cartilage roughens. In time, the cartilage may become completely worn and you may be left with bone rubbing against bone.

While the body tries to repair the damage from osteoarthritis, bone spurs (small growths known as osteophytes) may grow at the edge of the joint and small amounts of bone or cartilage may separate and drift in the joint. This triggers more pain.

Osteoarthritis (also called degenerative arthritis, degenerative joint disease, or osteoarthrosis) is a very common medical disorder. In the United States, it affects about 20 million people and accounts for about half of all cases of arthritis. Before midlife, it affects more men; after midlife, women are at far greater risk. Most often, osteoarthritis develops after the age of 45. Just about everyone over the age of 60 has some evidence of the disease.

Unlike some other forms of arthritis which spread throughout the body, osteoarthritis affects only the joints. Depending upon the location in the body, osteoarthritis acts in different ways. It is frequently found in joints in the fingers, knees, hips, and spine, and is rarely seen in joints in the shoulders, elbows, wrists, and jaw.

● Fingers: Osteoarthritis in fingers is more often seen in older women, and it is believed to have a genetic component. Bony knobs appear on the ends of joints. It commonly affects the first joint beyond the fingertips (Heberden's nodes), and it less often affects the second joint (Bouchard's nodes). Fingers become enlarged and gnarled. They tend to be stiff and ache, and sometimes they are numb. Osteoarthritis also often damages the base of the thumb.

● Knees: Osteoarthritic knees tend to become stiff, swollen, and painful. It may be hard to walk or climb stairs. When sitting down or standing, you may need to hold onto a support.

● Hips: Hips are a frequent target for osteoarthritis. Pain tends to develop slowly in the groin, on the outside of the hips, or in the buttocks. Sometimes, the pain spreads to the knee. If you have this disorder, you may rotate your leg to avoid pain, which will cause you to walk with a limp.

● Spine: Osteoarthritis may affect the cartilage in the disks that serve as cushioning between the bones in the spine. Or, it may affect the spine's moving joints. Sometimes, it affects both. There may be pain, muscle spasms, and reduced mobility. If nerves become pinched, there will be added pain. When osteoarthritis in the spine is advanced, there may be numbness and muscle weakness.

Causes and Risk Factors

Osteoarthritis is more likely to occur in older people. However, since osteoarthritic cartilage is chemically different from normal aged cartilage, osteoarthritis is not believed to be caused by aging. Instead, a number of other factors have been suggested. Osteoarthritis has a strong genetic component, so having close relatives with this disease places you at higher risk.

Have you injured a joint? Do you do physical work that involves repetitive stressful motions? These two factors increase risk. Also, excess weight places extra stress on weight-bearing joints. If you are obese, you are adding to your risk for osteoarthritis. Certain medications, such as corticosteroids, are associated with higher rates of osteoarthritis.

While most older people are at risk for osteoarthritis, there is some variability between ethnic groups. Whites are more likely than Asians to have osteoarthritis. Still, Asians have a higher incidence of osteoarthritis in the knee, and whites and Asians have an equal risk for osteoarthritis in the spine. African Americans have the highest overall risk for osteoarthritis.

Signs and Symptoms

Symptoms associated with osteoarthritis include aching pain in a joint or joints made worse by humid weather and excessive use of the joint, and stiffness after periods of inactivity, such as sleeping. The pain may come and go, and there may or may not be inflammation. When you move your knees, there may be a cracking noise.

Conventional Treatments
Exercise

Exercise is now viewed as a conventional treatment for osteoarthritis. It reduces pain and stiffness and increases muscle strength and flexibility. Without exercise, your joints will further stiffen. Consult with your doctor before beginning an exercise program. In general, you should include range-of-motion, strengthening, and aerobic exercises. If your doctor agrees, you may wish to meet with a physical therapist or personal trainer, who can design an exercise program that will meet your particular needs.

A Quick Guide to Symptoms

☐ Aching pain in a joint made worse by humid weather or excessive use
☐ Stiffness after periods of inactivity
☐ Pain that comes and goes
☐ Inflammation
☐ A cracking noise when you move your knees

Heat and Ice

Applying ice to an inflamed joint may bring a good deal of relief. Keep the ice on for about 20 to 30 minutes. If you don't have an ice pack, use a bag of frozen peas, which works equally well. If you have osteoarthritis in your hands, try hot soaks and warm paraffin applications.

Medications

Capsaicin. Made from the seeds of hot chili peppers, capsaicin (Zostrix, Capzasin-P) is a cream that reduces levels of substance P, an element in the nerve fibers that fosters the delivery of pain impulses to the brain. When using capsaicin, rub a small amount of cream on the affected area four times a day. During the first few days of use, you may have a localized feeling of warmth and stinging. That passes, and pain relief begins within 1 to 2 weeks.

COX-2 inhibitors. COX-2 inhibitors are

If you have high blood pressure, a severe circulation disorder, or kidney or liver problems, or if you are taking diuretics or oral hypoglycemics, and your doctor places you on NSAIDs for an extended period of time, then you need to be monitored carefully. Also, since NSAIDs reduce blood clotting, stop taking them a week before any scheduled surgery.

often effective. Examples are celecoxib (Celebrex) and meloxicam (Mobic). They suppress the enzyme cyclooxygenase-2, or COX-2, that causes joint inflammation and pain, while preserving the COX-1 enzyme, which protects the stomach lining. Patients taking COX-2 inhibitors tend to have fewer gastrointestinal concerns than those taking nonsteroidal anti-inflammatory drugs (NSAIDs). Nevertheless, many of those who take these medications do have gastrointestinal problems, and they may also experience other potential side effects such as headache, dizziness, and kidney problems. Those on anticoagulant drugs may be at greater risk for bleeding. And, in a small number of cases, higher doses of COX-2 have been related to hallucinations, a buildup of fluid, high blood pressure, and excess potassium in the blood.

Hyaluronic acid. If you have osteoarthritis in your knee, your doctor may try injecting hyaluronic acid, a natural substance found in the body. It makes the joint better able to absorb shock. Generally, it is given in a series of three to five injections.

Pain relievers. About 20 to 30 percent of people with osteoarthritis are helped by the pain reliever acetaminophen (Tylenol). Be aware that taking higher doses over an extended period of time increases your risk for kidney and liver damage. Heavy alcohol drinkers, people taking blood-thinning medications, and those with liver disease must use acetaminophen with caution.

Doctors commonly advise their patients with osteoarthritis to take NSAIDs. These include aspirin, ibuprofen (Motrin, Advil), and naproxen (Aleve, Naprosyn). It may take a week or two before you experience significant amounts of pain relief. While NSAIDs are quite effective in treating osteoarthritis, they frequently cause gastrointestinal problems such as ulcers, upset stomachs, and internal bleeding. This occurs even when these medications are injected intravenously. NSAIDs may also increase blood pressure, especially among those who already have hypertension. Other potential side effects include headaches, skin rashes, ringing in the ears, dizziness, and depression. There is some evidence that NSAIDs may damage cartilage and/or cause kidney damage. These medications should be used with caution—the longer they are used, the more likely they are to cause side effects.

For some people with severe osteoarthritic pain, narcotics may be an option. There are two types. Opiates (such as morphine and codeine) are derived from natural opium, while opioids such as oxycodone are synthetic drugs. Since these are highly addictive medications, those taking narcotics should be monitored carefully.

Another choice for severe pain is the use of corticosteroid injections to the affected area. These are used when pain is accompanied by inflammation. But they work only for relatively short periods of time, and no more than two or three injections should be given each year.

Surgery

Arthrodesis (joint fusion). If a joint needs to be stabilized but cannot be replaced, arthrodesis may be advised. During the procedure, bones are fused together. After healing, the joint may bear weight, but it is inflexible. The most common sites for this surgery are the wrist and ankle.

Arthroplasty (joint replacement). In this procedure, a surgeon reconstructs the joint with artificial or prosthetic implants. It may be advised when pain and immobility from an osteoarthritic joint have made normal functioning impossible. The most commonly replaced joints are the hip and knee, accounting for about 80 percent of such surgeries in the United States. But joints in the ankles, shoulders, elbows, and knuckles are also successfully replaced.

During the surgery, which is done under general anesthesia, the surgeon will open the joint and separate the tendons and ligaments. The surgeon removes the damaged portions of the joint and replaces them with plastic and/or metal prostheses. Sometimes, the prostheses are cemented into place. Then, the remainder of the joint parts, as well as the ligaments and tendons, are reattached. Since some blood loss is associated with arthroplasty, a month or two before your surgery, you may wish to donate one to three units of your own blood. If you require a transfusion, your blood may be used.

Depending on the type of surgery, expect to spend 3 to 7 days in the hospital, then a week or two in a rehabilitation facility. This will be followed by outpatient therapy.

The majority of people who have undergone joint replacements are thrilled with the pain relief and newfound independence. As with all surgeries, there are risks for complications. Infections, which occur in about

1 percent of all joint replacements, may require the removal of the implant. You may experience blood clots and damage to the nerves near the joint. A prosthesis may loosen or a joint may dislocate, and the replacement parts of weight-bearing joints may wear out and fail. Hips tend to last between 10 and 15 years, while you may have as many as 20 years with new knees.

Arthroscopic debridement. In general, arthroscopic surgery is performed to remove the bone and cartilage fragments in the knee that are causing pain and inflammation. The surgeon begins by making a small incision into which a sterile solution is injected. Since that makes the joint swell, it is easier for the surgeon to see. A lighted tube called an arthroscope is inserted into a second small incision. Entering through a third incision, the surgeon trims or stitches the damaged tissue. Typically, this procedure is done under local anesthetic. Recovery rarely takes more than a few weeks.

Joint lavage. In this procedure, which is also known as tidal irrigation, your physician uses a trocar or large-bore needle to infuse a joint with a salt-and-water combination. Joint fluid is then drained, which removes particles of cartilage debris and other substances. Improvements may last from months to years.

Osteotomy. If your osteoarthritis has caused a deformity in your knee or hip joints, your doctor may recommend an osteotomy. In this surgery, the physician opens the knee or hip and reshapes a wedge of bone, thereby correcting the weight-bearing problems you have been experiencing. This procedure is advised for heavier adults who are under the age of 60. It may provide pain relief, increased joint stability, and better range of motion.

Complementary Treatments

With proper care and attention, osteoarthritis may be controlled or even reversed. Approaches that allow the body to heal itself by assisting in the normal function of the cartilage and repairing the damage already done are beneficial. Practitioners will also address the underlying cause of the joint degeneration and try to relieve the pain and inflammation. Dietary changes are a significant factor in the healing process.

Acupuncture

Recent studies have shown acupuncture to be very effective in reducing the pain and inflammation associated with osteoarthritis. To locate an acupuncturist in your area, visit the Web site of the National Certification Commission for Acupuncture and Oriental Medicine (NCCAOM) at www.nccaom.org.

Ayurveda

Ayurvedic treatments vary according to physical constitution, emotional makeup, specific symptoms, dietary habits and preferences, present lifestyle, and sleeping habits. However, practitioners of Ayurvedic medicine believe that osteoarthritis is due to poor digestion, and will design a treatment to improve the digestive process. There is no professional organization that offers membership to Ayurvedic practitioners. However, the Ayurvedic Institute may provide the names of appropriate professionals in your area. The Institute may be contacted through its Web site: www.ayurveda.com.

Diet

The process of healing osteoarthritis begins on the cellular level. It is important to eat foods that aid in the destruction of damaging free radicals—molecules that bind to and kill healthy cells, damage the joints, and deplete the antioxidant nutrients necessary for the body to heal itself. The diet should be rich in fruits and vegetables, which contain the antioxidants beta-carotene, flavonoids, and vitamin C. Foods rich in vitamin E and selenium are also recommended, because these nutrients block the damaging effects of free radicals.

Vitamin C and beta-carotene are found in almost all fruits and vegetables, including dark green, leafy vegetables. Fruits rich in flavonoids are cherries, blackberries, and blueberries. Vitamin E may be found in vegetable oils, nuts, seeds, and wheat germ; smaller amounts are found in leafy vegetables and whole grains. Selenium is available in whole grains, red meat, chicken, broccoli, asparagus, egg yolks, milk, and onions. Juicing fresh fruits and vegetables is an excellent way to obtain these nutrients and to have them better absorbed by the body.

It is also useful to eat foods that have anti-inflammatory properties, such as wheat grass and barley, and sulfur-containing foods, such as onions, garlic, brussels sprouts, and cabbage. Sulfur repairs and rebuilds bones, cartilage, and connective tissues and assists in calcium absorption.

In people who are genetically susceptible to arthritis, nightshade vegetables (potatoes, eggplant, peppers, and tomatoes) have been known to increase inflammation and inhibit the repair of cartilage. It may be necessary to see a doctor who will test for allergies to these and other foods that may be causing or aggravating this condition.

Avoid fried foods and other foods high in trans fats, saturated fat, refined sugar products, and excess salt. Aside from having no nutritional benefit and increasing body weight, these foods contribute to osteoarthritis.

Feldenkrais Method

Practitioners teach individuals to become aware of their movement patterns. This improves body motion and corrects poor postural habits. It may relieve stiffness and inflammation, which may decrease pain. Feldenkrais practitioners may be found at the Web site www.feldenkrais.com.

Herbal Medicine

Because of their anti-inflammatory properties and their ability to relieve pain and rebuild bones, many herbal remedies have been used in the treatment of osteoarthritis.

Boswellia serrata. Boswellia is an anti-inflammatory herb that improves blood supply to the joint tissue. Boswellia is available in capsule, tincture, and ointment form. The recommended dose in capsule form is 400 milligrams three times a day. Look for products containing 60 percent boswellic acids.

Capsaicin. Since capsaicin interferes with pain messages, it is good for pain relief. It is available in cream form. Rub a small amount on the affected area.

Ginger. Ginger is an anti-inflammatory herb. Fresh ginger is best and may be taken as a tea or applied directly to the joint as a warm compress.

Proanthocyanidin bioflavonoids. Proanthocyanidin bioflavonoids, often referred to as PAC or grape seed extract, are antioxidants and free-radical scavengers that reduce inflammation. The typical recommended dose is a 100-milligram capsule three times a day of extract standardized to contain 92 to 95 percent PCOs.

Hydrotherapy

Warm water is an ideal medium for the treatment of the pain and stiffness associated with osteoarthritis. The gentle, rhythmic movements in the water may release toxins that build up in joints and may increase flexibility, coordination, balance, and circulation. This will improve joint mobility, strengthen muscles, and decrease pain and stiffness.

Electric heating pads and dry heat applications are not recommended for osteoarthritis. Moist heat packs applied over or near the affected area for 20 minutes will penetrate deeper and lessen stiffness and pain much better than dry heat.

Nutritional Supplements

Many nutritional supplements have anti-inflammatory properties and support healthy cellular structure.

- Multivitamin/mineral: Take as directed on the label. Should include A, C, E, beta-carotene, calcium, copper, magnesium, selenium, and zinc to aid in healthy cell structure and provide anti-inflammatory properties.

- B-complex vitamins: Take as directed on the label. B_5 levels may be low in people with osteoarthritis. B vitamins work best when taken together.

- Boron: 3 milligrams twice a day. Aids in the regulation of calcium.

- Bromelain: 500 milligrams daily. Enzyme found in pineapple with anti-inflammatory properties.

- Vitamin D: 400 IU daily. Essential for cartilage health, needed for absorption of calcium; deficiency linked to osteoarthritis.

- DLPA (DL-phenylalanine): 750 milligrams daily. Enhances body's ability to deal with pain. Requires 1 to 2 weeks to become effective. May raise blood pressure.

- Essential fatty acids—omega-3 (flaxseed and fish oil) and omega-6 (borage, evening primrose, and black currant seed oils): Available in oil and capsule form. Take as directed on the labels. Increase anti-inflammatory agents in the body.

- Glucosamine sulfate: 500 milligrams daily. Slows the breakdown, aids in the repair, and stimulates the growth of new cartilage. Pain relief may be initially slow, but results are extremely promising.

- MSM (methylsulfonylmethane): 1,000 milligrams daily. Effective against arthritis pain and inflammation.

- SAMe (S-adenosyl-methionine): Dose varies depending on symptoms. See your doctor for a starting point. Amino acid that helps lubricate joints and relieve pain and stiffness.

Shiatsu

The deep finger pressure of shiatsu massage may help release obstructions in the muscles and vital energy system. Shiatsu may be stimulating and relaxing, aiding in the relief of pain. To find a practitioner trained in shiatsu, visit the following Web sites: www.aobta.org (American Organization for Bodywork Therapies of Asia) and www.ncbtmb.org (National Certification Board for Therapeutic Massage and Bodywork).

Therapeutic Massage

Massage treatments may remove toxins that build up in the joints, causing inflammation and pain. Massage reduces muscular tension,

which places added stress on joints that are already stiff. It has an overall calming effect on the body and mind.

Lifestyle Recommendations

Consider magnet therapy. Preliminary studies have shown a reduction in pain when magnets are applied directly over the affected area for several hours. It is also thought that low-energy AC and DC fields may help stimulate the production of cartilage-building cells.

Lose weight. If your doctor has indicated that excess weight is contributing to your osteoarthritis, you will need to drop some of the pounds. Ask your doctor for some suggestions or a referral to a weight loss program.

Reduce stress. Stress and tension may aggravate and increase the severity of pain. Every day, find a way to reduce stress and relax your body and mind. Even 15 minutes of deep breathing exercises while listening to quiet music may have a healthy effect on the physical body and help reduce pain.

Preventive Measures

Both serious injury and repeated minor injuries may place your joints at greater risk. Try to avoid actions that may be injurious to your joints.

Parkinson's Disease

People with Parkinson's disease often have tremors and difficulty with walking. This happens because the disease causes a significant loss of the brain cells that produce the muscle-directing chemical known as dopamine. As a result, there is a slow, but progressive, loss of muscle control, coordination, and balance. The disease may also harm nerve endings that control the release of norepinephrine, a hormone that regulates pulse rate, perspiration, blood pressure, and other automatic responses to stress.

Parkinson's disease is far more common than most people realize. Though the exact figures are hard to determine, it is believed that at least 1 million Americans are living with this disorder. Each year, about 50,000 new cases are diagnosed.

Causes and Risk Factors

Parkinson's disease is frequently referred to as an idiopathic disorder, which means that the cause is unknown. No one has been able to determine the exact reason for the loss of dopamine. Parkinson's disease has, however, been linked to a number of genetic and environmental factors. Those who have a first-degree relative (parent, sibling, or child) with Parkinson's are three times more likely to develop the disorder. In addition, some people who have been exposed to herbicides and pesticides may have three times the risk. Exposure to other environmental toxins, such as manganese dust or the chemical MPTP, or to infectious agents may also place people at increased risk. It is believed that low levels of folate (folic acid), a B vitamin, may increase susceptibility.

When taken in excessive doses or consumed over an extended period of time, a number of medications may cause Parkinson's-type symptoms. These include metoclopramide (Reglan) and prochlorperazine (Compazine, Compro), which are used for nausea; haloperidol (Haldol, Halperon) and chlorpromazine (Thorazine, Sonazine), which are used for some psychiatric disorders; and valproate (Depakote), a medication for epilepsy.

The vast majority of cases of Parkinson's disease appear in people over the age of 50—the average age of onset is 55. But about 10 percent of cases are in people under the age of 40. After the age of 75, the incidence appears to decline and the very elderly are at low risk.

Genes seem to play a crucial role. So, those with a close relative who has been diagnosed with this disorder should be aware of their increased risk and watch for symptoms. Men may face up to twice the risk of women. Americans of European descent have a higher risk than those of African or Asian descent. Interestingly, people who smoke and/or drink coffee have lower rates of the disease.

Signs and Symptoms

During the earliest stages of Parkinson's disease, the symptoms may be rather subtle. When you walk, one of your arms may not swing. You may have trouble getting out of a chair, and you may feel shaky. You may speak softly, or your handwriting may be cramped or spidery. There may be mild tremors in the fingers of one hand or speech may be slightly mumbled. You may be tired, irritable, depressed, and have trouble sleeping. It may take you a little longer to complete routine tasks.

As the disease progresses, the symptoms become more obvious. Tremors that began in a finger spread to the entire arm. Hand tremors sometimes involve the back-and-forth rubbing of the thumb and forefinger, which is known as pill rolling. Tremors may also develop in other parts of the body, such as the head, lips, and feet. They tend to be more noticeable when you are under stress and disappear during sleep.

Many people with Parkinson's move more slowly, a condition known as bradykinesia. They may have a shuffling walk, an unsteady gait, and a stooped posture. There may be postural instability or impaired balance and coordination. On occasion, muscles may freeze. The digestive system may slow, resulting in problems with chewing, swallowing (dysphagia), and constipation. Bladder control and incontinence are frequent medical concerns, as are insomnia and sexual dysfunction.

Still other symptoms of Parkinson's disease include rigid muscles (akinesia), often in the limbs and neck, the loss of automatic movements such as blinking and smiling, and impaired speech. There may also be changes in temperature response, hot flashes, excessive sweating, and a sudden drop in blood pressure when standing (orthostatic hypotension), which results in dizziness and fainting. Many people with Parkinson's disease have an impairment of their sense of smell and/or vision loss, and the skin on the forehead and the sides of the nose tends to become quite oily. Some have a problem with drooling.

About 40 percent of those with Parkinson's disease experience depression. In approximately 25 percent of these people, the depression precedes the Parkinson's diagnosis by months or years. People with Parkinson's disease are also prone to other emotional changes, such as fear, insecurity, and a loss of motivation. There may be memory loss and slow thinking. Moreover, as many as one-third of those who have

A Quick Guide to Symptoms

- ☐ Tremors in the fingers of one hand
- ☐ Slightly mumbled speech
- ☐ Bradykinesia (slow movements)
- ☐ Impaired balance and coordination
- ☐ Slowed digestive system
- ☐ Insomnia
- ☐ Rigid muscles (akinesia)
- ☐ Changes in temperature response
- ☐ Impairment of sense of smell and/or vision loss
- ☐ Drooling
- ☐ Depression and other emotional changes
- ☐ Dementia

Parkinson's disease become demented—they experience memory loss, impaired judgment, and changes in their personality.

Conventional Treatments

Most treatments for Parkinson's disease begin with dietary changes, exercise, and physical therapy. Though these do not stop the progression of the disease, they will help build muscle strength and improve gait and balance. If you have speech problems, you may want to work with a speech therapist. When lifestyle changes provide insufficient relief, other treatments may be advised.

Medications

A number of medications that increase the brain's supply of dopamine are used to treat Parkinson's disease. (Unfortunately, since dopamine does not cross the body's blood-brain barrier, treatment with dopamine itself is ineffective.) Though they may have uncomfortable side effects, none of these medications should be discontinued without consulting your doctor.

Amantadine. Amantadine is an antiviral medication that is effective in reducing the symptoms of Parkinson's disease. Often used in the early stages of the disease, this medication's effectiveness wanes within a few months in about one-third to one-half of all people taking it. Potential side effects include blurred vision, confusion, swollen ankles, mottled skin, edema, and depression. Overdoses may result in life-threatening toxicity.

Anticholinergics. Anticholinergics, the main treatment for Parkinson's disease before the introduction of levodopa, are useful in controlling tremors in the early stages of the disease. Examples are trihexyphenidyl (Artane, Trihexy), benztropine (Cogentin), biperiden (Akineton), and procyclidine (Kemadrin). Potential side effects of anticholinergics are dryness of the mouth, nausea, urinary retention, constipation, and blurred vision. They may also cause mental problems such as memory loss, confusion, and hallucinations, and those who have glaucoma should use them with care.

Catechol-O-methyltransferase inhibitors. Catechol-O-methyltransferase (COMT) inhibitors block an enzyme that breaks down dopamine. In so doing, they prolong the effect of levodopa therapy. An example is tolcapone (Tasmar). Nevertheless, because they have

Treating the Complications of Parkinson's

Many people with Parkinson's disease suffer from depression and/or insomnia. Your doctor may recommend treating these problems. Similarly, if your medications have triggered psychotic symptoms, your doctor may recommend the drugs clozapine (Clozaril) and quetiapine (Seroquel). To combat daytime sleepiness, you may be placed on modafinil (Provigil), and to improve your voice loss, you may be given collagen injections in the neck. Shots of botulism toxin (Botox) have been found to be useful for drooling.

been associated with liver damage and liver failure, these medications are usually given only to those who have not responded to other therapies. Other potential side effects include involuntary muscle movements, cramps, headache, nausea and vomiting, mental confusion and hallucinations, urine discoloration, diarrhea, constipation, sweating, susceptibility to respiratory infection, and dry mouth.

Dopamine agonists. Dopamine agonists are medications that imitate the effects of dopamine in the brain. They cause the cells to react as if there were sufficient amounts of dopamine. The potential side effects include sudden drop in blood pressure upon standing (orthostatic hypotension), headache, nausea and constipation, nightmares, hallucinations, psychosis, sudden sleep attacks, and nasal congestion. They should be avoided by anyone who has experienced hallucinations or confusion. Examples of dopamine agonists are bromocriptine (Parlodel), pergolide (Permax), pramipexole (Mirapex), and ropinirole (Requip).

Levodopa. The most common medication for Parkinson's disease is levodopa (L-dopa), which is able to cross the blood-brain barrier. When levodopa is combined with the antinausea medication known as carbidopa (Sinemet), it is even better able to cross the blood-brain barrier, making it more effective. Levodopa tends to work best for rigidity and slowness. Less benefit may be obtained for problems with tremor, balance, and gait.

During the earlier stages of Parkinson's disease, the side effects of levodopa treatment are usually minimal. But as the medication is used for longer periods of time, potential side effects that may appear include a drop in blood pressure (especially when standing), abnormal heart rhythms (arrhythmia), nausea and gastrointestinal bleeding, hair loss, confusion, anxiety, vivid dreams, sleepiness and sleep attacks, and hallucinations. As the disease progresses, this therapy may be less effective, a process called the "wearing-off effect," and you may experience involuntary movements (dyskinesia). Moreover, each dose of the medication controls symptoms for shorter periods of time.

Selegiline. An adjunct to levodopa therapy, selegiline (Atapryl, Carbex, Eldepryl) helps stop the breakdown of dopamine. Potential side effects of selegiline include nausea, vomiting, diarrhea, insomnia, vivid dreams, confusion, and agitation. People taking this medication and other monoamine oxidase (MAO) inhibitors should not consume foods or beverages that contain tyramine, such as aged cheese, red wines, vermouth, dried meats and fish, canned figs, fava beans, and concentrated yeast products. Consuming such foods could seriously raise blood pressure. Some people who have taken this drug with meperidine (Demerol, Pethadol) have had toxic reactions.

Surgery

When medications fail to improve the symptoms of Parkinson's, surgery may be an option. There are several potential procedures. Though they may relieve symptoms, they are not a cure.

Deep-brain stimulation (DBS). With this procedure, a device known as a thalamic stimulator is implanted in a region of the brain known as the subthalamic nucleus.

Then, through a wire, a pacemaker-like chest unit sends electrical pulses to the implant. These pulses stop the signals that cause tremors. The pulse generator may be controlled by passing a magnet over the chest. Because it may be used in both sides of the thalamus, tremors in both sides of the body may be controlled. The device may also be placed in the thalamus or globus pallidus. About every 3 to 5 years, the generator must be replaced. Potential complications include bleeding in the brain, infection, and decrease in verbal memory and the ability to work on mental tasks involving visual-spatial functions.

In one study, 156 people with Parkinson's were divided into two treatment groups. One group was given deep-brain stimulation, and the other group was given medication. After 6 months, researchers determined that people with advanced Parkinson's disease who received deep-brain stimulation had better outcomes than those who received medication.

Pallidotomy. During a pallidotomy, which requires about 6 hours, an electric current kills a small amount of tissue in the pallidum (globus pallidus), the location in the brain that causes many of the Parkinson's symptoms. The procedure may result in an improvement in many symptoms, including tremors, rigidity, and slowed movement, as well as the involuntary movements caused by drug therapy. But the benefits may not last. The surgery has potential risks, such as disabling weakness, slurred speech, stroke, decline in memory capacity and verbal fluency, apathy, and vision problems. Individuals with dyskinesia (uncontrolled movements),

rigidity, and tremor are considered the best candidates for this procedure.

Thalamotomy. In a thalamotomy, a small section on one side of the thalamus, a portion of the brain, is destroyed. If the surgery is effective, it will relieve tremors on the opposite side of the body. Since operating on both sides of the thalamus poses a risk of speech loss and other complications, surgeons normally operate on only one side.

Complementary Treatments

Complementary medicine addresses the symptoms associated with Parkinson's disease through nutritional and dietary changes and by using approaches that help to increase coordination, balance, and muscle control.

Acupuncture

Acupuncture may alleviate muscle stiffness and soreness as well as address the tremors associated with Parkinson's disease. To locate an acupuncturist in your area, visit the Web site of the National Certification Commission for Acupuncture and Oriental Medicine (NCCAOM) at www.nccaom.org.

Aquatic Therapy

Resistive exercises in the water may increase strength and improve balance and flexibility. A heated pool provides a safe environment to do exercises for improving the symptoms of Parkinson's disease.

Craniosacral Therapy

Craniosacral therapy (CST) is the hands-on gentle manipulation of the craniosacral systom the brain, spinal cord, cerebrospinal fluid, dural membrane, cranial bones, and sacrum. Craniosacral therapy balances the cerebrospinal fluid, which may help to alleviate tremors. To search for a qualified therapist in your area, visit the Web site of the International Association of Healthcare Practitioners at www.iahp.com.

Diet

Many foods may interfere with the effectiveness and absorption of medications for Parkinson's disease. For this reason, you may need a specific diet that is closely watched. To create the best diet for your needs, consult with a registered or licensed dietitian or certified nutritional consultant. As studies have shown that individuals with Parkinson's disease are low in certain vitamins and minerals, you may also want to discuss nutritional supplementation. However, when taking prescription medications, caution must be used before embarking on a nutritional supplement regimen.

Feldenkrais Method

Since it helps to support the neuromuscular system and improves the autonomic motor response, Feldenkrais is an especially useful technique for people with Parkinson's disease. Practitioners teach individuals to become aware of their movement patterns. This improves body motion and corrects poor postural habits. It may relieve stiffness and inflammation, which may decrease pain. To locate a practitioner, visit the Web site of the Feldenkrais Educational Foundation of North America (FEFNA) at www.feldenkrais.com.

Nutritional Supplements

While studies have found that some individuals with Parkinson's disease have low levels of vitamin B_6, it is important to not supplement with B_6 if you are taking the medication L-dopa alone. Outside the brain, B_6 converts L-dopa to dopamine, thereby lowering the level of dopamine delivered to the brain. This does not happen when L-dopa is combined with carbidopa (Sinemet).

Because people with Parkinson's disease are usually deficient in essential fatty acids, it is recommended that evening primrose oil and flaxseed oil be taken daily. The recommended dose is 1 tablespoon, twice a day.

Tai Chi and Qigong

The gentle movement therapies of tai chi and qigong help improve balance, coordination, and flexibility and reduce anxiety.

Therapeutic Massage

Therapeutic massage, particularly deep muscle work, may stretch the connective tissue, relieve tension in tight muscles, and alleviate cramping. This may lead to an increase in joint range of motion, balance, and coordination. Massage also stimulates the lymphatic system. Because of the lack of mobility, a sluggish lymphatic system may be found in people with Parkinson's disease.

Trager Approach

The Trager Approach reeducates the nerves to control muscle movement and releases patterns of muscle tension and restriction, making it beneficial for people with Parkinson's disease. As it is a passive treatment, it is especially useful for people with limited mobility. Over time, the body's nervous system is reeducated to respond in the proper manner to relieve pain and discomfort. To locate a Trager therapist, visit www.trager-us.org (the Web site of the United States Trager Association) or www.ncbtmb.org (the Web site for the National Certification Board for Therapeutic Massage and Bodywork).

Lifestyle Recommendations

Be sure to get enough sun. Fifteen minutes of sunshine a day may provide an adequate amount of vitamin D. Since all people with Parkinson's disease are prone to osteoporosis, this is particularly important as vitamin D helps protect against this disorder.

Exercise. To improve the quality of your life and maintain productivity, you should exercise. You need exercises that will help retain your balance and reduce muscle freezing. Include exercises such as stretching, walking, and marching in place. A physical therapist or personal trainer may help create an exercise program designed for your particular needs and in keeping with your limitations.

Join a support group. You may benefit from talking to others who are also dealing with Parkinson's disease. You will derive psychological benefits and may learn additional coping mechanisms.

Limit protein. In the advanced stages of Parkinson's, higher levels of protein in the diet reduce the effectiveness of levodopa. Though you should not avoid protein, try to keep protein to about 12 percent of your total daily calories.

Prevent constipation. Since constipation is an ongoing problem for many people with Parkinson's disease, eat a diet that is high in fiber and water. You may wish to take a soluble-fiber supplement such as Metamucil. Psyllium seed husks have also been very effective in improving bowel function and eliminating constipation. It is important to maintain gastrointestinal health. Taking acidophilus, which are friendly bacteria, may be useful in preventing constipation and ensuring a healthy gastrointestinal tract.

Remain mentally active. Using your mind will help you retain the brain's dopamine. Learn a new hobby, especially one that requires finger and hand mobility. Or study a new language and keep up with the daily news.

Take a digestive enzyme. Since people with Parkinson's disease may not be able to utilize nutrients effectively, a digestive enzyme should be taken after each meal.

Preventive Measures

There is a direct link between pesticides and the development of Parkinson's disease. If you are going to continue to use pesticides, take precautions and wear protective clothing, gloves, and a mask.

Peripheral Neuropathy

People with peripheral neuropathy can experience anything from mild tingling to loss of feeling to intense pain. *Peripheral neuropathy* is a general term used to describe disorders of the peripheral nervous system, the complex network of nerves that link the spinal column to the other parts of the body. With this disorder, there is some form of damage to the nerves that communicate between your brain and your muscles, internal organs, skin, and blood vessels. When only one nerve is affected, it is called mononeuropathy. Yet, often many peripheral nerves are involved, and then it is called polyneuropathy.

Peripheral neuropathy is very common. It is believed that more than 2 million Americans have some form of this disorder.

Causes and Risk Factors

Damage to the peripheral nerves may occur in a number of ways. With mononeuropathy, the cause is normally trauma or some form of repetitive use. Thus, it may be the result of using crutches or typing at a computer keyboard. One such example is carpal tunnel syndrome. On the other hand, polyneuropathy is more often the result of a medical problem, such as diabetes, a condition called diabetic neuropathy. For some unknown reason, high levels of sugar in the blood appear to inhibit the ability of your nerves to transmit signals.

Peripheral neuropathy is also more frequently seen in those with autoimmune diseases, such as rheumatoid arthritis; in alcoholics; in people with compromised immune systems; and in people who take certain medications or who have specific vitamin deficiencies, such as low levels of vitamin B_{12}. Further, those who are dealing with liver and kidney disease and hypothyroidism are more likely to have peripheral neuropathy. It is believed that exposure to toxic substances, such as lead and mercury, may result in peripheral neuropathy. And an attack of acute Guillain-Barré syndrome may destroy the myelin sheath that covers nerve fibers, leaving an individual with a case of peripheral neuropathy.

Signs and Symptoms

People with peripheral neuropathy have a wide range of symptoms, which may vary dramatically in intensity. Sometimes, you may be hardly aware of your symptoms, while at other times you may find them unbearable. Symptoms from peripheral neuropathy include tingling, pain, numbness, burning, and a loss of feeling. These often begin gradually and then intensify. For example, you may have pain in your hands that travels up your arms or pain in your feet that extends up your legs. On occasion, the pain can be so intense that you may feel pain even from the light touch of a sheet that covers you at night. Often, there is numbness or a lack of feeling

A Quick Guide to Symptoms

☐ Tingling or burning
☐ Pain
☐ Numbness, loss of feeling
☐ Weakness or even paralysis
☐ Reduced ability to sweat, frequent constipation or diarrhea, bladder problems, or impotence
☐ Insomnia, depression, weight loss, or difficulty breathing or swallowing

in your hands or feet. Because people with diabetic neuropathy are prone to nerve damage and poor circulation in their feet and other parts of their bodies, they may develop ulcers or gangrene.

If your peripheral neuropathy has affected your motor nerves (such as in Guillain-Barré syndrome), you may have problems with the muscles controlled by those nerves. You may have weakness or even paralysis. If your condition has damaged nerves that control some autonomic nerve system functions, you may have reduced ability to sweat, frequent constipation or diarrhea, bladder problems, or impotence. Your stomach may empty too slowly, resulting in nausea, vomiting, and bloating. In some cases, when you stand after sitting or lying down, your blood pressure may drop and you may become lightheaded or faint. People with peripheral neuropathy may also have problems with insomnia, depression, weight loss, or difficulty breathing or swallowing.

Conventional Treatments

Treatments vary according to the underlying cause of your neuropathy. The goal of treatment is to manage the condition that is causing the neuropathy, thereby providing symptom relief. So, if your peripheral neuropathy is a result of high blood sugar levels, for example, then your doctor will want you to work to control them. If your symptoms are triggered by a vitamin B_{12} deficiency, you will receive injections of the vitamin. If you have pressure on a nerve, then treatment will center on ways to eliminate the pressure. Thus, if your keyboard is causing pain in your wrists, then you will be advised to use an ergonomically correct keyboard.

However, when there is no obvious cause of your peripheral neuropathy, you will be offered a number of pain-relieving alternatives.

Medications

Numerous over-the-counter pain medications may provide some relief. These include acetaminophen (Tylenol) and nonsteroidal anti-inflammatory drugs (NSAIDs) such as aspirin and ibuprofen (Advil, Motrin). If your pain is more severe, your doctor may prescribe stronger NSAIDs. NSAIDs taken in higher doses or over a long period of time may cause stomach pain and bleeding, nausea, and ulcers. Large doses may also result in kidney problems and heart failure.

Since they interfere with the chemical processes in the brain that cause you to feel pain, tricyclic antidepressants are often used for pain from peripheral neuropathy. Examples are amitriptyline (Elavil), nortriptyline (Pamelor), imipramine (Tofranil), and desipramine (Norpramin). These medications have potential side effects, including nausea, tiredness, dry mouth, dizziness, weight gain, and weakness. To reduce the chance that you will be forced to deal with these side effects, your doctor will probably start you on a low dose. If you have a good tolerance of the medication, then the dose may be increased.

If you are dealing with bouts of jabbing pain, your doctor may suggest an antiseizure medication, originally developed for those with epilepsy. Examples are gabapentin (Neurontin), phenytoin (Dilantin), and carbamazepine (Tegretol). Potential side effects include confusion and drowsiness. In a clinical trial, lamotrigine, an anticonvulsant, has been shown to be effective against moderate pain from peripheral neuropathy caused by diabetes or HIV. Minimal side effects were reported.

Still another medication is mexiletine (Mexitil), more commonly used for irregular heart rhythms. Potential side effects include nausea, lightheadedness, vomiting, shaking hands, or difficulty walking. If you have diabetes-related peripheral neuropathy, you may wish to try the topical ointment capsaicin (Capzasin-P, Zostrix). You may see results in a week or two. Potential side effects include mild skin irritation, tingling, or burning at the point of application.

Transcutaneous Electrical Nerve Stimulation (TENS)

Transcutaneous electrical nerve stimulation (TENS) uses low-level electrical pulses to reduce pain. Typically, 80 to 100 pulses per second are given for 45 minutes, three times per day. The sensations are barely felt. In a similar procedure, known as percutaneous electrical nerve stimulation (PENS), the pulses are applied in small needles to acupuncture points. While this approach appears to provide some relief for most people with pain, it tends to work better in men than in women.

Complementary Treatments

To determine the best treatment plan, complementary medicine practitioners seek to find the underlying cause of peripheral neuropathy. However, the symptoms of peripheral neuropathy may also be treated individually by various complementary medicine treatments.

Acupuncture

Acupuncture can help reduce the pain associated with peripheral neuropathy. To locate an acupuncturist in your area, visit the Web site of the National Certification Commission for Acupuncture and Oriental Medicine (NCCAOM) at www.nccaom.org.

Biofeedback

Biofeedback uses an electric monitoring device to obtain data on vital body functions.

During a session, you will be taught ways to use relaxation techniques to alter or slow the body's signals. Biofeedback can help teach individuals how to control the bodily responses that can help reduce pain. Various health care professionals incorporate biofeedback into their practice, including psychiatrists, psychologists, social workers, nurses, physical therapists, occupational therapists, speech therapists, respiratory therapists, exercise physiologists, and chiropractors.

Seek a health care practitioner who has been certified through the Biofeedback Certification Institute of America (BCIA). To locate a practitioner in your area, look on the BCIA Web site at www.bcia.org, check your local hospitals or medical clinics, or look in the Yellow Pages under the practitioners mentioned above.

Diet

Following a healthy, low-fat diet that includes lots of whole grains, fresh fruits, vegetables, and essential fatty acids may help reduce your risk of developing some forms of neuropathy. These foods are high in essential nutrients that feed the nerves and the brain and ensure proper communication between the two. They also support the immune system, which keeps the body healthy and fights viruses. If you have neuropathy that is caused by a particular medical condition, to ensure that the foods you are eating do not aggravate your condition, you should consult with your doctor.

Nutritional Supplements

To guarantee that you are receiving proper nutritional support, take a high-quality multivitamin/mineral supplement. Additional supplementation of vitamin B_{12} injections may also be a good idea. If injections are not available, take a 1,000-microgram tablet sublingually (under the tongue) daily.

Relaxation/Meditation

Relaxation/meditation techniques can help release the muscular tension that often leads to an increase in pain. A regular routine of guided imagery, meditation, yoga, or deep breathing exercises will promote relaxation, thus allowing the release of physical and emotional tension.

To practice deep breathing, lie flat on your back and place both hands on your abdomen. Slowly inhale through your nose, pushing your abdomen up as if you were blowing up a balloon. Then, exhale slowly through the mouth, and feel your abdomen deflate. Repeat this process 8 to 10 times, and practice this breathing process as often as possible.

Lifestyle Recommendations

Calm your burning hands and feet. Try soaking your hands and feet in cool water for 15 minutes, twice each day. After you finish, rub your hands and feet with petroleum jelly.

Exercise. Following an exercise program

will help you deal with your symptoms. Ask your doctor to suggest an exercise routine. A referral to a physical therapist who has special training in dealing with the symptoms of peripheral neuropathy is also a good idea.

Limit caffeine and alcohol. Caffeine and alcohol exacerbate peripheral neuropathy symptoms, so limit your intake.

Regularly massage your hands and feet. By massaging your hands and feet, you will improve circulation and stimulate the nerves, which may also relieve the pain.

Stop smoking. Smoking will only aggravate your peripheral neuropathy.

Take care of your feet. Don't wear tight shoes or socks. This is particularly important if you have diabetes. If your bedcovers are bothering your sensitive feet, purchase a semicircular hoop that holds the covers over your body. You can find this device in a medical supply store.

Preventive Measures

Avoid repetitive motions. People who engage in repetitive motions are more likely to suffer from peripheral neuropathy. Try to be proactive in avoiding repetitive motions, such as typing or other job-related activities.

Be careful with chemicals. Toxic chemicals may harm your nerves. Try to avoid using them, or if you must use them, wear protective clothing.

Manage your medical condition. If you have a medical condition, such as diabetes, that places you at increased risk for peripheral neuropathy, then you need to control it. In the case of diabetes, you need to manage your sugar levels.

Peripheral Vascular Disease

With peripheral vascular disease (PVD), the arteries that carry blood to the arms or legs become narrowed or clogged. Blood is unable to flow normally.

Also known as peripheral artery disease (PAD) or occlusive arterial disease, peripheral vascular disease is very common. Over the age of 50, about one out of every 20 people has this disorder. About 10 million Americans are affected, yet 2.5 million are undiagnosed.

Causes and Risk Factors

Most often, peripheral vascular disease is caused by atherosclerosis, which is also called hardening of the arteries. With atherosclerosis, cholesterol and scar tissue (plaque) build up inside the blood vessels, which become narrowed or clogged. However, blood clots in the arteries may also cause PVD.

A Quick Guide to Symptoms

☐ Painful cramping in the legs, calves, hips, or feet, especially when walking
☐ Erectile dysfunction
☐ Numbness, tingling, or weakness in the affected leg
☐ The skin of the affected legs and feet may seem cooler and change color
☐ Loss of hair on the legs
☐ Feet and toes may burn and ache
☐ Leg or foot sores that do not heal

Men are more likely than women to have PVD. People over the age of 50 have an increased risk, as do smokers, people with diabetes, and people who are overweight and do not exercise. High blood pressure, high cholesterol, and a family history of heart or vascular disease all raise the risk.

Signs and Symptoms

The most frequent symptom associated with peripheral vascular disease is painful cramping in the legs, calves, hips, or feet, especially when walking. This painful cramping, which is called intermittent claudication, is a result of inadequate bloodflow in the leg muscles. While the pain tends to disappear when you stop walking, as soon as you start walking again, it will likely reappear. Men may experience erectile dysfunction. Other common symptoms include numbness, tingling, or weakness in the affected legs. The skin of the affected legs and feet may seem cooler and change color. There may be a loss of hair on the legs. In the worst cases, your feet and toes may burn and ache, even when resting, and you may have leg or foot sores that do not heal. Sometimes, untreated PVD may lead to gangrene.

Conventional Treatments

Your treatment will probably begin with a review of your lifestyle. If you smoke, you will be told to stop. If you have diabetes, you'll need to maintain better control of your blood sugar. Do you have high blood pressure? If so, you need to lower it. Is your cholesterol too high? You must find ways to lower it.

Angioplasty

During an angioplasty, a surgeon places a tiny balloon in a blood vessel at the site of the blockage. When the balloon is inflated, the blockage opens. Sometimes, to keep a vessel open, a metal cylinder called a stent may be inserted.

Exercise

Regular exercise appears to be the most consistently effective treatment for peripheral vascular disease. If you participate in a regular exercise program, you will gradually be able to reduce your level of pain. Begin with brief walks, then slowly increase the amount of time that you walk.

Interventional Radiology Treatments

A number of interventional radiology treatments are available for PVD. These use catheters or tiny tubes and other miniaturized tools as well as x-rays.

Medications

A variety of medications may be prescribed for people with PVD. If you have high blood pressure or high cholesterol, you may get a prescription to treat those conditions. You might get a prescription for ticlopidine (Ticlid), which helps some people with PVD to walk longer distances. Still, the pharmacologic management of PVD has not been as successful as the pharmacologic treatment of coronary artery disease. Pentoxifylline (Trental) has been shown to increase the duration of exercise in individuals with claudication, but its efficacy has not been demonstrated consistently in clinical trials.

Surgery

In severe cases of PVD, surgery may be required. These procedures should be performed by a vascular surgeon.

Amputation. Without bloodflow, tissue dies and poses an extremely high risk for serious infection. An amputation is done only as a last resort, when there is little or no

Self-Testing

The following is a self-test for peripheral vascular disease. The more "yes" answers that you have, the more likely it is that you have this disorder.

☐ Do you have a history of cardiovascular (heart) problems, such as high blood pressure, heart attack, or stroke?
☐ Do you have diabetes?
☐ Do you have a family history of diabetes or cardiovascular problems with immediate family members (mother, father, sister, or brother)?
☐ Do you have aching or cramping in your legs when you walk or exercise? Does the pain stop when you rest?
☐ Do your feet and toes hurt at night?
☐ Do ulcers or sores on your feet heal slowly?
☐ Do you smoke?
☐ Did you previously smoke?
☐ Are you more than 25 pounds overweight?
☐ Do you eat fatty foods at least three times each week?
☐ Are you inactive?

Legs for Life

The Society of Interventional Radiology has created Legs for Life, a community screening program for PVD. People who are believed to have PVD are referred to their primary care physician for additional diagnosis. To determine when and where the screenings will be held, log on to the program's Web site at www.legsforlife.org.

bloodflow to the foot or leg, and when there are no other options.

Bypass grafts. In a bypass graft, a portion of vein is removed from another part of the body. It is then grafted onto the affected area, creating a detour around the blockage. Sometimes, rather than taking a vein from another part of the body, the surgeon uses a synthetic graft.

Thrombectomy. A thrombectomy is done only when PVD symptoms develop suddenly

In some uncommon instances, your doctor will advise against exercising. Before beginning any exercise program, check with your doctor.

from a blood clot. During this procedure, the surgeon inserts a balloon into the artery beyond the blood clot. The balloon is inflated and pulled back, thereby removing the clot.

Thrombolytic Therapy

If a clot is causing the blockage in an artery, an interventional radiologist may use a catheter to administer a clot-busting drug.

Thrombolytic therapy is often combined with another treatment, such as an angioplasty.

Complementary Treatments

The best complementary medicine treatment approach is prevention through dietary modification, nutritional supplementation, herbal therapies, and lifestyle changes.

Aquatic Therapy

Aquatic therapy is a gentle way to begin an exercise program. Water is an ideal environment to promote relaxation. The rhythmic movements and simple stretches help the mind and body to unwind and reduce stress. Aerobic exercise and relaxation techniques have been shown to lower blood pressure.

Diet

Eating a balanced and healthy diet is most beneficial for maintaining a healthy cardiovascular system. Your diet should include lots of vegetables, fruits, whole grains, and nuts and seeds (walnuts, almonds, and sesame seeds). Try to include a minimum of five servings of vegetables, four servings of fruit, and six servings of whole grains each day.

You should avoid trans fatty acids, fried foods, sugar, and other processed foods. Since the regular consumption of animal products increases the risk of cardiovascular problems, saturated fats and cholesterol-rich foods, such as fatty meats, egg yolks, milk fat, and margarine, should be eliminated from the diet.

Increase your intake of water-soluble fiber. By removing fat that has accumulated in the intestines and by decreasing the absorption of this fat, water-soluble fiber, which is contained in many healthy foods, may lower cholesterol and blood pressure. Also, reduce your intake of dairy products, as dairy has been linked to an increased risk of developing cardiovascular disease.

Foods rich in essential fatty acids and the antioxidants beta-carotene, the B vitamins, and vitamins C and E; magnesium; and selenium are all useful for heart health. Essential fatty acids are found in flaxseed oil, salmon, and other cold-water fish. Beta-carotene is contained in almost all fruits and vegetables. It is the substance that provides their color. Good sources of vitamin C also include almost all fruits and green vegetables, especially strawberries, cranberries, melons, oranges, mangoes, papayas, peppers, spinach, kale, broccoli, tomatoes, and potatoes.

Vitamin E may be found in vegetable oils, nuts, seeds, and wheat germ. Smaller amounts of vitamin E are in leafy vegetables and whole grains. The B vitamins are found in dark green, leafy vegetables; whole grains; oranges; avocados; beets; bananas; potatoes; dairy products; nuts; beans; fish; and chicken. Magnesium is found in green, leafy vegetables such as spinach, parsley, broccoli, chard, kale, and mustard and turnip greens. It is also in raw almonds, wheat germ, potatoes, and tofu. Selenium is contained in seafood, chicken, whole-grain cereals, and garlic.

Anthocyanosides are compounds that have antioxidant properties and are found in blueberries, cherries, raspberries, red or purple grapes, and plums. The European species of blueberry, the bilberry, has the highest level of anthocyanosides. Anthocyanosides help improve capillary circulation.

Garlic, onions, cayenne pepper, ginger, turmeric, and alfalfa all reduce cholesterol, thus aiding in the health of the heart. Garlic, onions, and cayenne pepper also thin the blood, thereby preventing clotting. And foods containing soy have been shown to drop elevated cholesterol levels.

To ensure that there is no interaction between medicines and the nutrients found in food, if you are taking any prescription medication for your heart, you should consult with your doctor.

Herbal Medicine

Garlic. Garlic, an antioxidant that lowers cholesterol, may also reduce high blood pressure and improve the elasticity of blood vessel walls. The daily dose of fresh garlic is two to three cloves per day, while the supplement dose is 500 milligrams. If you have a choice, select fresh garlic over supplements. The supplements contain concentrated extracts, which may increase the risk of excessive bleeding.

Ginkgo biloba. Ginkgo is an antioxidant that supports circulation; it is available in capsule form. The recommended daily dose is 120 milligrams, twice a day, of an extract standardized to 24 percent of flavone glycosides and 6 percent terpene lactones. The flavone glycosides give ginkgo its antioxidant benefits, while terpene lactones increase circulation and have a protective effect on nerve cells. If you are also taking prescription blood-thinning medications, be sure to check with a doctor before using ginkgo supplements.

Green tea. Green tea is a powerful antioxidant that helps to decrease cholesterol, lower blood pressure, and prevent the clogging of arteries. Green tea can be taken as a tea or in capsules. Drinking 3 cups of green tea per day provides 240 to 320 milligrams of polyphenols. In capsule form, standardized extract of EGCG (a polyphenol) may provide 97 percent polyphenol content, which is the equivalent of drinking 4 cups of tea per day.

Hawthorn. Like green tea, hawthorn works to decrease cholesterol and lower blood pressure. In addition, hawthorn helps to strengthen heart muscles, improve circulation, and rid the body of unnecessary fluid and salt. Hawthorn is available in capsule or tincture form, standardized to 2.2 percent total bioflavonoid content. It may take up to 2 months before you see the effects of this herb on your health. The recommended daily dose of hawthorn capsules varies widely, ranging from 100 to 300 milligrams, two to three times per day. Be aware that higher doses may significantly lower blood pressure, which may cause you to feel faint. When using the tincture, the recommended dose is 4 to 5 milliliters, three times per day.

Nutritional Supplements

The following nutritional supplements are very beneficial to maintaining a healthy vascular system.

- B-complex vitamins: Take as directed on the label. Help prevent the arteries from getting clogged and prevent inappropriate blood clot formation.

- Vitamin B_6: 50 milligrams daily in divided doses of 25 milligrams. Helps with absorption of calcium, magnesium, and vitamin C.

- Vitamin C: 1,000 milligrams daily in divided doses of 500 milligrams. Essential for heart health. Vitamin C converts cholesterol into bile, strengthens the arterial walls, and stops the buildup of cholesterol.

- Calcium: 1,500 milligrams daily in divided doses of 750 milligrams. Lowers total cholesterol and increases HDL cholesterol.

- Chromium: 200 micrograms daily. Aids in the prevention of the buildup of cholesterol and increases HDL.

- Coenzyme Q_{10}: 200 milligrams daily in divided doses of 100 milligrams. Increases oxygen to the heart tissue and may help lower blood pressure and prevent oxidation of LDL ("bad") cholesterol.

- Vitamin E: 400 IU daily. Stops the oxidation of LDL cholesterol, prevents damage to the arterial lining, improves circulation, and fortifies the immune system. Vitamin E may thin the blood. If you are taking blood-thinning medication, consult your doctor before taking this supplement. If there are no contraindications, take vitamin E with selenium for best absorption.

- L-carnitine: 500 milligrams daily in divided doses of 250 milligrams. Effective for intermittent claudication (leg cramps). Lowers total cholesterol and increases HDL cholesterol.

- Magnesium: 800 milligrams daily in divided doses of 400 milligrams. Helps to lower total cholesterol and increases HDL cholesterol.

• Selenium: 400 micrograms daily in divided doses of 200 micrograms. Helps prevent heart disease and future heart attacks by thinning the blood. However, if you are taking blood-thinning medication, consult your doctor before taking this supplement. Selenium should not be taken at the same time as vitamin C as they interfere with each other's absorption.

Relaxation/Meditation

Many practitioners recommend relaxation/meditation techniques to help people reduce stress, control their emotions, and lower blood pressure. Clinical trials have shown that by combining biofeedback, yoga, and meditation, you will improve your ability to lower blood pressure. A 2006 study showed that practicing mental relaxation or slow breathing can reduce blood pressure and heart rate. Other effective techniques for reducing stress include qigong, tai chi, yoga, deep breathing exercises, and visualization.

Lifestyle Recommendations

If you have peripheral vascular disease, you may be tempted to stop exercising. Work together with your doctor to develop an exercise plan. In general, you should start with something as brief as a 5-minute walk, then gradually increase the length of your exercise routine. By reducing blood pressure and decreasing resting heart rate, exercise improves the bloodflow in the arteries. Further, exercise helps you lose weight and manage stress. So, over time, it reduces the symptoms of PVD.

Preventive Measures

A healthy weight, lipid profile, and blood pressure are a good start to preventing peripheral vascular disease.

Avoid excess salt consumption. Sodium causes the body to retain fluid, creating more work for the heart.

Control the stress in your life. Find some means to reduce the stress in your life. Consider meditating or some other way to calm yourself.

Decrease coffee consumption. Coffee increases stress hormones, which puts coffee drinkers at greater risk for heart problems. However, studies have failed to prove a link between atherosclerosis and caffeine intake.

Reduce alcohol consumption. Alcohol may raise blood pressure and overtax the liver, interfering with the liver's ability to detoxify foods. This may result in a buildup of cholesterol. Studies have shown that red wine may be beneficial for the cardiovascular system, as the flavonoids in the wine help stop the buildup of fatty deposits in blood vessels. The recommended daily intake is one 5-ounce glass for women, and no more than two 5-ounce glasses for men.

Stop smoking. Smoking is a major risk factor in the development of PVD. Smoking can also interfere with the treatment of the disease. The carbon monoxide produced from cigarette smoking decreases the oxygen in the blood, causing the heart to work harder. Smoking also causes blood platelets to stick together, which blocks the arteries. In some instances, smoking may interfere with your prescription medications.

Prostate Enlargement

Prostate enlargement shows up in men as they age. The older you are, it seems, the more likely you'll be dealing with problems of the prostate gland. Located in front of the rectum and just below the bladder, the walnut-size prostate gland squeezes fluid into the urethra as sperm move through during ejaculation. When the prostate first begins to enlarge, a condition also called benign prostatic hyperplasia (BPH) or benign prostatic hypertrophy, it rarely causes any problems. However, eventually, it presses against the urethra, resulting in the bladder becoming thicker and irritated. The bladder may contract when it contains only a small amount of urine. More frequent urination becomes necessary, but since the bladder may be unable to empty itself fully, urine may remain in the bladder after urination.

Prostate enlargement is a common disorder. Though rare before the age of 40, more than half of all men who are in their sixties have prostate enlargement. Almost all men in their seventies and eighties have evidence of this problem.

Causes and Risk Factors

Though there is no clear cause for prostate enlargement, it is known that married men develop the disorder more often than single men. It is more common in American and European men than Asian men. And genetics appears to play a role. If members of your family tend to have prostate enlargement, then you are at increased risk.

Signs and Symptoms

Only about half of the men with prostate enlargement are so significantly bothered by their symptoms that they seek medical care. Symptoms include difficulty starting urination, stopping and starting while urinating, dribbling at the end of urination, urgent need to urinate, frequent need to urinate, weak urine stream, and increased rate of nighttime urination (nocturia).

Conventional Treatments

If an enlarged prostate has caused no symptoms, then no treatment will be recommended. However, if you do have symptoms, a number of treatments are available. The recommended treatment will depend upon the type of symptoms you are experiencing.

Medications

If you have moderate symptoms, there is a good chance that your treatment will begin with medication. There are two types of medications used for prostate enlargement, alpha-blockers and finasteride.

Alpha-blockers. Although originally developed to treat high blood pressure, alpha-blockers have been found useful for other medical problems, including an enlarged prostate. They relax the muscles at the neck of the bladder, thereby making it easier to urinate. Examples of alpha-blockers approved for prostate enlargement are tamsulosin (Flomax), terazosin (Hytrin), and doxazosin (Cardura).

Effective in about 75 percent of the men who take them, alpha-blockers begin working in a day or two. Men will note that they need to urinate less often, and that there is an increase in the urinary flow. Potential side effects include headaches, dizziness, lightheadedness, and tiredness. It is recommended that you take the medication before bedtime. In some instances, the medication may cause low blood pressure when standing, as well as erectile dysfunction (impotence). Tamsulosin, which is the newest of these medications, tends to cause less dizziness, but it may result in abnormal ejaculation.

Finasteride. Finasteride, which actually shrinks the prostate, works best for men with large prostate glands. It is not as effective for those with moderately enlarged prostate glands, in which it may result in an obstruction. Examples are Proscar and Propecia. Unfortunately, finasteride takes a while to work. While you may have some improvement within 3 months, it often requires up to a year. In addition, finasteride lowers your baseline PSA level, which could interfere with a proper determination of your risk for prostate cancer. (PSA, or prostate-specific antigen, is a protein made by cells in the prostate gland. High levels are considered a marker for prostate cancer.)

Nonsurgical Therapies

Nonsurgical therapies for prostate enlargement focus on widening the urethra, thus making it easier to urinate.

Heat therapy. With heat therapy, heat energy, which is delivered via the urethra, is used to destroy excess prostate tissue. It is better than medications for prostate enlarge-

If you find that you are unable to pass any urine, you may have a serious medical problem known as acute urinary retention. You need to seek emergency medical assistance.

ment that is causing moderate to severe symptoms, and it has fewer side effects than surgery. Though heat therapy is usually performed on an outpatient basis, you may need to spend the night at the hospital.

Microwave therapy. Transurethral microwave therapy (TUMT) uses computer-controlled heat in the form of microwave energy to destroy excess tissue in the enlarged gland. During the procedure, you will be given a local anesthetic. Then, a urinary catheter (a tube that has a tiny microwave device) will be used to heat enlarged prostate cells and destroy them. You will probably feel some heat in the prostate and bladder area, and you will have a strong desire to urinate. You may also have bladder spasms. Most likely, you will need to wear a urinary catheter for a few days. As you recover, you may have periods when you have

A Quick Guide to Symptoms

- ☐ Difficulty starting urination
- ☐ Stopping and starting while urinating
- ☐ Dribbling at the end of urination
- ☐ Urgent need to urinate
- ☐ Frequent need to urinate
- ☐ Weak urine stream
- ☐ Increased rate of nighttime urination (nocturia)

urgent, frequent urination and blood in your urine, and there may be changes in the semen you ejaculate. You should not have TUMT if you have a pacemaker or any metal implants.

Radiofrequency therapy. With transurethral needle ablation (TUNA), radio waves are sent through needles inserted into the prostate gland. This heats and destroys the tissue. TUNA tends to be less effective than surgery in reducing symptoms and improving the flow of urine, and it is not as useful for men with large prostates. Among the potential side effects are painful urination, blood in the urine, urine retention, and a slight risk for retrograde ejaculation, a condition in which part of the semen goes backward into the bladder.

Electrovaporization. During a transurethral electrovaporization of the prostate (TVP), a metal instrument that emits a high-frequency electrical current is used to cut and vaporize excess prostate tissue. To prevent bleeding, tissue is sealed. This procedure is particularly useful for men at higher risk for bleeding, such as those who take blood-thinning medications.

Laser therapy. With laser therapy, heat from lasers is used to destroy prostate tissue. Transurethral evaporation of the prostate (TUEP) is similar to electrovaporization. It is considered quite safe and results in only a small amount of bleeding. Urine flow tends to improve fairly quickly. Noncontact visual laser ablation (VLAP) uses laser energy to damage excess prostate cells, which are eliminated over an extended period of time. As a result of the swelling and slow wearing away of the tissue, urine is often retained, and you will probably

need to wear a catheter for several days. You may also have burning during urination for days or even weeks. Interstitial laser therapy sends laser energy inside prostate growths, resulting in moderate reductions in the size of the prostate and moderate improvements in urine flow. It appears to be useful for men with large prostates, but there tends to be a lot of postsurgical inflammation, so you may require a catheter for up to 3 weeks, and infections are fairly common.

Surgery

Years ago, surgery was frequently used for an enlarged prostate. Because of the other available options, it is now used most often for those who have the most severe symptoms or complicating factors such as bleeding through the urethra, kidney damage from urinary retention, frequent urinary tract infections, and stones in the bladder. Unless no other therapy is effective, it tends not to be used for men with serious lung, kidney, or heart conditions; uncontrolled diabetes; cirrhosis of the liver; or major psychiatric disorder.

Transurethral resection of the prostate (TURP). With TURP, while you are either under general anesthesia or anesthetized from the waist down, part of the prostate is removed. The surgeon inserts a narrow instrument known as a resectoscope into the urethra. The resectoscope has an electrical loop that may be used to remove prostate tissue and seal blood vessels. Potential complications from TURP surgery include blood in the urine, a sense of urgency to urinate, short-term difficulty controlling urine, and problems with sexual function. Some men develop retrograde or dry ejaculation—in this condition, part of the semen goes backward into the bladder. In up to 10 percent of cases, prostate tissue grows back, and a second surgery may be required.

Transurethral incision of the prostate (TUIP). If you are not considered a good candidate for TURP, your doctor may recommend TUIP. As with TURP, several instruments are inserted through the urethra. However, rather than remove prostate tissue, the urethra is enlarged. While there are fewer side effects from this procedure, it is not as effective and it frequently must be repeated.

Open prostatectomy. If you have extreme prostate enlargement or a complicating factor such as bladder damage, bladder stones, or urethral strictures, your doctor may advise an open prostatectomy, the removal of the inner portion of your prostate via an incision in your lower abdomen. Potential complications tend to be the same as with TURP, though they are often more severe.

Complementary Treatments

Dietary changes and nutritional and herbal supplementation have been shown to be effective in reducing and eliminating prostate enlargement.

Diet

To avoid prostate enlargement, it is extremely beneficial to maintain a healthy diet low in saturated fats. By substituting soy protein for animal protein, you may quickly and effectively reduce cholesterol. Essential fatty acids have also been shown to be useful to prevent prostate enlargement. Good food sources are seafood (particularly bluefish, herring, salmon, and tuna), almonds, peanuts, walnuts, and sunflower seeds. Although seafood is, in fact, animal protein, the essential fatty acid content is so beneficial that including it in your diet is a good thing.

Herbal Medicine

Pygeum and stinging nettle. Along with saw palmetto, pygeum and stinging nettle are diuretics, which increase the secretion and flow of urine and reduce irritation of the bladder and urethra. Both are available in tincture form. Pygeum, in particular, has been shown to aid males who have trouble initiating urination, and it also supports the complete emptying of the bladder. The typical recommended daily dose for pygeum is 50 milligrams twice a day of extract

Recovering from Surgery

During your surgical procedure, a catheter will be inserted through the penis into the bladder. It will enable urine to be collected into a collection bag. You will probably be required to wear this catheter for several days. In some instances, it may cause painful bladder spasms. These should go away fairly quickly. Most likely, there will be blood in your urine. Be sure to drink lots of water, which helps flush the bladder and aids in healing. After surgery, you should not do any heavy lifting for several weeks.

standardized to 13 percent total sterols; for stinging nettle, the recommended daily dose is 250 milligrams of nettle root twice a day.

Saw palmetto. Clinical studies have shown saw palmetto to be useful for the relief of symptoms of an enlarged prostate. Saw palmetto is available in capsules containing 160 milligrams of extract standardized to 85 to 95 percent fatty acids and sterols. The typical recommended daily dose is 320 milligrams. Though you may notice symptom relief within 30 days, you should continue to take the supplement.

Naturopathy

There is a link between food sensitivity and prostate problems. A naturopathic physician may test for food allergies or sensitivities. To find a naturopathic practitioner in your area, contact the American Association of Naturopathic Physicians at www.naturopathic.org.

Nutritional Supplements

Nutritional supplements are beneficial in shrinking an enlarged prostate.

- Omega-3 fatty acids: 1 tablespoon of flaxseed oil or fish oil capsules as directed on the label. May prevent the prostate from swelling.

- Zinc: 30 milligrams daily. Effective in shrinking an enlarged prostate and enhancing the immune system.

Lifestyle Recommendations

Empty your bladder. When you void, try to urinate as much as possible. Some men void more effectively when they sit on the toilet.

Keep warm. You are more likely to retain urine when you are cold. And you are also more likely to experience an urgency to urinate when you are cold.

Limit alcohol intake. Alcohol irritates the bladder and increases urine production.

Limit your evening beverage intake. While you should drink a good deal of water during the day, reduce the amount of water you drink in the evening to lessen your need to urinate while you sleep.

Stay active. Inactivity may trigger urine retention.

Take care with over-the-counter decongestants. In some instances, decongestants may cause the urethral sphincter (the band of muscles that controls urine flow) to tighten, making urination more difficult.

Preventive Measures

Eat a healthy diet. Beans and legumes contain pectin, a water-soluble fiber that helps move cholesterol out of the body. It is recommended to eat one serving of beans ($1\frac{1}{2}$ cups) each day. Especially good choices are soybeans, lima beans, kidney beans, navy beans, pinto beans, black-eyed peas, and lentils. Fruits also contain pectin and should be eaten regularly. Carrots, cabbage, broccoli, and onions have pectin in the form of calcium pectate, which also helps move cholesterol. Starting your day with half a grapefruit and eating two raw carrots at lunch is an ideal way to begin lowering your cholesterol. A compound found in skim milk may actually inhibit cholesterol production in the liver.

Maintain a healthy cholesterol level. It is best to keep your total cholesterol level below 220.

Prostatitis

Prostatitis is inflammation of the prostate gland. The doughnut-shaped, walnut-size prostate gland, which is found only in men, is located behind the pubic bone and in front of the rectum. It produces most of the fluids in semen.

Though rarely discussed, prostatitis is one of the most common medical problems faced by men. Every year, men make about 2 million visits to doctors because of this medical problem.

There are three types of prostatitis: acute bacterial prostatitis, chronic bacterial prostatitis, and nonbacterial prostatitis. Acute bacterial prostatitis develops quickly; you immediately know you are sick. It is not uncommon for this type of prostatitis to require hospitalization. The progression of chronic bacterial prostatitis and nonbacterial prostatitis is slower and more subtle.

Causes and Risk Factors

Many cases of prostatitis are caused by a bacteria-induced infection. Generally, the bacteria travel to the prostate from other parts of the urinary tract, such as the kidneys or bladder. But they may also be transmitted through the urethra during sexual activity. And bacteria found in the large intestine may also be a culprit. Only infrequently are the bacteria spread through the bloodstream. It is well known that the insertion of a catheter into the urethra has the potential to introduce bacteria and trigger an infection. And calcified stones that may form in the prostate gland may attract bacteria.

However, most cases of prostatitis are not a result of bacteria. In these instances, there is no evidence of bacteria in the urine or prostate fluid. Nevertheless, elevated white blood cells in urine specimens will usually indicate inflammation. Though researchers are not certain what causes nonbacterial prostatitis, they have a number of theories. Some think it may be related to inflammation of the urethra or a sexually transmitted disease, such as gonorrhea or chlamydia. There is speculation that it may be connected to a reduction in sexual activity or an undetected infectious agent. Further, it has been theorized that men who start and stop their urination instead of allowing the urine to flow freely may cause a backing up of urine, which irritates the prostate.

Other hypotheses focus on anxiety and stress or lifting heavy objects with a full bladder. Occupations that subject the prostate to a good deal of vibrations—such as riding on heavy equipment—may place men at risk. And recreational bikers and joggers may irritate their prostate glands.

Men who are over 50 who have benign enlargement of the prostate are at increased risk of urinary tract infections, and that increased risk places them at greater risk for prostatitis. Also, men who have suffered a bout of acute bacterial prostatitis are at greater risk for a recurrence, as well as the development of chronic bacterial prostatitis.

Certain behaviors, such as excess alcohol consumption, are believed to cause congestion in the prostate gland. A congested prostate gland is a good environment for bacteria to thrive.

Signs and Symptoms

With acute bacterial prostatitis, symptoms may be rather dramatic: a spiking fever, chills, sweating, cloudy urine, and lower back pain. There may be pain behind the scrotum, pain in the testicles, and pain with urination or bowel movements. You may be unable to urinate and empty the bladder, or you may feel the need to urinate frequently. Urine may contain blood or smell bad, and ejaculation may be painful.

The symptoms of chronic bacterial prostatitis and nonbacterial prostatitis tend to develop more slowly. While not as severe as acute bacterial prostatitis, they are definitely worrisome. Among the many possible symptoms are pain or burning during urination, mild lower back pain, aching sensation in the middle to lower abdomen, pain in the penis and scrotum, frequent urination, blood in the semen, low-grade fever, and painful ejaculation. In chronic bacterial prostatitis, there are bacteria in the urine or in the fluid from the prostate. There are no detectable bacteria in nonbacterial prostatitis.

A Quick Guide to Symptoms

Acute bacterial prostatitis
- [ ] Spiking fever
- [ ] Chills
- [ ] Sweating
- [ ] Cloudy, bloody, or foul-smelling urine
- [ ] Pain in the lower back, behind the scrotum, or in the testicles
- [ ] Pain with urination or bowel movements
- [ ] Inability to urinate and empty the bladder, or the need to urinate frequently
- [ ] Painful ejaculation

Chronic bacterial prostatitis
- [ ] Pain or burning during urination
- [ ] Lower back pain
- [ ] Aching sensation in the middle to lower abdomen
- [ ] Pain in the penis and scrotum
- [ ] Frequent urination
- [ ] Blood in the semen
- [ ] Low-grade fever
- [ ] Painful ejaculation

Conventional Treatments

Treatments vary according to the type of prostatitis. Prostatitis does not always respond well to treatments, so a number of different options may be needed.

Medications

Though it may make you quite ill, acute bacterial prostatitis is the easiest form of prostatitis to treat. Depending upon the type of bacteria that is found, your doctor will prescribe an antibiotic. You'll likely also get an antibiotic for chronic bacterial prostatitis, and you will probably take it for a longer period of time.

In general, antibiotics that penetrate the prostate are preferred. Typically, they are prescribed for 4 weeks. These antibiotics include the fluoroquinolones, such as ciprofloxacin and levofloxacin. In addition, trimethoprim-sulfamethoxazole has been found to be effective for treating chronic bacterial prostatitis.

Further, some doctors prescribe antibiotics for their patients with nonbacterial prostatitis. And in certain cases, it does help with the symptoms, although it is not known why this occurs.

If an obstruction in the urinary tract is causing you to have difficulty with urination, your doctor may prescribe an alpha-blocker such as terazosin. This medication relaxes the prostate and bladder neck, which improves the flow of urine. Since the urine will flow more easily, you may not need to urinate as often during the night. If you are experiencing pain during bowel movements, a stool softener such as Colace may be advised.

To help you cope with discomfort and pain, your doctor may recommend a pain reliever. Since you may be taking it over an extended period of time, be sure to review potential side effects.

Physical Therapy

The symptoms of prostatitis may be relieved by learning how to stretch and relax the lower pelvic muscles. A physical therapist may teach you specific exercises as well as ways to heat muscles, thereby making them more limber. In addition, a physical therapist may provide instruction in the use of biofeedback to relax muscles.

Surgery

If you have ongoing pain and complications from chronic bacterial prostatitis, surgery to remove part of the prostate gland may be an option. For the surgery, which is known as a transurethral resection of the prostate (TURP), you will either be under general anesthesia or be anesthetized from the waist down. The surgeon inserts a narrow instrument known as a resectoscope into the urethra. The resectoscope has an electrical loop that may be used to remove prostate tissue and seal blood vessels. Potential complications from TURP include blood in the urine, a sense of urgency to urinate, short-term difficulty controlling urine, and problems with sexual function. Some men develop retrograde or dry ejaculation. In this condition, part of the semen goes backward into the bladder.

If you have an obstruction to the bladder neck, it may be relieved with surgery. The surgery usually is successful in increasing the rate of urine flow.

Warm Baths

Many men find that sitting in a warm tub or sitz bath relieves pain and relaxes muscles. Consider making time for regular warm baths.

Complementary Treatments

Herbal remedies and nutritional supplements may help boost recovery from infection.

Therapies and lifestyle changes that strengthen the immune system may be effective in controlling prostatitis.

Diet

Increase your intake of fluids, which will cause you to urinate more often and flush bacteria from the bladder. Studies have shown that zinc deficiency may lead to prostate problems. Zinc may be found in pumpkin and sunflower seeds, so try to include them in your diet.

Avoid foods that tend to irritate the bladder, such as hot or spicy foods and citrus juices. Also, stay away from foods and supplements containing caffeine. Since sugar impairs the ability of white blood cells to kill bacteria and alcohol robs the body of zinc, avoid both sugar and alcohol.

Herbal Medicine

Goldenseal. Goldenseal is an herb with antiseptic and diuretic properties. Although effective in fighting infection, it should be used only for short periods of time. The body may build up an immunity to it, and in higher doses it may be irritating to the throat, mouth, and skin and cause diarrhea and nausea. Goldenseal contains the alkaloid berberine, its most extensively researched constituent. In capsule form, goldenseal may contain 0.5 percent to 6 percent berberine. As dosage may vary depending upon the percentage of berberine in the bottle, take as directed on the label. In tincture form, the daily dose is 4 to 6 milliliters.

Pygeum and stinging nettle. Along with saw palmetto, pygeum and stinging nettle are diuretics, which increase the secretion and flow of urine and reduce irritation of the bladder and urethra. Pygeum, in particular, has been shown to aid males who have trouble initiating urination, and it also supports the complete emptying of the bladder. The typical recommended daily dose for pygeum is 50 milligrams twice a day of extract standardized to 13 percent total sterols. For stinging nettle, the recommended daily dose is 250 milligrams of nettle root twice a day. Both herbs are available in tincture form.

Saw palmetto. Clinical studies have shown saw palmetto to be useful for the relief of symptoms of an inflamed prostate. Saw palmetto is available in capsules containing 160 milligrams of extract standardized to 85 to 95 percent fatty acids and sterols. The typical recommended dose is 320 milligrams. Though you may notice symptom relief within 30 days, you should continue to take the supplement.

Nutritional Supplements

Nutritional supplements are beneficial in shrinking an inflamed prostate.

- Omega-3 fatty acids: 1 tablespoon of flaxseed oil or fish oil capsules as directed on the label. May prevent the prostate from swelling.

- Zinc: 30 milligrams daily. Effective in shrinking an inflamed prostate and enhancing the immune system.

Lifestyle Recommendations

Limit your evening beverage intake. While you should drink a good deal of water during the day, reduce the amount of water you drink in the evening to lessen your need to urinate while you sleep.

Practice yoga. The gentle movement and postures of yoga may increase circulation to the groin area and ease prostate problems.

Preventive Measures

Begin walking. Walking is the most effective exercise for relieving prostatitis. Avoid bicycling, running, rowing, or any other activity that puts pressure on the groin area.

Maintain a healthy cholesterol level. High cholesterol has been linked to prostate problems.

Practice good genital hygiene. Especially if you are uncircumcised, you must keep yourself clean. Also, after a bowel movement, wash your hands before touching your penis. This will reduce the chance of spreading *E. coli* organisms from the rectal area to the genitourinary tract, lessening the likelihood of developing prostatitis.

Engage in safer sex. If you are not in a committed long-term relationship, use a condom during sexual intercourse. This will decrease the risk for sexually transmitted diseases and prostatitis.

Treat urinary infections. Do not delay treatment for a potential urinary infection. And be sure to take the full course of medication recommended by your doctor.

Rosacea

With rosacea, the facial skin becomes inflamed and tends to redden and flush. The facial blood vessels remain dilated, and your face may have small, red, pus-filled bumps or pustules. Though rosacea is often referred to as adult acne or acne rosacea, it actually has little in common with the acne that affects teens.

Rosacea is not infectious. There is no evidence that it spreads from one person to another. Still, when untreated, rosacea tends to worsen over time. In most people, it is cyclic. It appears for a period of time and then goes away until there is a flare-up.

Rosacea is quite common. An estimated 13 million Americans have this skin condition.

Causes and Risk Factors

While the exact cause of rosacea is unknown, there are a few theories. One view is that rosacea is related to a blood vessel disorder. Another hypothesis is that it is associated with an infection of the stomach caused by *Helicobacter pylori*. Other possible causes include microscopic skin mites (demodex), a malfunction of connective tissue under the skin, and a fungus. Some believe that it has a psychological derivation. The cause may be a combination of factors.

Since there is a strong hereditary component to rosacea, individuals who have a relative with this disorder are at greater risk. In addition, in the United States, those who are of Irish, English, Scandinavian, Scottish, Welsh, or Eastern European descent have an increased risk. Rosacea tends to affect those with fair skin who are between the ages of 30 and 60, and it is usually more severe in men.

Signs and Symptoms

Normally, rosacea appears in different phases. During the earliest stages, you may blush more easily. Then, there may be redness in the center of the face, especially the nose. The redness is caused by the dilation of blood vessels that are close to the surface of the skin. This phase of the disorder is called prerosacea.

As the disorder progresses, you may develop vascular rosacea. With this, small blood vessels on your cheeks and nose become visible. In some instances, the skin may be dry and sensitive. In other cases, it may be oily, and you may have dandruff. With time, you may have red bumps or pustules across the nose, cheeks, forehead, and chin. This condition is called inflammatory rosacea. In the worst cases, the oil or sebaceous glands in your nose and/or cheeks may enlarge and result in a buildup of tissue on and around the nose. This complication, which is called rhinophyma, occurs far more often in men than it does in women.

About half of those with rosacea experience a burning and gritty feeling in the eyes, known as ocular rosacea. And rosacea may cause an inflammation or scaling of the inner skin of the eyelids, which is called conjunctivitis.

Conventional Treatments

There is no cure for rosacea. Nevertheless, there are a number of helpful treatments. Generally, more than one treatment is required.

Antibiotics

For mild cases of rosacea, your doctor may prescribe a topical antibiotic cream, such as metronidazole. It is applied directly to the skin. If you appear to have a more difficult case of rosacea, you may get a prescription for an oral antibiotic, such as tetracycline, minocycline, doxycycline, or erythromycin. Antibiotics are quite useful for treating the papules and pustules, but less useful for the redness and flushing. In some cases, both topical and oral antibiotics are called for. Frequently, after you have completed taking the oral antibiotics, you will be asked to use a topical antibiotic once each day, which may prevent future flare-ups.

Glycolic Acid Peel

To accelerate the rate of healing, you may receive a glycolic acid peel along with antibiotics. Peels, which take only 3 to 5 minutes, may be performed every 2 to 4 weeks. After the procedure, your skin will be red for several hours. During this time, you should not use makeup. The peels may be combined with

A Quick Guide to Symptoms

- ☐ **Redness in the center of the face, especially the nose**
- ☐ **Dry, sensitive skin or oily skin with dandruff**
- ☐ **Red bumps or pustules across the nose, cheeks, forehead, and chin**
- ☐ **Rhinophyma (a buildup of tissue on and around the nose)**
- ☐ **Burning and gritty feeling in the eyes**
- ☐ **Conjunctivitis**

glycolic acid washes and topical creams.

Laser Therapy

Laser therapy, which reduces redness and removes visible blood vessels, may be a valuable tool in the treatment of rosacea. Normally, you will require at least three treatments. Though the removed vessels do not reappear, after treatment new vessels may emerge. Laser therapy may also be used to slow the buildup of excess tissue or to remove unwanted tissue.

Other Treatments

If you have a severe case of rosacea, you may receive a prescription for isotretinoin (Accutane), which inhibits the production of oil by the sebaceous glands. However, there may be serious side effects from isotretinoin, so you will need to be carefully monitored. Eye problems from rosacea are treated with oral antibiotics, especially tetracycline and doxy-cycline. You may be asked to practice eyelid hygiene with an over-the-counter eyelid cleaner and warm compresses. When the eyes are severely affected, steroid eye drops may be used.

Complementary Treatments

In order to find the best treatment, people with rosacea should be individually assessed. However, dietary changes, supplementation with certain vitamins and minerals, strength-ening of the immune system, and herbal rem-edies taken internally and/or used topically may be helpful in eliminating or reducing the symptoms and flare-ups of rosacea.

Acupuncture

By toning the meridian of the liver and elimi-nating waste material from the body, acu-puncture is effective in the treatment of certain skin conditions such as rosacea. The accumulation of waste material in the body may irritate the skin, causing inflammation and flare-ups of rosacea.

Diet

The diet plays an important role in the condi-tion of the skin. It is essential to eat a diet high in nutrients, consisting of fruits, vegeta-bles, and whole grains. Try to include a mini-mum of five servings of vegetables, four servings of fruit, and six servings of whole grains each day. Since it may reduce the inflammation, the magnesium found in dark green, leafy vegetables is especially useful for this condition. These vegetables also contain other nutrients beneficial to the health of the skin. Juicing is an easy way to obtain a sub-stantial amount of these vegetables in your system every day. Since less digestive break-down is required, juices allow the body to begin absorbing the nutrients immediately.

Food allergies, low stomach acid, and a low level of digestive enzymes, particularly pancreatic enzymes, may contribute to rosa-cea flare-ups. In the area of food, an allergy or intolerance to yeast is a likely culprit. See a doctor who can evaluate your particular situation. People with low stomach acid have trouble absorbing nutrients. Your body will better absorb nutrients if your diet is health-ier. It's possible that low stomach acid allows more toxins into the body, which may cause a rosacea flare-up.

As saturated fat causes inflammation, sat-urated fats such as fried and processed foods should be eliminated. Saturated fats and trans fatty acids are also difficult to digest. People with rosacea who also have digestive problems should be particularly vigilant in avoiding saturated fat. If you eat meat, con-sume only the leanest cuts.

Because it supplies the essential fatty acids necessary for healthy skin, flaxseed oil is use-ful for people with rosacea. Take 1 teaspoon daily.

Naturopathy

By identifying food intolerances through an elimination diet, strengthening the immune system, assessing nutritional deficiencies, and making dietary and nutritional supplementation recommendations, naturopathic physicians have been successful in treating rosacea. Lifestyle factors may also be addressed.

A naturopath may prescribe azelaic acid cream, which should be applied topically. Azelaic acid is a natural substance found in barley, rye, and wheat. Preliminary studies have shown it to be useful in mild to moderate cases of rosacea. Since studies have shown that people with rosacea produce less of the digestive enzyme lipase, naturopathic physicians may further address the need for lipase.

Nutritional Supplements

The following nutrients protect against free radicals, support the immune system, and are beneficial for maintaining healthy skin.

- Vitamin A: 10,000 IU daily. Beneficial for healing and the development of new skin tissue.

- B-complex vitamins: Take as directed on the label. Antistress vitamins that help reduce anxiety, which can aggravate rosacea flare-ups.

- Vitamin C: 1,000 milligrams daily in divided doses of 500 milligrams. Supports the immune system as well as the capillaries.

- Vitamin E: 400 IU daily. Antioxidant that protects against free radicals and helps strengthen the immune system.

- Essential fatty acids—omega-3 (flaxseed and fish oil) and omega-6 (borage, evening primrose, and black currant seed oils): Available in oil and capsule form. Take as directed on the labels. Help maintain healthy skin.

- Evening primrose oil: 3,000 milligrams daily in divided doses of 1,000 milligrams each to provide 240 milligrams of GLA (gamma-linolenic acid). Helps heal skin tissue.

Lifestyle Recommendations

Avoid triggers. Trigger factors vary from person to person. While avoiding trigger factors

Other Supplements to Consider

When low stomach acid is addressed, rosacea symptoms and flare-ups may greatly improve. Hydrochloric acid capsules are the recommended treatment for people with low stomach acid. Before taking these capsules, you will need a gastric analysis. The unsupervised dosing and use of hydrochloric acid supplementation could cause an ulcer. It has been found that taking acidophilus (healthy bacteria) capsules along with the hydrochloric acid is especially effective.

Pancreatic digestive enzymes have also been found to be useful in reducing symptoms and rosacea flare-ups. Some studies have shown that individuals with rosacea produce less pancreatic lipase, a digestive enzyme. In order to determine if you are, in fact, low in pancreatic lipase, consult with your doctor before taking digestive enzyme supplementation.

will not prevent rosacea, if you are able to identify your trigger factors, you may help mitigate the symptoms and reduce the probability of a flare-up. The following are some of the reported trigger factors: heated beverages, hot baths, alcohol, spicy foods, heavy exercise, corticosteroids, drugs that dilate the blood vessels, caffeine withdrawal, emotional stress, sun exposure, hot or cold weather, wind, and some skin care products.

Be gentle with your skin. Use a mild soap or cleanser to wash your skin and stay away from grainy or abrasive products. Ask your doctor for suggestions. While you can use a soft pad or washcloth, you should not use rough products such as sponges or brushes. After you wash your skin, dry it with a soft towel. Before applying topical medication, allow your skin several minutes to dry. Further, give your skin 5 to 10 minutes to absorb the antibiotic ointment before applying other skin care products.

Don't be discouraged. Rosacea responds slowly to treatment. It may take a few months before you see significant improvement.

Drink water. Drinking plenty of purified water helps remove excess waste products from the body and reduces the buildup of toxins. Drink at least 8 glasses of water per day.

Keep a food journal. To determine which foods may be triggering a rosacea flare-up, keep a food diary. Eliminating the offending foods may greatly improve your condition.

Limit your alcohol consumption. While alcohol may not be the cause of rosacea, since it causes the blood vessels to dilate, it may definitely have an effect on the reddening of the skin.

Stop smoking. Because nicotine constricts blood vessels and deprives the skin of necessary nutrients and oxygen, smoking can irritate this condition.

Use sunscreen. If you have rosacea, it is particularly important for you to use a sunscreen that protects against ultraviolet rays (both UVA and UVB). It should have an SPF of 15 or higher. Remember to use it every day and in all types of weather.

Preventive Measures

There is no proven method to prevent rosacea. If rosacea runs in your family, you may want to be periodically checked. Your treatments will be most effective if they begin early in the progression of the disease.

Excess stress and worry may lead to digestive imbalance, which may be a cause of rosacea. It is important to find some way to reduce the stress in your life. Regular exercise in moderation and the practice of yoga, tai chi, and qigong are all beneficial. Deep breathing exercises, meditation, or simply finding the time to be alone and quiet are all good ways to unwind and reduce stress.

Shingles

If you had chickenpox as a kid, the virus that caused that itchy, unpleasant disease could revisit you in your later years. Only this time, what happens is a lot worse than chickenpox. The virus (varicella zoster) causes shingles, also known as herpes zoster, which begins with pain and tingling in the trunk area of the body. This early period, which is known as prodrome, may be accompanied by flulike symptoms. Though it may sometimes take longer, normally within a few days there will be blisters. The disorder is then called active shingles.

Shingles are very common. At some point, about 20 percent of the population who previously had chickenpox is affected. In those who live until the age of 80, about 50 percent will deal with a bout of shingles. It is estimated that each year about 1 million Americans become ill with this disorder.

In some people, shingles may involve the nerves in the face and ears. This is called Ramsey Hunt syndrome or herpes zoster oticus. There may be severe pain, facial paralysis, loss of taste, dizziness, hearing loss, and mild inflammation of the brain. While most of the symptoms pass, the facial paralysis may be permanent. If shingles affects the eye, the cornea may become infected, which may cause temporary or permanent blindness.

Shingles may lead to a complication, known as postherpetic neuralgia (PHN), which is pain that continues for more than a month. It is most likely to occur in those who had shingles with many blisters and severe pain. If you have PHN, you no longer have shingles. However, shingles damaged your nervous system, which is now sending exaggerated pain messages to the brain. When PHN occurs, it tends to take one of three forms. It may result in continuous burning or aching pain, you may have periodic intense pain, or you may have pain from very light stimulation, such as the touch of clothing.

PHN is usually worse at night, and it may be affected by temperature changes. The pain may even extend beyond the area in which you had blisters. About 200,000 Americans have PHN, and approximately 25 percent of people over the age of 50 who have shingles will develop it. The older you are, the longer the PHN will tend to last, but most cases resolve within a year.

> **Doctors sometimes refer** to the three syndromes associated with shingles (prodrome, active shingles, and PHN) with a single term, *zoster-associated pain (ZAP)*.

Causes and Risk Factors

If you never had chickenpox, you cannot develop shingles. But anyone who has had chickenpox is considered at risk. When you had chickenpox, it was not completely destroyed by the immune system. The leftover virus entered the nervous system and remained latent near the spinal cord. Many years or decades later, some trigger causes the virus to reemerge and travel along nerve pathways to the skin. The vast majority of cases of shingles occur in people over the age of 50.

People with weakened immune systems from illness, age, stress, and medications (such as chemotherapy or immunosuppressant drugs) are most vulnerable. A small percentage of those who have shingles, between 1 percent and 5 percent, may experience a recurrence. Shingles tends to recur in those who have compromised immune systems. The seriousness of shingles in people with compromised immune systems should not be minimized—it may be a life-threatening illness.

Avoid Spreading the Infection

During an outbreak of shingles, the shingles lesions in your skin contain virus particles. As a result, you can spread chickenpox to someone who has never had the disease. On the other hand, if you are in contact with someone who has already had chickenpox, you cannot give that person shingles. If you have shingles, you should avoid the following people.

☐ **Newborns (who have immature immune systems)**
☐ **Pregnant women (you may harm the fetus)**
☐ **Any person who has not had chickenpox or who has a compromised immune system**

Signs and Symptoms

Shingles begins with pain, burning, tingling, and/or itching in a localized area of the body, most often the trunk. There may also be headache, fever, stomach upset, and muscle aches. Most often, within 1 to 3 days, a painful rash with reddish bumps and blisters appears. The rash spreads and becomes fluid-filled. It is similar to the rash you had with chickenpox, but you will have more pain and less itching. The rash tends to wrap around the middle of your body, following the nerve distribution. However, the rash and blisters may appear on the face, scalp, around one eye, inside the mouth, or down an arm or leg. Usually, shingles is limited to a relatively small area on one side of the body.

After 2 to 3 weeks, scabs cover the rash. During this time, you may have a good deal of discomfort. Fortunately, most cases of shingles heal within a month. However, after the scabs fall off, you may notice changes in the color of your skin. In the more difficult cases, the color changes may remain.

Conventional Treatments

There are a number of preliminary treatments that you may try to relieve discomfort. You may soak in cool baths or place cold compresses that have been soaked in Burrow's solution (an over-the-counter preparation that relieves itching) on the blisters. Take care not to break the blisters, which could cause infection. Avoid warm treatments, as they may intensify the itching. You might also try taking an oatmeal bath or using a topical antihistamine, such as Benadryl.

Medications

Antidepressants. If you have severe pain from shingles or PHN, you may require prescription medication. Tricyclic antidepressants are used for the related pain and depression. Examples of these are amitriptyline (Elavil, Endep), desipramine (Norpramin), and nortriptyline (Pamelor, Aventyl). It may take several weeks before you feel the full effects. Potential side effects include blurred vision, dry mouth, difficulty with urination, dizziness, disturbances in heart rhythm, and constipation. When moving from a sitting to standing position, the medications may cause a sudden drop in blood pressure, which could make you feel faint.

Anti-epileptic drugs. Anti-epileptic drugs are used for people with PHN who experience episodes of severe pain. Examples are gabapentin (Neurontin), carbamazepine (Tegretol), valproic acid (Depakene, Depakote), and phenytoin (Dilantin). Potential side effects include headache, increased risk for infection, sleepiness, and upset stomach. When the drug levels are at their highest, some people have ringing in the ears, agitation, visual disturbances, and odd movements.

Antivirals. You will probably be given medication to fight the viral infection. The nucleoside analogues, which block viral production, are the most effective drugs for varicella zoster. Acyclovir (Zovirax), famciclovir (Famvir), and valacyclovir (Valtrex)

If you suspect shingles around an eye, you should see your doctor immediately. Without treatment, shingles may damage your vision or lead to a case of glaucoma later in life.

have been approved for shingles. Each is taken for 7 days. If you are able to begin taking these medications within 72 hours of the onset of shingles, they may markedly reduce symptoms and lower the risk of developing PHN. While these medications appear to be well tolerated, potential side effects include nausea, vomiting, headache, fatigue, rash, tremor, and (in rare instances) seizure.

Pain medications. To deal with the pain, you may wish to try capsaicin ointment (Zostrix), which contains an active ingredient from hot chili peppers. But this ointment may not be used until the blisters have dried and fallen off. Apply with a gloved hand three or four times each day. Initially, you will feel a burning sensation, but it will subside. You

A Quick Guide to Symptoms

☐ Pain, burning, tingling, or itching in a localized area of the body, most often the trunk

☐ Painful rash with reddish bumps and blisters

☐ The rash and blisters may appear on the face, scalp, around one eye, inside the mouth, or down an arm or leg may also want to take acetaminophen (Tylenol) or ibuprofen (Motrin).

If pain fails to respond to these medications, your doctor my prescribe opioids, such as oxycodone. Since there is the potential for addiction, oxycodone should be carefully monitored. Or, you may be given an injection of an anesthetic or steroid to block the nerves. Other pain-relieving options include a patch that contains the anesthetic lidocaine (Lidoderm) and a spray that has a combination of ethyl chloride (Chloroethane) and Fluorimethane, which cools the blood vessels in the skin.

Procedures

Some people with PHN obtain relief from transcutaneous electrical nerve stimulation (TENS) treatments, which suppress pain with low-level electrical pulses. Generally, individuals are given 80 to 100 pulses per second for 45 minutes, three times a day. Another procedure known as iontophoresis uses direct electrical current to deliver ions of medication through the skin. Laser therapy has also been used for PHN. Because it carries a high risk for permanent damage, surgery on the brain or spinal cord to reduce pain is used only as a last resort and only for intolerable pain.

Complementary Treatments
Acupuncture

Acupuncture may accelerate the healing process, cool the body, and aid in the reduction of pain. To locate an acupuncturist in your area,

visit the Web site of the National Certification Commission for Acupuncture and Oriental Medicine (NCCAOM) at www.nccaom.org.

Diet

Eating a diet full of whole grains, legumes, and fresh fruits and vegetables is beneficial in recovering from shingles. Try to include a minimum of five servings of vegetables, four servings of fruit, and six servings of whole grains each day. Whole grains, legumes, eggs, and fish contain B vitamins that help protect nerve endings. Fruits and vegetables contain vitamins A and C, which aid in the healing of skin lesions. Foods high in vitamin A are apricots, cantaloupes, carrots, mangoes, pumpkin, romaine lettuce, spinach, and sweet potatoes. Vitamin C may be found in apricots, broccoli, cabbage, cantaloupes, kiwifruit, oranges, pineapple, plums, spinach, tomatoes, and watermelon.

Calcium and magnesium are also beneficial to nerve health. They may be found in green, leafy vegetables. Lysine is an amino acid that may actually prevent the virus from replicating. It is also useful in reducing the severity of a shingles outbreak and speeds the recovery process. Lysine may be found in nonfat dairy products such as yogurt.

Herbal Medicine

A number of herbal remedies may be valuable in treating shingles.

Chamomile and valerian root. When taken as a tea at bedtime, chamomile and valerian root may promote a restful night of sleep.

These teas are available at health food stores. Follow the directions on the package.

Lemon balm. Lemon balm may have an antiviral effect. It should be applied to the affected area several times a day with a cotton ball. Steep 2 teaspoons of the dried leaf of lemon balm per cup of boiling water.

Licorice. Licorice is an immune booster as well as an antiviral herb. If you do not have high blood pressure, you may drink it as a tea up to three times a day. (Those with high blood pressure should avoid it.) There is also a licorice gel that may be applied to the affected area to fight the infection.

Homeopathy

Homeopathy has been shown to be effective for the pain associated with shingles, and it aids in the recovery process. While homeopathic remedies are not harmful and may be used for self-treatment, to ensure that you are using the remedy and dose best suited for your symptoms, you may wish to seek the advice of a homeopathic practitioner. The remedy chosen should most closely match your symptoms, and dosing may range from taking a remedy several times an hour to a couple of times each day. With the appropriate homeopathic remedy, your recovery may progress faster. To find a practitioner trained in homeopathy, visit the Web site of the National Center for Homeopathy at www.homeopathic.org.

Hydrotherapy

In the early stages of a shingles outbreak, cool down the area with ice. Apply ice for 5 minutes and then remove it for 5 minutes. Repeat this procedure two more times and then again every few hours. The cold from the ice confuses the nerves and helps break the pain cycle. If you are unable to tolerate the ice, try a cold compress. Soak a washcloth in very cold water, squeeze out the excess water, and apply directly to the affected area until the washcloth feels warm. Repeat this throughout the day. Soaking in a lukewarm bath for 20 to 30 minutes is also a way to calm the nervous system.

Naturopathy

Since they provide dietary, nutritional supplement, herbal, and homeopathic recommendations, naturopathic physicians may be a valuable resource when dealing with shingles. To find a naturopathic practitioner in your area, contact the American Association of Naturopathic Physicians at www.naturopathic.org.

Nutritional Supplements

Complications of shingles generally occur in people with weakened immune systems, so supplements that boost the immune system and protect the nerves are essential in combating a shingles outbreak.

- Multivitamin/mineral: Take as directed on the label. Should include calcium, magnesium, and vitamin D.

- B-complex vitamins: Take as directed on the label. Essential for nerve function.

- Vitamin B_{12}: Injections or 1,000-microgram sublingual tablet daily. Useful in preventing nerve damage. Injections are recommended. If not, sublingual tablets.

- Vitamin C: 2,000 milligrams daily in divided doses of 500 milligrams each. Acts as an antiviral agent, destroying the herpes virus.

- Vitamin E: 400 IU daily. Helps prevent scar tissue from forming.

- Beta-carotene: 25,000 IU daily. Protects against infection.

- Lysine: 1,000 milligrams daily in divided doses of 500 milligrams. Symptoms, severity, and duration of outbreak may be greatly reduced when taken at onset.

- Zinc: 30 milligrams daily. Antioxidant that boosts the immune system.

Lifestyle Recommendations

Avoid heat. Because they become more irritated with heat, keep blisters cool. Keep your baths lukewarm.

Consider visiting several doctors. If you have a debilitating case of shingles or if you are left with PHN, you may benefit from visits with a pain specialist and/or a psychiatrist.

Reduce stress. Excess stress has been known to trigger an outbreak of shingles as well as increase the severity of an outbreak. Stress impairs the immune system and prevents it from fighting off illness. Try a number of stress-reduction techniques, such as deep breathing exercises, meditation, guided imagery, or visualization. Yoga, tai chi, and qigong are movement exercises that may calm the mind and reduce stress.

Take an oatmeal bath. Taking a lukewarm bath with colloidal oatmeal right before bedtime may enable you to feel more comfortable and help you to sleep. Colloidal oatmeal is available at your local pharmacy.

Wear loose clothing. You will feel more comfortable if your clothing does not rub against the area of pain and blisters.

Preventive Measures

Get a vaccine. In 2006, the FDA approved the shingles vaccine known as Zostavax for people 60 years and older. Studies have shown that the vaccine can prevent shingles in about half the people vaccinated. About 20 percent of individuals who have had chickenpox will develop shingles during their lifetime. Speak to your physician to see if you are able to receive the vaccine.

Sleep Apnea

In sleep apnea, there are brief breathing interruptions, usually greater than 10 seconds, during sleep. In some instances, these interruptions (called involuntary breathing pauses or apneic events) may occur 20 to 30 times per hour. Though it is possible to have sleep apnea without snoring, usually there is snoring between the breathing interruptions. There may also be choking. Because the sleep pattern is so interrupted, people with sleep apnea are unable to obtain sufficient amounts of deep, restorative sleep. They tend to have morning headaches and excessive daytime sleepiness.

Sleep apnea is very common. It may affect as many as 12 to 25 million Americans, but only about 1 million are aware that they have this disorder.

Because there are sudden drops in blood oxygen levels, sleep apnea is viewed as a serious medical problem. It strains the cardiovascular system. About half of those with this disorder develop high blood pressure, which increases the risk for heart failure and stroke. Sleep apnea has also been associated with diabetes, gastroesophageal reflux disease (GERD), kidney failure, peripheral nerve damage, and eye disorders. And people dealing with sleep apnea are often depressed.

According to a study completed at Yale University and published in the *New England Journal of Medicine*, sleep apnea may lead to stroke. The study found that in participants over the age of 50, obstructive sleep apnea more than doubles the risk of stroke or death. Further, severe cases of sleep apnea may triple the risk for stroke or death.

Causes and Risk Factors

There are two types of sleep apnea, each with a different cause. With obstructive sleep apnea, the more common form, while you are sleeping, the muscles in the walls of the throat (pharynx) relax and impede the flow of air. As seconds pass and there is no exchange of air, you enter a lighter level of sleep. The muscles regain their muscle tone, and then you breathe. Many people with this form of sleep apnea are unaware that they have a problem.

With central sleep apnea, the brain sends

A Quick Guide to Symptoms

- ☐ Episodes of stopped breathing during the night
- ☐ Severe daytime sleepiness
- ☐ Awakening with a dry mouth or throat
- ☐ Irritability
- ☐ Problems with concentration and memory
- ☐ Depression
- ☐ Frequent nighttime urination
- ☐ Heartburn
- ☐ Impotence
- ☐ Morning headaches
- ☐ Snoring

improper signals to the throat muscles that are involved with breathing. When breathing is interrupted, the amount of carbon dioxide in your blood rises, which may cause you to

Because of their breathing disorder, people with sleep apnea have increased risks when undergoing major surgery. If you have sleep apnea, be sure to share this information with your surgeon.

awaken. If you have central sleep apnea, you are more likely to be aware that you have a problem.

A number of factors place you at greater risk for sleep apnea. Most cases occur in people between the ages of 40 and 70. Men have a greater risk than women. Other factors that increase risk include excess weight, especially around the neck; enlarged tonsils or adenoids; physical abnormality in the nose; a narrow throat; use of alcohol, sedatives, or tranquilizers; an overbite; receding chin; larger tongue; long lower part of the face; narrow upper jaw; soft palate in the throat; and a family history of the disorder. Smokers and alcohol users have higher rates, and African Americans appear to have the highest risk of any ethnic group.

Signs and Symptoms

Though many people with sleep apnea are unaware they have a problem, the disorder is associated with a number of symptoms. These include severe daytime sleepiness, episodes of breathing stoppage during the night, awakening with a dry mouth or throat, irritability, problems with concentration and memory, depression, frequent nighttime urination, heartburn, impotence, and morning headaches. Sleep apnea may be present with or without snoring.

Conventional Treatments

Your doctor will recommend that you stop sleeping on your back. If you are overweight, you should also lose excess weight. In some instances, the change in position and weight loss will be sufficient to correct the sleep apnea. You will also be told to avoid alcohol, tobacco, and sleep medications. However, you may need to consider additional options.

Devices and Machines

Your dentist can fit you with a device that brings your jaw forward. Called a mandibular advancement device (MAD), it opens your throat and may relieve mild cases of apnea. Potential MAD side effects include pain, dry lips, tooth discomfort, and excessive salivation.

For moderate or severe cases of sleep apnea, you might use a nasal continuous positive airway pressure (nCPAP) system. With an nCPAP, a machine delivers air through a mask that is placed over your nose. The pressure keeps your airway passages open. In some instances, you will be asked to use a humidifier with your nCPAP. While some people find the systems to be cumbersome and the mask claustrophobic, they often bring dramatic improvements in symptoms. Potential side effects include irritation in the nose and throat and over the bridge of the nose, upper respiratory infections, eye irritation or conjunctivitis, and mild chest muscle discomfort. Rare side effects include heart rhythm disorders, severe nosebleeds, and air pockets in the skull.

Clinical studies have demonstrated that nCPAP may improve sleep quality and reduce both daytime sleepiness and cognitive impairment (caused by obstructive sleep apnea). In a few studies, nCPAP has also reduced blood pressure in people with both normal and high blood pressure who have obstructive sleep apnea.

If you are having trouble tolerating an nCPAP, your doctor may recommend a bilevel positive airway pressure (BiPAP) device. It reduces the air pressure when a person exhales and appears to be more comfortable than the nCPAP. However, it tends to be significantly more expensive than nCPAP.

Surgery

Uvulopalatopharyngoplasty (UPPP) is the most common surgical procedure used to treat sleep apnea and snoring. During UPPP, tissue is removed from the top of the throat and the rear of the mouth. Normally, the tonsils and adenoids are also removed. However, tissue that is farther down the throat may continue to block your air passage. This sur-

Self-Testing

If you suspect that you have sleep apnea, you should evaluate yourself with the following Epworth Sleepiness Scale. Rate the following eight activities from 0 to 3. A "0" means that you would never doze; "1" means that there is a slight chance you would doze; "2" indicates that there is a moderate chance you would doze; and a "3" means that there is a high chance you may doze. If you score 9 or more, you should visit your doctor.

1. Sitting and reading
2. Watching TV
3. Sitting inactive in a public place
4. Sitting as a passenger in a car for an hour without a break
5. Lying down to rest in the afternoon
6. Sitting and talking to someone
7. Sitting quietly after a lunch without alcohol
8. Sitting in a car while stopped for a few minutes in traffic

Also, consider keeping a sleep journal. Every morning, record how you slept and how you are feeling. Share the journal with your doctor.

gical procedure requires a general anesthetic. After surgery, expect a severe sore throat, and you will only be able to eat soft foods until you heal. Allow yourself about a month to recover fully. Frequent complications include impaired sense of smell, swallowing problems, mucus in the throat, infection, reduced functioning of the soft palate and throat muscles, and regurgitation of fluids through the mouth or nose.

Depending upon what your doctor finds, you may have surgery to remove nasal polyps or to align the partition between your nostrils (a condition known as a deviated nasal septum). You may have surgery to move your tongue and jaw forward or surgery that removes only the tonsils and/or adenoids.

If all previous treatments have failed and if you are experiencing life-threatening sleep apnea, your doctor may advise a tracheostomy. During this procedure, a surgeon creates an opening in your neck and inserts a tube that enables you to breathe. When you are awake, the opening is covered. When you sleep, it is uncovered, thereby allowing air to pass in and out of the lungs.

Complementary Treatments

To reduce and eliminate sleep apnea and its associated symptoms, practitioners of complementary medicine recommend lifestyle and dietary changes.

Acupuncture

Acupuncture has been found to increase serotonin levels in the body. Low levels of serotonin have been linked to sleep apnea. To find a practitioner in your area, contact the National Certification Commission for Acupuncture and Oriental Medicine (NCCAOM) at www.nccaom.org.

Diet

Eating a well-balanced diet that limits the amount of sugar, caffeine, and processed foods may help you maintain a healthy weight, which reduces your risk of developing sleep apnea. Also, calcium, magnesium, and vitamins B_6 and B_{12} are all useful nutrients for their ability to calm the nervous system, which may aid in getting a restful night's sleep. Foods high in calcium and magnesium are tofu, shrimp, almonds, black beans, potatoes, and green leafy vegetables, such as spinach, kale, or broccoli. Meat, fish, and eggs are foods that naturally contain vitamin B_{12}. B_{12} is often added to breakfast cereals as well. Poultry and fish are the best natural sources for vitamin B_6.

Naturopathy

To detect potential food allergies, it may be useful to see a naturopathic physician who may start you on a food elimination diet. These allergies have been linked to blockages in the air passageway. A naturopath may also use other techniques such as homeopathy and nutritional supplementation to treat sleep apnea.

Nutritional Supplements

5-HTP is a precursor to serotonin. To release serotonin and produce a more restful night's sleep, it may be useful to take 100 milligrams of 5-HTP at bedtime. Studies have found it to be useful for sleep apnea and the associated symptoms, such as daytime sleepiness and depression. Serotonin receptors are also responsible for controlling the hormone cortisol, which regulates the muscles needed for breathing.

Lifestyle Recommendations

Avoid alcohol. In addition to relaxing the muscles in the back of the throat, alcohol consumption, especially within 4 to 6 hours of bedtime, may increase the frequency and severity of sleep apnea. It has been found that alcohol is a trigger for sleep apnea, even in individuals who might otherwise only snore.

Avoid tranquilizers and sleeping medications. Since these drugs may relax the muscles in the back of the throat, they can interfere with breathing.

Exhale. When people are awakened from their sleep because they momentarily stop breathing, the initial response is to gasp and inhale quickly. This will only make the condition worse. Instead, try to remember to first sharply exhale and then inhale slowly. Repeat until breathing becomes natural and relaxed.

Gargle before bed. Gargle before bed with warm water and salt. This can help shrink your tonsils.

Keep your nasal passages open when you sleep. Experiment with nasal decongestants, which may help keep nasal passages clear.

Lose excess weight. If you have been carrying excess weight, you may improve your sleep apnea by dropping some pounds. Losing weight tends to relieve the constriction in your throat. Even a small loss may make a big difference.

Raise the head of the bed or mattress. To raise the entire top half of your body, elevate the head of the bed with 4- to 6-inch blocks or a wedge support. Don't attempt to accomplish this goal with pillows, as this will only further interrupt your breathing.

Relax before bed. Before getting into bed, try some relaxation techniques. One way to relax is to lie on your bed without pillows and with your legs and arms spread wide apart. Tilt your head slightly back. Take a long, deep breath through the nose and exhale slowly through the mouth for as long as you can. The exhale should be longer than the inhale. Get into a rhythm and continue until you feel the muscles of your body relax. When you are ready to get under the blankets and use a pillow, turn on your side. Try to maintain this long and relaxed way of breathing as you drift off to sleep.

Try sleeping on your side. When you sleep on your back, your tongue and soft palate lie against the back of your throat, thereby blocking the airway. If you are a back sleeper and need some assistance training yourself to sleep on your side, try placing a thick pillow behind your back after you get into bed and lie on your side. This may prevent you from rolling over onto your back.

Preventive Measures

Live a healthier lifestyle. People who maintain a healthier weight and don't smoke are less likely to develop sleep apnea.

Stop smoking. Smoking may swell the throat tissue and increase mucus buildup, interfering with the ability of air to pass through without obstruction.

Source Notes

INTEGRATIVE MEDICINE: THE BEST OF ALL WORLDS

Kim DH, et al. CT colonography versus colonoscopy for the detection of advanced neoplasia. *New England Journal of Medicine*, October 4, 2007: 1403-1412.

ANGINA

Yeghiazarians Y, et al. Unstable angina pectoris. *New England Journal of Medicine*, January 13, 2000: 101-114.

ATHEROSCLEROSIS

Howard G, et al. Cigarette smoking and progression of atherosclerosis: The Atherosclerosis Risk in Communities (ARIC) Study. *JAMA*, January 14, 1998: 119-124.

BACK PAIN

Brinkhaus B, et al. Acupuncture in patients with chronic low back pain: a randomized controlled trial. *Archives of Internal Medicine*, February 27, 2006: 450-457.

Carragee EJ. Clinical practice. Persistent low back pain. *New England Journal of Medicine*, May 5, 2005: 1891-1898.

Hayden JA, et al. Meta-analysis: exercise therapy for nonspecific low back pain. *Annals of Internal Medicine*, May 3, 2005: 765-775.

CARDIOVASCULAR CONDITIONS

Andersen LF, et al. Consumption of coffee is associated with reduced risk of death attributed to inflammatory and cardiovascular diseases in the Iowa Women's Health Study. *American Journal of Clinical Nutrition*, May 2006: 1039-1046.

Greenberg JA, et al. Caffeinated beverage intake and the risk of heart disease mortality in the elderly: a prospective analysis. *American Journal of Clinical Nutrition*, February 2007: 392-398.

Hansson GK. Inflammation, atherosclerosis, and coronary artery disease. *New England Journal of Medicine*, April 21, 2005: 1685-1695.

Jayadevappa R, et al. Effectiveness of transcendental meditation on functional capacity and quality of life of African Americans with congestive heart failure: a randomized control study. *Ethnicity & Disease*, Winter 2007: 72-77.

Johnsen SP, et al. Intake of fruit and vegetables and the risk of ischemic stroke in a cohort of Danish men and women. *American Journal of Clinical Nutrition*, July 2003: 57-64.

Joshipura KJ, et al. Fruit and vegetable intake in relation to risk of ischemic stroke. *JAMA*, October 6, 1999: 1233-1239.

Joshipura KJ, et al. The effect of fruit and vegetable intake on risk for coronary heart disease. *Annals of Internal Medicine*, June 19, 2001: 1106-1114.

Khatta M, et al. The effect of coenzyme Q_{10} in patients with congestive heart failure. *Annals of Internal Medicine*, April 18, 2000: 636-640.

Lee IM, et al. Relative intensity of physical activity and risk of coronary heart disease. *Circulation*, March 4, 2003: 1110-1116.

Manson JE, et al. Walking compared with vigorous exercise for the prevention of cardiovascular events in women. *New England Journal of Medicine*, September 5, 2002: 716-725.

Mink PJ, et al. Flavonoid intake and cardiovascular disease mortality: a prospective study in postmenopausal women. *American Journal of Clinical Nutrition*, March 2007: 895-909.

Whooley MA. Depression and cardiovascular disease: healing the broken-hearted. *JAMA*, June 28, 2006: 2874-2881.

Wilkinson IB, et al. Oral vitamin C reduces arterial stiffness and platelet aggregation in humans. *Journal of Cardiovascular Pharmacology*, November 1999: 690-693.

Yochum LA, et al. Intake of antioxidant vitamins and risk of death from stroke in postmenopausal women. *American Journal of Clinical Nutrition*, August 2000: 476-483.

CATARACTS

Chasan-Taber L, et al. A prospective study of carotenoid and vitamin A intakes and risk of cataract extraction in US women. *American Journal of Clinical Nutrition*, October 1999: 509-516.

Christen WG, et al. Fruit and vegetable intake and the risk of cataract in women. *American Journal of Clinical Nutrition*, June 2005: 1417-1422.

Hankinson SE, et al. A prospective study of cigarette smoking and risk of cataract surgery in women. *JAMA*, August 26, 1992: 994-998.

Schaumberg DA, et al. Relations of body fat distribution and height with cataract in men. *American Journal of Clinical Nutrition*, December 2000: 1495-1502.

Taylor A, et al. Long-term intake of vitamins and carotenoids and odds of early age-related cortical and posterior subcapsular lens opacities. *American Journal of Clinical Nutrition*, March 2002: 540-549.

Taylor A, et al. Relations among aging, antioxidant status, and cataract. *American Journal of Clinical Nutrition*, December 1995: 1439S-1447S.

Valero MP, et al. Vitamin C is associated with reduced risk of cataract in a Mediterranean population. *Journal of Nutrition,* June 2002: 1299-1306.

CELIAC DISEASE

Catassi C, et al. Risk of non-Hodgkin lymphoma in celiac disease. *JAMA,* March 20, 2002: 1413-1419.

Dahele A, Ghosh S. Vitamin B_{12} deficiency in untreated celiac disease. *American Journal of Gastro-enterology,* March 2001: 745-750.

Murray JA, et al. Effect of a gluten-free diet on gastrointestinal symptoms in celiac disease. *American Journal of Clinical Nutrition*, April 2004: 669-673.

COLON POLYPS

Chan AT, et al. Aspirin and the risk of colorectal cancer in relation to the expression of COX-2. *New England Journal of Medicine,* May 24, 2007: 2131-2142.

Lieberman DA, et al. Risk factors for advanced colonic neoplasia and hyperplastic polyps in asymptomatic individuals. *JAMA*, December 10, 2003: 2959-2967.

DEPRESSION

Eich H, et al. Acupuncture in patients with minor depressive episodes and generalized anxiety. Results of an experimental study. *Fortschritte der Neurologie–Psychiatrie*, March 2000: 137-144.

Rush AJ, et al. Bupropion-SR, sertraline, or venlafaxine-XR after failure of SSRIs for depression. *New England Journal of Medicine*, March 23, 2006: 1231-1242.

DIABETES

Belcaro G, et al. Diabetic ulcers: microcirculatory improvement and faster healing with pycnogenol. *Clinical and Applied Thrombosis/Hemostasis,* July 2006: 318-323.

Hu FB, et al. Walking compared with vigorous physical activity and risk of type 2 diabetes in women: a prospective study. *JAMA*, October 20, 1999: 1433-1439.

Jenkins DJ, et al. Type 2 diabetes and the vegetarian diet. *American Journal of Clinical Nutrition*, September 2003: 610S-616S.

McGinnis RA, et al. Biofeedback-assisted relaxation in type 2 diabetes. *Diabetes Care,* September 2005: 2145-2149.

Meisinger C, et al. Body fat distribution and risk of type 2 diabetes in the general population: are there differences between men and women? The MONICA/KORA Augsburg cohort study. *American Journal of Clinical Nutrition*, September 2006: 483-489.

Meyer KA, et al. Carbohydrates, dietary fiber, and incident type 2 diabetes in older women. *American Journal of Clinical Nutrition*, April 2000: 921-930.

Nathan DM, et al. Intensive diabetes treatment and cardiovascular disease in patients with type 1 diabetes. *New England Journal of Medicine*, December 22, 2005: 2643-2653.

Nissen SE, Wolski K. Effect of rosiglitazone on the risk of myocardial infarction and death from cardiovascular causes. *New England Journal of Medicine,* June 14, 2007: 2457-2471.

Pham AQ, et al. Cinnamon supplementation in patients with type 2 diabetes mellitus. *Pharmacotherapy,* April 2007: 595-599.

Pittas AG, et al. Vitamin D and calcium intake in relation to type 2 diabetes in women. *Diabetes Care*, March 2006: 650-656.

Salmerón J, et al. Dietary fat intake and risk of type 2 diabetes in women. *American Journal of Clinical Nutrition*, June 2001: 1019-1026.

Vuksan V, et al. American ginseng (Panax quinquefolius L) reduces postprandial glycemia in nondiabetic subjects and subjects with type 2 diabetes mellitus. *Archives of Internal Medicine*, April 10, 2000: 1009-1013.

EMPHYSEMA

Fishman A., et al. A randomized trial comparing lung-volume-reduction surgery with medical therapy for severe emphysema. *New England Journal of Medicine,* May 22, 2003: 2059-2073.

Gigliotti F, et al. Breathing retraining and exercise conditioning in patients with chronic obstructive pulmonary disease (COPD). a physiological approach. *Respiratory Medicine*, March 2003: 197-204.

ERECTILE DYSFUNCTION

Aydin S, et al. Acupuncture and hypnotic suggestions in the treatment of non-organic male sexual dysfunction. *Scandinavian Journal of Urology and Nephrology*, June 1997: 271-274.

Bacon CG, et al. Sexual function in men older than 50 years of age: results from the Health Professionals Follow-up Study. *Annals of Internal Medicine*, August 5, 2003: 161-168.

Chen J, et al. Effect of oral administration of high-dose nitric oxide donor L-arginine in men with organic erectile dysfunction: results of a double-blind, randomized, placebo-controlled study. *BJU International,* February 1999: 269-273.

Dorey G, et al. Pelvic floor exercises for erectile dysfunction. *BJU International,* September 2005: 595-597.

Esposito K, et al. Effect of lifestyle changes on erectile dysfunction in obese men: a randomized controlled trial. *JAMA,* June 23, 2004: 2978-2984.

Hong B, et al. A double-blind crossover study evaluating the efficacy of Korean red ginseng in patients with erectile dysfunction: a preliminary report. *Journal of Urology,* November 2002: 2070-2073.

Kho HG, et al. The use of acupuncture in the treatment of erectile dysfunction. *International Journal of Impotence Research,* February 1999: 41-46.

Thompson IM, et al. Erectile dysfunction and subsequent cardiovascular disease. *JAMA,* December 21, 2005: 2996-3002.

ESSENTIAL TREMOR
Louis ED. Clinical practice. Essential tremor. *New England Journal of Medicine,* September 20, 2001: 887-891.

GASTROESOPHAGEAL REFLUX DISEASE (GERD)
Jacobson BC, et al. Body-mass index and symptoms of gastroesophageal reflux in women. *New England Journal of Medicine,* June 1, 2006: 2340-2348.

Lagergren J. Body measures in relation to gastroesophageal reflux. *Gut,* June 2007: 741-742.

Spechler SJ, et al. Long-term outcome of medical and surgical therapies for gastroesophageal reflux disease: follow-up of a randomized, controlled trial. *JAMA,* May 9, 2001: 2331-2338.

GLAUCOMA
Alward WL. Medical management of glaucoma. *New England Journal of Medicine,* October 29, 1998: 1298-1307.

GOUT
Choi HK, et al. Pathogenesis of gout. *Annals of Internal Medicine,* October 4, 2005: 499-516.

GUM DISEASE
Staudte H, et al. Grapefruit consumption improves vitamin C status in periodontitis patients. *British Dental Journal,* August 27, 2005: 213-217.

Tomar SL, Asma S. Smoking-attributable periodontitis in the United States: findings from NHANES III. National Health and Nutrition Examination Survey. *Journal of Periodontology,* May 2000: 743-751.

Vandana KL, Reddy MS. Assessment of periodontal status in dental fluorosis subjects using community periodontal index of treatment needs. *Indian Journal of Dental Research,* April-June 2007: 67-71.

HEARING LOSS
Dobie RA. Folate supplementation and age-related hearing loss. *Annals of Internal Medicine,* January 2, 2007: 63-64.

Durga J, et al. Effects of folic acid supplementation on hearing in older adults: a randomized, controlled trial. *Annals of Internal Medicine,* January 2, 2007: 1-9.

Houston DK, et al. Age-related hearing loss, vitamin B_{12}, and folate in elderly women. *American Journal of Clinical Nutrition,* March 1999: 564-571.

Mizoue T, et al. Combined effect of smoking and occupational exposure to noise on hearing loss in steel factory workers. *Occupational and Environmental Medicine,* January 2003: 56-59.

Rueter A. Nutrients might prevent hearing loss in war zones, concert halls and workplaces, new animal study suggests. www.med.umich.edu/opm/newspage/2007/hearingloss.htm. March 28, 2007.

HEART PALPITATIONS
Zimetbaum P, Josephson ME. Evaluation of patients with palpitations. *New England Journal of Medicine,* May 7, 1998: 1369-1373.

HIGH BLOOD PRESSURE
Beulens JW, et al. Alcohol consumption and risk for coronary heart disease among men with hypertension. *Annals of Internal Medicine,* January 2, 2007: 10-19.

Burgess E, et al. Lifestyle recommendations to prevent and control hypertension. 6. Recommendations on potassium, magnesium and calcium. Canadian Hypertension Society, Canadian Coalition for High Blood Pressure Prevention and Control, Laboratory Centre for Disease Control at Health Canada, Heart and Stroke Foundation of Canada. *Canadian Medical Association Journal,* May 4, 1999: S35-S45.

Cabrera C, et al. Beneficial effects of green tea—a review. *Journal of the American College of Nutrition,* April 2006: 79-99.

Chiu YJ, et al. Cardiovascular and endocrine effects of acupuncture in hypertensive patients. *Clinical and Experimental Hypertension,* October 1997: 1047-1063.

Choudhury A, Lip GY. Exercise and hypertension. *Journal of Human Hypertension,* August 2005: 585-587.

Hagberg JM, et al. The role of exercise training in the treatment of hypertension: an update. *Sports Medicine,* September 2000: 193-206.

Hulsman CA, et al. Blood pressure, arterial stiffness, and open-angle glaucoma: the Rotterdam study. *Archives of Ophthalmology,* June 2007: 805-812.

Kaushik RM, et al. Effects of mental relaxation and slow breathing in essential hypertension. *Complementary Therapies in Medicine,* June 2006: 120-126.

Laterza MC, et al. Exercise training restores baroreflex sensitivity in never-treated hypertensive patients. *Hypertension,* June 2007: 1298-1306.

Messerli FH, et al. Essential hypertension. *Lancet,* August 18, 2007: 591-603.

Peluso MR. Flavonoids attenuate cardiovascular disease, inhibit phosphodiesterase, and modulate lipid homeostasis in adipose tissue and liver. *Experimental Biology and Medicine,* September 2006: 1287-1299.

Peppard PE, et al. Prospective study of the association between sleep-disordered breathing and hypertension. *New England Journal of Medicine,* May 11, 2000: 1378-1384.

Welty FK, et al. Effect of soy nuts on blood pressure and lipid levels in hypertensive, prehypertensive, and normotensive postmenopausal women. *Archives of Internal Medicine,* May 28, 2007: 1060-1067.

HIGH CHOLESTEROL

Kodama S, et al. Effect of aerobic exercise training on serum levels of high-density lipoprotein cholesterol: a meta-analysis. *Archives of Internal Medicine,* May 28, 2007: 999-1008.

Nissen SE, et al. Statin therapy, LDL cholesterol, C-reactive protein, and coronary artery disease. *New England Journal of Medicine,* January 6, 2005: 29-38.

Welty FK, et al. Effect of soy nuts on blood pressure and lipid levels in hypertensive, prehypertensive, and normotensive postmenopausal women. *Archives of Internal Medicine,* May 28, 2007: 1060-1067.

INDIGESTION

Holtmann G, et al. A placebo-controlled trial of itopride in functional dyspepsia. *New England Journal of Medicine,* February 23, 2006: 832-840.

INFLUENZA

Barak V, et al. The effect of Sambucol, a black elderberry-based, natural product, on the production of human cytokines: I. Inflammatory cytokines. *European Cytokine Network,* April-June 2001: 290-296.

Barrett BP, et al. Treatment of the common cold with unrefined echinacea. A randomized, double-blind, placebo-controlled trial. *Annals of Internal Medicine,* December 17, 2002: 936-946.

Cabrera C, et al. Beneficial effects of green tea—a review. *Journal of the American College of Nutrition,* April 2006: 79-99.

Fortes C, et al. The effect of zinc and vitamin A supplementation on immune response in an older population. *Journal of the American Geriatrics Society,* January 1998: 19-26.

Moscona A. Neuraminidase inhibitors for influenza. *New England Journal of Medicine,* September 29, 2005: 1363-1373.

INSOMNIA

Cerny A, Schmid K. Tolerability and efficacy of valerian/lemon balm in healthy volunteers (a double-blind, placebo-controlled, multicentre study). *Fitoterapia,* June 1, 1999: 221-228.

Lin Y. Acupuncture treatment for insomnia and acupuncture analgesia. *Psychiatry and Clinical Neurosciences,* May 1995: 119-120.

Silber MH. Clinical practice. Chronic insomnia. *New England Journal of Medicine,* August 25, 2005: 803-810.

KIDNEY STONES

Hollingsworth JM, et al. Medical therapy to facilitate urinary stone passage: a meta-analysis. *Lancet,* September 30, 2006: 1171-79.

MACULAR DEGENERATION

de Jong PT. Age-related macular degeneration. *New England Journal of Medicine,* October 5, 2006: 1474-1485.

Krinsky NI, et al. Biologic mechanisms of the protective role of lutein and zeaxanthin in the eye. *Annual Review of Nutrition,* 2003;23: 171-201.

Mares JA, Moeller SM. Diet and age-related macular degeneration: expanding our view. *American Journal of Clinical Nutrition,* April 2006: 733-734.

Seddon JM. Multivitamin-multimineral supplements and eye disease: age-related macular degeneration and cataract. *American Journal of Clinical Nutrition,* January 2007: 304S-307S.

MALE MENOPAUSE

Federman DD. The biology of human sex differences. *New England Journal of Medicine,* April 6, 2006: 1507-1514.

MEMORY LOSS

Wilson RS, et al. Chronic distress and incidence of mild cognitive impairment. *Neurology,* June 12, 2007: 2085-2092.

METABOLIC SYNDROME

Ford ES, et al. Prevalence of the metabolic syndrome among US adults: findings from the third National Health and Nutrition Examination Survey. *JAMA,* January 16, 2002: 356-359.

Lakka HM, et al. The metabolic syndrome and total and cardiovascular disease mortality in middle-aged men, *JAMA,* December 4, 2002: 2709-2716.

Wannamethee SG, et al. Metabolic syndrome vs Framingham Risk Score for prediction of coronary heart disease, stroke, and type 2 diabetes mellitus. *Archives of Internal Medicine,* December 12-26, 2005: 2644-2650.

MUSCLE CRAMPS

Thompson PD, et al. Statin-associated myopathy. *JAMA,* April 2, 2003: 1681-1690.

NAIL FUNGUS

Buck DS, et al. Comparison of two topical preparations for the treatment of onychomycosis: Melaleuca alternifolia (tea tree) oil and clotrimazole. *Journal of Family Practice,* June 1994: 601-605.

Gupta AK, et al. Ciclopirox nail lacquer topical solution 8% in the treatment of toenail onychomycosis. *Journal of the American Academy of Dermatology,* October 2000: S70-S80.

OBESITY

Jakicic JM, et al. Effect of exercise duration and intensity on weight loss in overweight, sedentary women: a randomized trial. *JAMA,* September 10, 2003: 1323-1330.

Sjöström L, et al. Effects of bariatric surgery on mortality in Swedish obese subjects. *New England Journal of Medicine,* August 23, 2007: 741-752.

Stenlöf K, et al. Topiramate in the treatment of obese subjects with drug-naive type 2 diabetes. *Diabetes, Obesity and Metabolism,* May 2007: 360-368.

Wansink B, Chandon P. Meal size, not body size, explains errors in estimating the calorie content of meals. *Annals of Internal Medicine,* September 5, 2006: 326-332.

Wing RR, Hill JO. Successful weight loss maintenance. *Annual Review of Nutrition,* 2001;21: 323-341.

OSTEOARTHRITIS

Berman BM, et al. Effectiveness of acupuncture as adjunctive therapy in osteoarthritis of the knee: a randomized, controlled trial. *Annals of Internal Medicine,* December 21, 2004: 901-910.

Geis GS. Arthrotec: a therapeutic option in the management of arthritis. *European Journal of Rheumatology and Inflammation,* January 1993: 25-32.

Han A, et al. Tai chi for treating rheumatoid arthritis. *Cochrane Database of Systematic Reviews,* 2004: CD004849.

Kulkarni B, et al. Arthritic pain is processed in brain areas concerned with emotions and fear. *Arthritis and Rheumatism,* April 2007: 1345-1354.

NCCAM, National Institutes of Health. Acupuncture found to be of benefit in knee osteoarthritis. *CAM at the NIH—Focus on Complementary and Alternative Medicine,* Winter 2005, Volume XII, Number 1.

Nicklas BJ, et al. Diet-induced weight loss, exercise, and chronic inflammation in older, obese adults: a randomized controlled clinical trial. *American Journal of Clinical Nutrition,* April 2004: 544-551.

Olsen NJ, Stein CM. New drugs for rheumatoid arthritis. *New England Journal of Medicine,* May 20, 2004: 2167-2179.

Sharma L, et al. Quadriceps strength and osteoarthritis progression in malaligned and lax knees. *Annals of Internal Medicine,* April 15, 2003: 613-619.

Towheed TE, Anastassiades TP. Glucosamine and chondroitin for treating symptoms of osteoarthritis: evidence is widely touted but incomplete. *JAMA,* March 15, 2000: 1483-1484.

Trock DH. Electromagnetic fields and magnets. Investigational treatment for musculoskeletal disorders. *Rheumatic Disease Clinic of North America,* February 2000: 51-62.

van Baar ME, et al. Effectiveness of exercise therapy in patients with osteoarthritis of the hip or knee: a systematic review of randomized clinical trials. *Arthritis and Rheumatism,* July 1999: 1361-1369.

Witt C, et al. Acupuncture in patients with osteoarthritis of the knee: a randomised trial. *Lancet,* July 9-15, 2005: 136-143.

PARKINSON'S DISEASE

Deuschl G, et al. A randomized trial of deep-brain stimulation for Parkinson's disease. *New England Journal of Medicine,* August 31, 2006: 896-908.

Dick FD, et al. Environmental risk factors for Parkinson's disease and parkinsonism: the Geoparkinson study. *Occupational and Environmental Medicine,* October 2007: 666-672.

PERIPHERAL NEUROPATHY

Mendell JR, Sahenk Z. Clinical practice. Painful sensory neuropathy. *New England Journal of Medicine,* March 27, 2003: 1243-1255.

PROSTATE ENLARGEMENT

Wilt TJ, et al. Saw palmetto extracts for treatment of benign prostatic hyperplasia: a systematic review. *JAMA,* November 11, 1998: 1604-1609.

PROSTATITIS

Schaeffer AJ. Clinical practice. Chronic prostatitis and the chronic pelvic pain syndrome. *New England Journal of Medicine,* October 19, 2006: 1690-1698.

ROSACEA

Chiu AE, et al. Double-blinded, placebo-controlled trial of green tea extracts in the clinical and histologic appearance of photoaging skin. *Dermatologic Surgery,* July 2005: 855-860.

Hsu S. Green tea and the skin. *Journal of the American Academy of Dermatology,* June 2005: 1049-1059.

SHINGLES

Irwin MR, et al. Augmenting immune responses to varicella zoster virus in older adults: a randomized, controlled trial of Tai Chi. *Journal of the American Geriatrics Society,* April 2007: 511-517.

SLEEP APNEA

Basner RC. Continuous positive airway pressure for obstructive sleep apnea. *New England Journal of Medicine,* April 26, 2007: 1751-1758.

Wang XH, et al. Clinical observation on effect of auricular acupoint pressing in treating sleep apnea syndrome. *Zhongguo Zhong Xi Yi Jie Hc Za Zhi,* October 2003: 747-749.

Yaggi HK, et al. Obstructive sleep apnea as a risk factor for stroke and death. *New England Journal of Medicine,* November 10, 2005: 2034-2041.

Index

Underscored page references indicate boxed text.

Abdominal discomfort, as symptom of
  celiac disease, 41, 42
  diverticulitis, 74–75, 75
  indigestion, 156, 156
ACE inhibitors. *See* Angiotensin-converting enzyme
    inhibitors
Acetyl-L-carnitine, for memory loss, 193
Acid blockers, 98, 157
Acid reflux, 96–101
Actisite, for gum disease, 118
Acupressure, 4
  for treating
    angina, 14
    back pain, 29
    insomnia, 169
Acupuncture, 4
  for appetite control, 211
  for treating
    angina, 13
    back pain, 29
    celiac disease, 42
    depression, 61
    diabetes, 72
    erectile dysfunction, 88
    glaucoma, 108
    hearing loss, 127
    high blood pressure, 143
    insomnia, 169
    male menopause, 187
    osteoarthritis, 218
    Parkinson's disease, 226
    peripheral neuropathy, 231
    rosacea, 252
    shingles, 258
    sleep apnea, 264
Acute urinary retention, 241
Adenomatous colon polyps, 45, 46–47
Agave nectar, as sugar substitute, 70
ALA. *See* Alpha-lipoic acid
Alcohol
  erectile dysfunction from, 85, 91
  essential tremor and, 92, 95
  limiting, with
    atherosclerosis, 22
    depression, 63
    GERD, 101
    gout, 114
    high blood pressure, 147
    insomnia, 172
    male menopause, 187
    memory loss, 194
    peripheral neuropathy, 233

prostate enlargement, 244
  rosacea, 254
  sleep apnea, 265
  macular degeneration and, 184
  peripheral vascular disease and, 239
Alexander Technique (AT), 4
  for treating
    back pain, 31
    hearing loss, 127
Aloe vera, for treating
  colon polyps, 46
  gum disease, 120
Alpha-blockers, for treating
  high blood pressure, 141–42
  prostate enlargement, 240–41
  prostatitis, 247
Alpha-glucosidase inhibitors, for diabetes, 66–67
Alpha-lipoic acid (ALA), for treating
    diabetes, 71
    metabolic syndrome, 197
Alpha-2 adrenergic agonists, for glaucoma, 104
Alprostadil, for erectile dysfunction, 86
Alzheimer's disease, 190, 191
Amantadine, for Parkinson's disease, 224
American ginseng, for diabetes, 70–71
Amputation, for peripheral vascular disease, 235–36
Amsler grid, for monitoring macular degeneration,
    180, 182
Anal itching and burning, from hemorrhoids, 134, 134
Andropause, 186–89
Angina, 10–16
  with atherosclerosis, 17, 18
  with coronary artery disease, 48, 49, 49, 50
Angioplasty, 13, 235
Angiotensin-converting enzyme (ACE) inhibitors
    diabetes and, 66
    for treating
      atherosclerosis, 18
      high blood pressure, 141
Angiotension II receptor blockers, for high blood
    pressure, 142
Antacids, 98, 157–58
Anthocyanosides, for treating
  cataracts, 38
  coronary artery disease, 52
  macular degeneration, 183
  peripheral vascular disease, 237
Antiangiogenesis drugs, for macular degeneration, 181
Antianxiety drugs, for depression, 58
Antibiotics, for treating
  emphysema, 81
  gum disease, 118–19

Antibiotics, for treating (*cont.*)
 indigestion, 158
 influenza-related complications, 162
 prostatitis, 246–47
 rosacea, 251, 252
Anticholinergics, for Parkinson's disease, 224
Anticoagulants
 back pain from, 24
 COX-2 inhibitors and, 26
 for treating
  angina, 11
  heart palpitations, 131
Antidepressants, for treating
 back pain, 27
 depression, 59, 60
 peripheral neuropathy, 231
 shingles, 257
Antifungal medication, for nail fungus, 204
Antihyperuricemic drugs, for gout, 111–12
Anti-inflammatory drugs. *See also* Nonsteroidal
    anti-inflammatory drugs (NSAIDs)
 for treating
  emphysema, 81
  gout, 112
Antioxidants. *See also specific antioxidants*
 for preventing cataracts, 37, 38–39
 for treating
  atherosclerosis, 20
  emphysema, 83
  memory loss, 192–93
Antipsychotic medications, for depression, 59
Antiseizure medications, for treating
  depression, 58–59
  essential tremor, 93
  peripheral neuropathy, 231
  shingles, 257
Antiviral medications, for treating
 influenza, 162
 shingles, 257
Aquatic therapy, 4
 for treating
  back pain, 29
  high blood pressure, 143
  Parkinson's disease, 226
  peripheral vascular disease, 236
Arterial plaque. *See* Plaque, arterial
Arthritis, 214–21
Arthrodesis, for osteoarthritis, 217
Arthroplasty, for osteoarthritis, 217–18
Arthroscopic debridement, for osteoarthritis,
    218
Asian ginseng, for treating
 erectile dysfunction, 89
 male menopause, 188
Aspirin
 for preventing colon polyps, 47
 for treating
  angina, 11
  atherosclerosis, 18

 coronary artery disease, 49
 heart palpitations, 131
Astragalus, for influenza, 163, 165
AT. *See* Alexander Technique
Atherectomy, 18–19, 50
Atherosclerosis, 17–22, 48, 149, 234
Athlete's foot, 205
Atrial fibrillation, 131
Atridox, for gum disease, 118
Autogenic training, for heart palpitations, 133
Ayurveda, 4–5
 for treating
  angina, 13–14
  atherosclerosis, 19
  coronary artery disease, 51
  diabetes, 69
  gum disease, 119
  insomnia, 169
  osteoarthritis, 218–19
 for weight loss, 211

Back pain, 23–34
Bacterial endocarditis, <u>117</u>
Balloon angioplasty, 18, 50
Barrett's esophagus, 96, 97, 99
Bed elevation, for treating
 angina, 16
 sleep apnea, 265
Behavior modification therapy, for obesity, 207
Beta-blockers
 side effects of, 11–12
 for treating
  angina, 11–12
  atherosclerosis, 18
  coronary artery disease, 49
  essential tremor, 93
  glaucoma, 104
  heart palpitations, 131
  high blood pressure, 142
Beta-carotene, for treating
 coronary artery disease, 51
 glaucoma, 106, 107
 memory loss, 192
 osteoarthritis, 219
 peripheral vascular disease, 237
 shingles, 260
Biguanides, for diabetes, 67
Bilberry and bilberry extract, for treating
 cataracts, 38
 diabetes, 71
 glaucoma, 107
 gout, 113
 macular degeneration, 183, 184
Bile-acid binding resins, for high cholesterol, 152
Biofeedback, 5
 for treating
  essential tremor, 94–95
  gum disease, 119
  peripheral neuropathy, 231–32

Bioflavonoids, for preventing muscle cramps, 200
Bipolar disorder, 55, 57, 59, 60
Black cohosh, for hearing loss, 128
Blood glucose, in diabetes, 64–73
Blood pressure
    controlling, for glaucoma prevention, 108
    high (*see* High blood pressure)
    measuring, 138, 141
Blood pressure medications, for angina, 13
Bloodroot, for gum disease, 120
Body mass index (BMI), 208
Bodywork, 5
Bone grafting, for gum disease, 117
Boron, for osteoarthritis, 220
Boswellia serrata, for osteoarthritis, 219–20
Botox injections, for essential tremor, 93
Bowel resection with colostomy, for diverticulitis, 76
Brace, for back pain, 25
Breathing stoppage during sleep, from sleep apnea, 261, 261, 262
Breathing techniques. *See* Deep breathing exercises
Bromelain, for treating
    back pain, 32
    GERD, 100–101
    gout, 113–14
    indigestion, 160
    osteoarthritis, 220
Bronchodilators, for treating
    emphysema, 81
    essential tremor, 93–94
Butcher's broom, for hemorrhoids, 136
B vitamins. *See also specific B vitamins*
    for health support with celiac disease, 43
    for preventing
        cataracts, 38
        kidney stones, 177
    for treating
        atherosclerosis, 19–20, 21
        coronary artery disease, 52, 53
        depression, 62
        diabetes, 71
        erectile dysfunction, 90
        gout, 113
        hearing loss, 127, 129
        insomnia, 171
        male menopause, 189
        memory loss, 193
        osteoarthritis, 220
        peripheral vascular disease, 237, 238
        rosacea, 253
        shingles, 259
Bypass grafts, for peripheral vascular disease, 236
Bypass surgery, coronary, 13, 50

CAD. *See* Coronary artery disease
Caffeine
    erectile dysfunction and, 89
    essential tremor from, 92, 95
    limiting, with
        angina, 14
        atherosclerosis, 22
        coronary artery disease, 54
        heart palpitations, 133
        high blood pressure, 147
        insomnia, 172
        male menopause, 187
        peripheral neuropathy, 233
Calcium
    kidney stones and, 178
    for preventing muscle cramps, 200, 201
    for treating
        angina, 15
        atherosclerosis, 21
        colon polyps, 47
        coronary artery disease, 53
        diabetes, 72
        gum disease, 120
        heart palpitations, 132
        high blood pressure, 146
        high cholesterol, 154
        insomnia, 169, 171
        metabolic syndrome, 197
        peripheral vascular disease, 238
        shingles, 258
        sleep apnea, 264
Calcium-channel blockers, for treating
    angina, 12
    coronary artery disease, 49
    heart palpitations, 131
    high blood pressure, 142–43
Calf pain
    during exercise, with atherosclerosis, 17, 18
    with peripheral vascular disease, 234, 234
Capsaicin, for treating
    back pain, 31
    osteoarthritis, 216, 220
    peripheral neuropathy, 231
    shingles, 257
Carbohydrates, avoiding, with metabolic syndrome, 197
Carbonic anhydrase inhibitors, for glaucoma, 104
Cataracts, 35–39, 71
Catechol-O-methyltransferase inhibitors, for Parkinson's disease, 224–25
Cayenne pepper
    for peripheral vascular disease, 237
    for weight loss, 211
Celiac disease, 40–44, 156
Centrally acting drugs, for high blood pressure, 143
Chamomile, for treating
    diverticulosis/diverticulitis, 76
    GERD, 100
    indigestion, 159
    insomnia, 170
    nail fungus, 204
    shingles, 258–59
Chest illness, acute, with emphysema, 80, 81

Chest pain
  as emergency, 12
  as symptom of
    angina, 10–16
    atherosclerosis, 17, 18
    coronary artery disease, 48, 49, 49
    GERD, 97, 97
    heart attack, 48, 131, 157
Chiropractic, 5, 30, 127
Chocolate, for coughs, 164
Cholesterol
  controlling, for prevention of
    prostate enlargement, 244
    prostatitis, 249
  foods lowering, 52
  HDL, 149, 151, 153, 155
  high, 149–55
    erectile dysfunction from, 91, 189
    macular degeneration and, 184
    medications lowering (see Cholesterol-lowering
      medications)
  LDL, 149, 151, 152
Cholesterol-lowering medications
  foods interacting with, 52
  muscle cramps from, 199
  for treating
    angina, 13
    atherosclerosis, 18
    coronary artery disease, 49
    high cholesterol, 152–53
    metabolic syndrome, 196
    peripheral vascular disease, 235
Chromium
  for treating
    atherosclerosis, 21
    coronary artery disease, 53
    diabetes, 70, 72
    metabolic syndrome, 197–98
    peripheral vascular disease, 238
  for weight loss, 212
Chymopapain injection, for back pain, 28
Cialis, for erectile dysfunction, 87
Cinnamon, for diabetes, 71
Clinical trials, for essential tremor medications, 95
Cochlear implant, for hearing loss, 126–27
Coenzyme Q₁₀, for treating
  angina, 15
  atherosclerosis, 21
  coronary artery disease, 53
  high blood pressure, 146
  metabolic syndrome, 198
  peripheral vascular disease, 238
Coffee. See also Caffeine
  avoiding
    with glaucoma, 106, 108
    for preventing peripheral vascular disease, 239
  for gout, 114
Cognitive-behavioral therapy, for depression, 57–58

Colchicine, for gout, 112
Cold treatments
  for back pain, 25, 33
  for gout, 111
  for hemorrhoids, 135
  for osteoarthritis, 216
Colon polyps, 45–47
Coltsfoot, for emphysema, 83
Complementary medicine, 1, 3–9
Constipation
  with diverticulosis, 75, 75
  hemorrhoids from, 134, 137
  with Parkinson's disease, 228
Conventional incisional surgery, for glaucoma, 105
Conventional medicine, 1–2, 3
Copper
  for preventing cataracts, 38
  for treating macular degeneration, 184
Coriander, for GERD, 100
Coronary artery disease (CAD), 11, 48–54, 56
Coronary bypass surgery, 13, 50
Corticosteroids, for treating
  emphysema, 81
  gout, 112
  osteoarthritis, 217
Coughs, with influenza, 164, 165
Counseling. See Psychotherapy
COX-2 inhibitors, for treating
  back pain, 26
  gout, 112
  osteoarthritis, 216
Cramps
  muscle, 199–202
  from peripheral vascular disease, 234, 234
Craniosacral therapy, 5
  for treating
    back pain, 29–30
    hearing loss, 127
    Parkinson's disease, 226–27
Cravings for sweets, with metabolic syndrome, 195, 196

Damiana, for treating
  erectile dysfunction, 89
  male menopause, 188
DASH diet, 143–44, 150
DBS. See Deep-brain stimulation
DDD. See Degenerative disk disease
Decongestants, 244, 265
Deep-brain stimulation (DBS), for treating
  essential tremor, 94
  Parkinson's disease, 225–26
Deep breathing exercises
  with emphysema, 83
  for preventing muscle cramps, 202
  for relaxation, 72, 171
  for treating
    heart palpitations, 133
    insomnia, 171

osteoarthritis, 221
    peripheral neuropathy, 232
Degenerative disk disease (DDD), 23–24, 28, 32
Dementia, 190, 191, 223, 224
Dental care products, choosing, 117, 121
Dental floss, 117, 121
Dental implants, 118
Depression, 55–63
    coronary artery disease and, 48, 56
    insomnia from, 166, 167
    with Parkinson's disease, 223, 223, 224
Dermatitis herpetiformis, 41
Devil's claw, for treating
    GERD, 100
    gout, 113
DHEA, for treating
    diabetes, 72
    erectile dysfunction, 90
Diabetes, 64–73
    atherosclerosis with, 17
    metabolic syndrome and, 195
    from obesity, 207
    peripheral neuropathy with, 229, 230, 233
    peripheral vascular disease with, 234–35
Diabetic ketoacidosis, 66
Diarrhea, with diverticulosis, 75, 75
Diet
    for preventing
        cataracts, 37
        colon polyps, 46
        diabetes, 73
        GERD, 97, 101
        glaucoma, 108
        hemorrhoids, 137
        high blood pressure, 147–48
        high cholesterol, 155
        indigestion, 160
        influenza, 165
        kidney stones, 177
        muscle cramps, 200
        obesity, 213
        prostate enlargement, 243, 244
    for treating
        angina, 14
        atherosclerosis, 19–20
        back pain, 30
        celiac disease, 41–42, 43
        coronary artery disease, 51–52
        depression, 61
        diabetes, 69–70
        diverticulosis/diverticulitis, 76
        emphysema, 82
        erectile dysfunction, 88–89
        glaucoma, 106–7
        gout, 112–13
        gum disease, 119
        hearing loss, 127–28
        heart palpitations, 131–32

hemorrhoids, 134, 135–36
high blood pressure, 143–44
high cholesterol, 150–51, 153–54
indigestion, 158–59
influenza, 162–63
insomnia, 169–70
kidney stones, 177
macular degeneration, 182–83
male menopause, 187
memory loss, 192–93
metabolic syndrome, 196–97
osteoarthritis, 219
Parkinson's disease, 227
peripheral neuropathy, 232
peripheral vascular disease, 236–37
prostatitis, 248
rosacea, 252
shingles, 258
sleep apnea, 264
    vegetarian, 70, 147–48
    for weight loss, 207–8, 211
    well-balanced, description of, 4
Digestive enzymes, for rosacea, 253
Discectomy, for back pain, 28
Diuretics
    for high blood pressure, 143
    muscle cramps from, 202
Diverticulosis/diverticulitis, 74–79
Dizziness, with atherosclerosis, 17, 18
DLPA, for osteoarthritis, 220
Dopamine agonists, for Parkinson's disease, 225
Dysthymia, 55, 57

Earwax removal, 125
Echinacea. See also Echinacea and goldenseal
    for preventing influenza, 165
    for treating
        influenza, 163
        nail fungus, 204–5
Echinacea and goldenseal, for treating
    gum disease, 120
    hearing loss, 128
ECT, for depression, 58
ED, 85–91
Elderberry, for influenza, 163
Electroconvulsive therapy (ECT), for depression, 58
Electrothermal surgery, for back pain, 28
Electrovaporization, for prostate enlargement, 242
Elyzol, for gum disease, 118
Emphysema, 80–84
Energy balancing, for back pain, 30–31
Erectile dysfunction (ED), 85–91
    with atherosclerosis, 17, 18, 85
    as diabetes symptom, 65
    in male menopause, 186, 189
    from peripheral vascular disease, 234, 234
Esophagitis, 96, 99

Essential fatty acids. *See also* Fish oil; Omega-3
    fatty acids
  for preventing prostate enlargement, 243
  for treating
    angina, 14
    atherosclerosis, 19
    back pain, 32
    diabetes, 69
    osteoarthritis, 220–21
    Parkinson's disease, 227
    peripheral vascular disease, 237
    rosacea, 252, 253
Essential tremor, 92–95
ESWL, for kidney stones, 175–76
Evening primrose oil, for rosacea, 253
Exercise
  calf pain during, 17, 18
  after eating, indigestion from, 160
  fluids and, 202
  for health support with celiac disease, 43–44
  for preventing
    back pain, 34
    cataracts, 39
    colon polyps, 47
    diabetes, 73
    erectile dysfunction, 91
    GERD, 101
    gout, 114
    hemorrhoids, 137
    high blood pressure, 148
    high cholesterol, 155
    kidney stones, 178
    muscle cramps, 201, 202
    obesity, 213
    prostatitis, 249
  preventing muscle cramps from, 200
  for treating
    angina, 16
    atherosclerosis, 22
    back pain, 26, 32
    coronary artery disease, 54
    depression, 63
    diabetes, 70
    diverticulosis/diverticulitis, 77, 79
    glaucoma, 108
    hearing loss, 129
    hemorrhoids, 137
    high blood pressure, 146
    high cholesterol, 151
    insomnia, 171
    macular degeneration, 184
    male menopause, 187–88
    memory loss, 194
    metabolic syndrome, 198
    osteoarthritis, 215
    Parkinson's disease, 228
    peripheral neuropathy, 232–33
    peripheral vascular disease, 235, 236, 239
  for weight loss, 208

Extracorporeal shock wave lithotripsy (ESWL), for
    kidney stones, 175–76
Eye drops, for glaucoma, 103–4, 105

Feldenkrais Method, 5–6
  for treating
    back pain, 31
    osteoarthritis, 219
    Parkinson's disease, 227
Fennel seeds, for treating
  GERD, 100
  indigestion, 159
Fiber. *See also* Fiber supplements
  foods containing, 78
  lack of, diverticulosis from, 74
  for preventing
    colon polyps, 46, 47
    diverticulosis, 79
    high cholesterol, 155
  for treating
    atherosclerosis, 19
    diverticulosis, 75, 76, 78
    hemorrhoids, 134, 135
    high cholesterol, 153
    peripheral vascular disease, 236–37
  for weight loss, 207–8
Fiber supplements, for treating
  constipation with Parkinson's disease, 228
  diverticulosis/diverticulitis, 77
  hemorrhoids, 136–37
  high cholesterol, 155
Finasteride, for prostate enlargement, 241
Fish oil, for treating
  coronary artery disease, 51
  diverticulosis/diverticulitis, 77
  glaucoma, 107
5-HTP, for treating
  depression, 62
  sleep apnea, 264
Flavonoids, for osteoarthritis, 219
Flaxseed and charcoal poultice, for gout, 113
Flu, 161–65
Fluids. *See also* Water
  exercise and, 202
  insomnia and, 172
  for preventing
    gout, 114
    kidney stones, 178
    nail fungus, 205
  prostate enlargement and, 244
  prostatitis and, 248, 249
  for treating
    hemorrhoids, 135–36
    influenza, 162–63
Fluoride, gum disease and, 121
Flu vaccine, 164–65, 164
Folic acid, for treating
  gout, 114
  hearing loss, 127

Foot care
   with diabetes, 73, 233
   with peripheral neuropathy, 233
Foot reflexology, for cataracts, 37–38
Forgetfulness, 190–94
Fungus, nail, 203–5

Garlic, for treating
   atherosclerosis, 20
   coronary artery disease, 52
   diabetes, 70
   diverticulosis/diverticulitis, 77
   emphysema, 82–83
   erectile dysfunction, 89
   hearing loss, 127–28
   high blood pressure, 144–45
   high cholesterol, 154
   influenza, 163
   nail fungus, 205
   peripheral vascular disease, 237
Gastric bypass, for weight loss, 210
Gastroesophageal reflux disease (GERD), 96–101, 156
GERD, 96–101, 156
Ginger, for treating
   back pain, 31
   coughs, 165
   diverticulosis/diverticulitis, 76
   GERD, 100
   hearing loss, 128
   osteoarthritis, 220
Gingivectomy and gingivoplasty, for gum disease, 117
Gingivitis, 115, 116
Ginkgo biloba, for treating
   angina, 15
   atherosclerosis, 20
   cataracts, 38
   coronary artery disease, 52
   erectile dysfunction, 89–90
   glaucoma, 107
   hearing loss, 128
   high blood pressure, 145
   macular degeneration, 183
   male menopause, 188
   memory loss, 193
   peripheral vascular disease, 237–38
Glaucoma, 36–37, 102–8
Glucomannan, for metabolic syndrome, 198
Glucosamine sulfate, for osteoarthritis, 221
Gluten intolerance, in celiac disease, 40–44
Glycolic acid peel, for rosacea, 251
Goldenseal. *See also* Echinacea and goldenseal
   for preventing influenza, 165
   for treating
      indigestion, 159
      nail fungus, 204
      prostatitis, 248
Gout, 109–14, 152
Grapefruit juice, kidney stones and, 177
Grapefruit seed extract, for nail fungus, 205

Grape juice, for treating
   high blood pressure, 147
   high cholesterol, 155
   influenza, 162–63
Grape seed extract, for treating
   gout, 113
   high blood pressure, 145
Green tea, for treating
   angina, 15
   atherosclerosis, 20
   coronary artery disease, 52–053
   high blood pressure, 145
   high cholesterol, 154
   peripheral vascular disease, 238
Guided-tissue regeneration, for gum disease, 117–18
Gum disease, 115–22
Gum problems, with diabetes, <u>64</u>, 65, 73

Hand washing, for preventing influenza, 165
Hardening of the arteries, 17–22
Hawthorn, for treating
   angina, 15
   atherosclerosis, 20–21
   coronary artery disease, 53
   heart palpitations, 132
   high blood pressure, 145
   high cholesterol, 154
   peripheral vascular disease, 238
HDL cholesterol, <u>149</u>, 151, 153, 155
Health insurance, 2, 3
Hearing aids, types of, 125–26
Hearing loss, 123–29
Heart attacks
   from coronary artery disease, 48
   depression after, 56
   from high blood pressure, 139
   from metabolic syndrome, 195
   symptoms of, <u>48</u>, <u>131</u>, <u>157</u>
Heartburn, as symptom of GERD, 96, 97, <u>97</u>
Heart disease. *See also* Angina; Atherosclerosis;
      Coronary artery disease (CAD); Heart attacks
   erectile dysfunction and, <u>85</u>
   high blood pressure and, 138–39
Heart palpitations, <u>10</u>, 11, 130–33
Heat stroke, 202
Heat therapy, for prostate enlargement, 241
Heat treatments
   for back pain, 25
   for kidney stones, 177
   for osteoarthritis, 216, 220
Helicobacter pylori, 156, 158, 250
Hemorrhoid banding or rubber band ligation, 135
Hemorrhoids, 134–37
Herbal medicine, 6. *See also specific herbs*
Hiatal hernia, 97, 99
Hibiscus, for high blood pressure, 145–46
High blood pressure, 138–48
   atherosclerosis with, 17
   with diabetes, 73

High blood pressure (*cont.*)
    macular degeneration and, 184
    with metabolic syndrome, 195, 196
    from obesity, 207
High blood pressure medications, for treating
    atherosclerosis, 18
    peripheral vascular disease, 235
High cholesterol. *See* Cholesterol, high
Homeopathy, 6
    for treating
      cataracts, 38
      hemorrhoids, 136
      indigestion, 159–60
      influenza, 164
      insomnia, 170
      muscle cramps, 200–201
      shingles, 259
Honey, for coughs, 165
Hoodia, for weight loss, 211–12
Hops, for insomnia, 170
Horse chestnut, for hemorrhoids, 136
Horsetail, for gum disease, 120
Hyaluronic acid, for osteoarthritis, 216
Hydrochloric acid supplements, for rosacea, 253
Hydrotherapy, 6
    for treating
      GERD, 100
      glaucoma, 107
      indigestion, 160
      muscle cramps, 201
      osteoarthritis, 220
      peripheral neuropathy, 232
      prostatitis, 247
      shingles, 256–57, 259
Hyperparathyroidism, kidney stones from, 176
Hypertension, 138–48
Hypnotherapy, 6–7
    for treating
      depression, 62
      erectile dysfunction, 90
      male menopause, 189
Hypoglycemia, 64

Impotence. *See* Erectile dysfunction
Indigestion, 156–60
Influenza, 161–65
Insomnia, 166–72
Insulin, for diabetes, 67
Insulin resistance syndrome, 195–98
Integrative medicine, 1–9
Interventional radiology treatments, for peripheral vascular disease, 235
Iron, for preventing muscle cramps, 200
Irregular heartbeat, with coronary artery disease, 49, 49
Itopride, for indigestion, 158

Joint fusion, for osteoarthritis, 217
Joint lavage, for osteoarthritis, 218

Joint pain, from osteoarthritis, 214–21
Joint replacement, for osteoarthritis, 217–18
Juniper berries, for gout, 113

Kegel exercises, for erectile dysfunction, 90
Kidney stones, 173–78
Knee pain
    with gout, 110, 111
    with osteoarthritis, 214

Lactase enzyme, for indigestion, 160
Lactobacillus acidophilus, for diverticulosis/diverticulitis, 77
Laminectomy or laminotomy, for back pain, 29
Laparoscopic fundoplication, for GERD, 99
Lap-band, for weight loss, 210
L-arginine, for treating
    erectile dysfunction, 90
    male menopause, 189
Laser ablation, for coronary artery disease, 50
Laser surgery, for macular degeneration, 181–82
Laser therapy, for treating
    prostate enlargement, 242
    rosacea, 251
    shingles, 258
Laser trabeculoplasty, for glaucoma, 105–6
L-carnitine
    for treating
      angina, 15
      atherosclerosis, 21
      coronary artery disease, 53
      metabolic syndrome, 198
      peripheral vascular disease, 238
    for weight loss, 212
LDL cholesterol, 149, 151, 152
Leg pain. *See* Calf pain
Lemon balm, for shingles, 259
Lemon juice, for kidney stones, 177
LES repair, for GERD, 100
Levitra, for erectile dysfunction, 87
Levodopa, for Parkinson's disease, 225
L-glutamine, for diverticulosis/diverticulitis, 77
Licorice, for treating
    GERD, 100
    shingles, 259
Light therapy, for seasonal affective disorder, 60–61
Lithium, for bipolar disorder, 59–60
Lower esophageal sphincter (LES) repair, for GERD, 100
Lung volume reduction surgery, for emphysema, 82
Lutein, for eye health, 37, 39, 106, 183, 184
Lysine, for shingles, 258, 260

Maca, for treating
    erectile dysfunction, 90
    male menopause, 188–89
Macular degeneration, 179–85

MAD, for sleep apnea, 262
Magnesium
  for preventing
    cataracts, 39
    kidney stones, 177
    muscle cramps, 200, 201
  for treating
    angina, 14, 15–16
    atherosclerosis, 20, 21
    colon polyps, 47
    coronary artery disease, 52, 53
    diabetes, 72
    glaucoma, 106, 107
    heart palpitations, 132
    high blood pressure, 146
    high cholesterol, 154–55
    insomnia, 169, 171
    metabolic syndrome, 198
    peripheral vascular disease, 237, 238
    rosacea, 252
    shingles, 258
    sleep apnea, 264
Magnet therapy, for osteoarthritis, 221
Major depression, 55, 57
Male menopause, 186–89
Mandibular advancement device (MAD), for sleep
    apnea, 262
MAOIs, for depression, 60
Massage, therapeutic. See Therapeutic massage
Meat, colon polyps and, 44, 46
Medications. See also specific medications
  interacting with lithium, 59
  side effects from
    cataracts, 39
    depression, 56
    erectile dysfunction, 85, 91
    GERD, 98
    gout, 110
    hearing loss, 124
    high blood pressure, 139
    indigestion, 157
    memory loss, 194
    Parkinson's-type symptoms, 222
    weight gain, 206
Meditation. See Relaxation/meditation
Mediterranean diet, for high cholesterol, 150
Meglitinides, for diabetes, 67
Melatonin, for treating
  insomnia, 170–71, 193
  memory loss, 193
Memory loss, 190–94, 223, 224
Menopause, male, 186–89
Metabolic syndrome, 195–98
Mexiletine, for peripheral neuropathy, 231
Microvascular angina, 10
Microwave therapy, for prostate enlargement, 241–42
Milk thistle, for metabolic syndrome, 197
Mind-body connection, 1, 3

Miotics, for glaucoma, 104
Monoamine oxidase inhibitors (MAOIs), for
    depression, 60
Mood stabilizers, for depression, 60
MSM, for osteoarthritis, 221
Mullein, for emphysema, 83
Multivitamin/mineral supplement
  for health support with
    back pain, 32
    celiac disease, 43
    depression, 62
    emphysema, 83
    gout, 113
    gum disease, 120
    heart palpitations, 132
    male menopause, 189
    memory loss, 193
    osteoarthritis, 220
    peripheral neuropathy, 232
    shingles, 259
    weight loss, 212
  for preventing influenza, 165
Muscle cramps, 199–202
Muscle relaxants, for treating
  back pain, 27
  muscle cramps, 200

Nail fungus, 203–5
Narcotics, for treating
  back pain, 27–28
  osteoarthritis, 217
Nasal continuous positive airway pressure (nCPAP)
    system, for sleep apnea, 262–63
Naturopathy, 7
  for treating
    celiac disease, 43
    diabetes, 71
    kidney stones, 177
    prostate enlargement, 244
    rosacea, 252–53
    shingles, 259
    sleep apnea, 264
  for weight loss, 212
nCPAP, for sleep apnea, 262–63
Niacin, for high cholesterol, 155
Nicotinic acid, for high cholesterol, 152, 153
Nitrates
  side effects of, 13
  for treating
    angina, 12–13
    atherosclerosis, 18
    coronary artery disease, 49–50
Nitroglycerin. See Nitrates
Nonsteroidal anti-inflammatory drugs (NSAIDs)
  caution about, 216
  for treating
    back pain, 25, 27
    gout, 112

Nonsteroidal anti-inflammatory drugs (NSAIDs) (*cont.*)
   for treating (*cont.*)
      osteoarthritis, 216–17
      peripheral neuropathy, 230
NSAIDs. *See* Nonsteroidal anti-inflammatory drugs
Numbness
   from peripheral neuropathy, 229–30, <u>230</u>
   from peripheral vascular disease, 234, <u>234</u>
Nutritional counseling
   with celiac disease, 44
   with kidney stones, 177
   for weight loss, 212
Nutritional deficiencies, causes of, 7
Nutritional supplements, 7. *See also specific*
    supplements

Oatmeal bath, for shingles, 257, 260
Obesity, 96–97, 195, 206–13. *See also* Weight loss
Omega-3 fatty acids
   for preventing macular degeneration, 183
   for treating
      diverticulosis/diverticulitis, 77
      gout, 114
      high blood pressure, 146
      male menopause, 189
      metabolic syndrome, 197, 198
      prostate enlargement, 244
      prostatitis, 248
Onions, for treating
   coronary artery disease, 52
   diabetes, 70
   peripheral vascular disease, 237
Open flap curettage, for gum disease, 118
Open Nissen fundoplication, for GERD, 99–100
Open prostatectomy, for prostate enlargement, 243
Ornish program, for high cholesterol, 151
Osteoarthritis, 214–21
Osteotomy, for osteoarthritis, 218
Overweight. *See* Obesity
Oxygen therapy, for emphysema, 81

Pain patch, for back pain, 25
Pain relievers. *See also specific pain relievers*
   for treating
      back pain, 25
      osteoarthritis, 216–17
      peripheral neuropathy, 230
      shingles, 257–58
Pallidotomy, for Parkinson's disease, 226
Palpitations. *See* Heart palpitations
Papain, for indigestion, 160
Parkinson's disease, <u>92</u>, 222–28
Passionflower, for insomnia, 170
Penile implants, for erectile dysfunction, 87
Peppermint, for treating
   diverticulosis/diverticulitis, 76–77
   emphysema, 83
   indigestion, 159

Percutaneous nephrolithotomy, for kidney stones, 176
PerioChip, for gum disease, 118
Periodontitis, 115, 116–17
Peripheral neuropathy, 229–33
Peripheral vascular disease (PVD), 234–39
Peritonitis, from diverticulitis, <u>76</u>
Personal fitness training, for back pain, 32
PHN. *See* Postherpectic neuralgia
Phototherapy, for seasonal affective disorder, 60–61
Physical therapy, for treating
   essential tremor, 94
   prostatitis, 247
Physicians, in conventional medicine, 1, 2
Pine bark extract, for diabetes, 71
Plaque, arterial
   atherosclerosis from, 17, 149
   coronary artery disease from, 48
Polyps, colon, 45–47
Postherpectic neuralgia (PHN), 255, 257, 260
Potassium
   for preventing muscle cramps, 200
   for treating heart palpitations, 132
PPIs, 98, 158
Primary bowel resection, for diverticulitis, 76
Proanthocyanidin bioflavonoids, for treating
   macular degeneration, 183
   osteoarthritis, 220
Progressive muscle relaxation, for insomnia,
   167–68
Prokinetics, for indigestion, 158
Prostaglandin analogues, for glaucoma, 104
Prostate cancer, 187
Prostatectomy, open, for prostate enlargement, 243
Prostate enlargement, 240–44
Prostatitis, 245–48
Protein
   kidney stones and, 177
   for metabolic syndrome, 197
   Parkinson's disease and, 228
   for weight loss, 208
Protein therapy, for emphysema, 81
Proton-pump inhibitors (PPIs), 98, 158
Psychosis, 59
Psychotherapy
   for treating
      depression, 57–58, 61
      erectile dysfunction, 87
      essential tremor, 94
      memory loss, 193
   for weight loss, 212
Pulmonary rehabilitation program, for emphysema,
   81–82
Purines, gout from, 109, 112–13
PVD, 234–39
Pycnogenol, for diabetes, 71
Pygeum, for treating
   prostate enlargement, 243–44
   prostatitis, 248

Qigong, 7
  for treating
    back pain, 31
    Parkinson's disease, 227
Quercetin, for treating
  GERD, 100–101
  gout, 114

Radiation, for macular degeneration, 182
Radiofrequency therapy, for prostate enlargement, 242
Ranexa, for angina, 13
Ranolazine, for angina, 13
Rash, with shingles, 255–60
Rectal bleeding
  from colon polyps, 45, 45
  from diverticulosis, 74, 75
  from hemorrhoids, 134, 134
Reflexology, 7, 30
Reiki, 7–8
  for treating
    back pain, 31
    depression, 62–63
Relaxation, progressive muscle, for insomnia, 167–68
Relaxation/meditation, 8
  for preventing
    erectile dysfunction, 91
    GERD, 101
    glaucoma, 108
    high blood pressure, 148
    insomnia, 172
    kidney stones, 178
    metabolic syndrome, 198
  for treating
    angina, 16
    atherosclerosis, 21–22
    back pain, 32
    coronary artery disease, 54
    depression, 63
    diabetes, 72
    essential tremor, 95
    heart palpitations, 132–33, 133
    high blood pressure, 146
    indigestion, 160
    memory loss, 194
    peripheral neuropathy, 232
    peripheral vascular disease, 239
    sleep apnea, 265
Rolfing, 8, 30
Rosacea, 250–54
Rosemary, for nail fungus, 205

SAD. See Seasonal affective disorder
Sage, for treating
  gum disease, 120
  nail fungus, 205
SAMe, for treating
  depression, 62
  osteoarthritis, 221

Sarsaparilla, for treating
  erectile dysfunction, 90
  male menopause, 189
Saw palmetto, for treating
  prostate enlargement, 244
  prostatitis, 248
Scaling and root planing (SRP), for gum disease, 117
Sciatica, 24, 25, 28
Seasonal affective disorder (SAD), 55, 57, 60–61
Selective serotonin reuptake inhibitors (SSRIs), for depression, 60
Selegiline, for Parkinson's disease, 225
Selenium
  for preventing cataracts, 39
  for treating
    atherosclerosis, 21
    coronary artery disease, 52, 53–54
    glaucoma, 108
    macular degeneration, 184
    memory loss, 193
    osteoarthritis, 219
    peripheral vascular disease, 237, 239
Shiatsu, 8
  for treating
    angina, 14
    back pain, 30
    osteoarthritis, 221
Shingles, 255–60
Shortness of breath, as symptom of
  angina, 10, 11
  coronary artery disease, 49, 49
  emphysema, 80–81, 81
Siberian ginseng, for erectile dysfunction, 90
Sildenafil, for erectile dysfunction, 86–87
Sitz bath, for treating
  hemorrhoids, 135
  prostatitis, 247
Skin redness, from rosacea, 250–54
Sleep
  for back pain, 25, 33
  GERD and, 101
  memory loss and, 194
Sleep apnea, 168, 261–65
Sleep difficulty, 166–72
Sleeping pills, 167, 168–69, 265
Sleep position, with sleep apnea, 265
Sleep restriction therapy, for insomnia, 168
Slippery elm, for treating
  diverticulosis/diverticulitis, 77
  indigestion, 159
Smoking. See also Smoking cessation
  emphysema from, 80
  erectile dysfunction from, 85, 91, 189
  essential tremor from, 92, 95
  macular degeneration from, 180, 185

Smoking cessation. *See also* Smoking
　for preventing
　　back pain, 34
　　cataracts, 39
　　colon polyps, 47
　　diabetes complications, 73
　　GERD, 101
　　glaucoma, 108
　　gout, 114
　　gum disease, 122
　　hearing loss, 129
　　indigestion, 160
　　influenza, 165
　　insomnia, 172
　　macular degeneration, 185
　　metabolic syndrome, 198
　　peripheral vascular disease, 239
　　sleep apnea, 265
　for treating
　　angina, 16
　　atherosclerosis, 22
　　coronary artery disease, 54
　　emphysema, 81
　　heart palpitations, 133
　　high blood pressure, 147
　　high cholesterol, 155
　　peripheral neuropathy, 233
　　peripheral vascular disease, 234
　　rosacea, 254
Snoring, with sleep apnea, 261, <u>261</u>, 262
Social interaction, for preventing high blood pressure, 147
Sodium restriction
　with angina, 14
　with high blood pressure, 144, <u>144</u>
　with kidney stones, 178
　with metabolic syndrome, 198
　for preventing peripheral vascular disease, 239
Spinal fusion, for back pain, 29
SRP, for gum disease, 117
SSRIs, for depression, 60
St. John's wort, for treating
　depression, 61–62
　hemorrhoids, 136
Statins. *See also* Cholesterol-lowering medications
　for high cholesterol, 152–53
Stereotactic thalamotomy, for essential tremor, 94
Stevia, as sugar substitute, 71
Stinging nettle, for treating
　gout, 113
　prostate enlargement, 243, 244
　prostatitis, 248
Stress reduction
　for preventing
　　GERD, 101
　　gum disease, 122
　　high blood pressure, 148
　　high cholesterol, 155
　　influenza, 165

　　metabolic syndrome, 198
　　peripheral vascular disease, 239
　　rosacea, 254
　relaxation/meditation for (*see* Relaxation/ meditation)
　for treating
　　celiac disease, 44
　　erectile dysfunction, 91
　　glaucoma, 108
　　heart palpitations, 133
　　male menopause, 189
　　osteoarthritis, 221
　　shingles, 260
Stretches
　with back pain, 33
　for preventing muscle cramps, <u>201</u>, 202
Sulfonylureas, for diabetes, 67–68
Sun exposure, Parkinson's disease and, 228
Sun protection
　for preventing
　　cataracts, 39
　　glaucoma, 108
　　macular degeneration, 185
　with rosacea, 254
Supplements, nutritional, 7. *See also specific supplements*
Support groups, 34, 44, 95, 228
Swallowing difficulty, with GERD, 97, <u>97</u>

Tadalafil, for erectile dysfunction, 87
Tai chi, 8, 31, 227
Talk therapy. *See* Psychotherapy
TCM. *See* Traditional Chinese medicine
Tea. *See also* Green tea
　for cholesterol control, 155
　herbal
　　for influenza, 163–64
　　for insomnia, 170
Tea tree oil, for treating
　gum disease, 120
　nail fungus, 205
TENS. *See* Transcutaneous electrical nerve stimulation
Testosterone replacement therapy (TRT), for treating
　erectile dysfunction, 88
　male menopause, 187
Thalamotomy, for Parkinson's disease, 226
Therapeutic massage, 8
　for preventing muscle cramps, 201
　for treating
　　back pain, 30, 32–33
　　depression, 63
　　heart palpitations, 133
　　insomnia, 171
　　osteoarthritis, 221
　　Parkinson's disease, 227
Therapeutic touch, 8–9, 31
Thiazolidinediones, for diabetes, 68
Thirst, as diabetes symptom, <u>64</u>, 65, 66
Thrombectomy, for peripheral vascular disease, 236

Thrombolytic therapy, for peripheral vascular disease, 236

Thyme, for nail fungus, 205

TIAs, with atherosclerosis, 17, 18

Ticlopidine, for peripheral vascular disease, 235

Tingling, as symptom of
    peripheral neuropathy, 229, 230
    peripheral vascular disease, 234, 234
    shingles, 256, 257

Tinnitus, 123, 124, 128, 129

TLC diet, for high cholesterol, 151

Toe pain, with gout, 110, 111

Tongue scraper, for preventing gum disease, 122

Tonic water, for muscle cramps, 202

Tooth brushing technique, for preventing gum disease, 121, 122

Total disk replacement, for back pain, 29

Trabeculectomy, for glaucoma, 105

Trabeculoplasty, laser, for glaucoma, 105–6

Tracheostomy, for sleep apnea, 264

Traditional Chinese medicine (TCM), 9
    for diabetes, 72
    for glaucoma, 108

Trager Approach, 9
    for treating
        back pain, 31
        Parkinson's disease, 227–28

Transcutaneous electrical nerve stimulation (TENS), for treating
    back pain, 25
    macular degeneration, 184
    peripheral neuropathy, 231
    shingles, 258

Transient ischemic attacks (TIAs), with atherosclerosis, 17, 18

Transmyocardial laser revascularization, for coronary artery disease, 50

Transplant surgery, for emphysema, 82

Transurethral electrovaporization of the prostate (TVP), 242

Transurethral incision of the prostate (TUIP), 243

Transurethral needle ablation (TUNA), for prostate enlargement, 242

Transurethral resection of the prostate (TURP), 242–43, 247

Tremor(s)
    essential, 92–95
    in Parkinson's disease, 222–28

Trigger point therapy, 9, 30

TRT. See Testosterone replacement therapy

TUIP, for prostate enlargement, 243

TUNA, for prostate enlargement, 242

Turmeric, for GERD, 100

TURP, for prostate problems, 242–43, 247

TVP, for prostate enlargement, 242

TZDs, for diabetes, 68

Ulcers, 156, 158

UPPP, for sleep apnea, 263

Ureteroscopic stone removal, for kidney stones, 176

Uric acid, in gout, 109, 110

Urinary infections, prostatitis and, 249

Urination, frequent, as diabetes symptom, 64, 65, 66

Urination problems, from prostate enlargement, 240–44

Uvulopalatopharyngoplasty (UPPP), for sleep apnea, 263

Vaccinations
    for diabetics, 73
    flu, 164–65, 164
    shingles, 260

Vacuum devices, for erectile dysfunction, 88

Valerian root, for treating
    insomnia, 170
    shingles, 258–59

Vardenafil, for erectile dysfunction, 87

Variant angina, 10

Vascular surgery, for erectile dysfunction, 87–88

Vegetarian diet, 70, 147–48

Venous flow controllers, for erectile dysfunction, 88

Vervain, for insomnia, 170

Viagra, for erectile dysfunction, 86–87

Vision problems
    from cataracts, 35, 36
    with diabetes, 64, 65, 73
    from glaucoma, 102–8
    from macular degeneration, 179–85

Vitamin A
    for preventing cataracts, 38
    for treating
        emphysema, 83
        glaucoma, 106, 107
        hearing loss, 129
        rosacea, 253
        shingles, 258

Vitamin B_6
    Parkinson's disease and, 227
    for treating
        angina, 15
        coronary artery disease, 53
        insomnia, 169, 170
        peripheral vascular disease, 238
        sleep apnea, 264

Vitamin B_{12}, for treating
    glaucoma, 106, 107
    hearing loss, 127, 129
    insomnia, 169–70
    memory loss, 193
    peripheral neuropathy, 230, 232
    shingles, 259–60
    sleep apnea, 264

Vitamin C
    kidney stones and, 177–78
    for preventing
        cataracts, 37, 38
        influenza, 165
        muscle cramps, 201

Vitamin C (*cont.*)
  for treating
    angina, 14, 15
    atherosclerosis, 20, 21
    coronary artery disease, 51, 53
    diabetes, 71
    emphysema, 83
    glaucoma, 106, 107
    gum disease, 119, 120
    hemorrhoids, 136
    high cholesterol, 154
    influenza, 164
    macular degeneration, 183–84
    memory loss, 192, 193
    metabolic syndrome, 197
    osteoarthritis, 219
    peripheral vascular disease, 237, 238
    rosacea, 253
    shingles, 258, 260
Vitamin D
  for preventing
    colon polyps, 47
    gum disease, 122
    macular degeneration, 184–85
    muscle cramps, 202
  for treating
    diabetes, 71
    hearing loss, 129
    osteoarthritis, 220
    Parkinson's disease, 228
Vitamin E
  for preventing
    cataracts, 38
    muscle cramps, 200, 201
  for treating
    angina, 15
    atherosclerosis, 20, 21
    coronary artery disease, 52, 53
    diabetes, 71
    emphysema, 83
    glaucoma, 106, 107
    hemorrhoids, 136
    high cholesterol, 154
    macular degeneration, 184
    memory loss, 193
    metabolic syndrome, 197
    osteoarthritis, 219
    peripheral vascular disease, 237, 238
    rosacea, 253
    shingles, 260

Walking
  with emphysema, 83
  for GERD, 101
Water
  for improving memory, 194
  for preventing
    diverticulosis, 79
    kidney stones, 178

  for treating
    emphysema, 82
    gum disease, 121
    rosacea, 254
Weight control
  with emphysema, 83
  for preventing cataracts, 39
Weight gain
  as diabetes symptom, 64, 65
  with metabolic syndrome, 195, 196
  in obesity, 206–13
Weight loss
  as diabetes symptom, 64, 65
  methods of, 207–13
  for preventing
    diabetes, 73
    GERD, 101
    high blood pressure, 148
    kidney stones, 178
  for treating
    angina, 16
    gout, 114
    high cholesterol, 151–52
    metabolic syndrome, 198
    osteoarthritis, 221
    sleep apnea, 265
Weight loss products and medications, 208–9,
    212–13
Weight loss programs, 210–11
Wild cherry bark, for emphysema, 83
Wine, for macular degeneration, 184
Witch hazel, for hemorrhoids, 136

Yoga, for prostatitis, 249

Zeaxanthin
  for preventing cataracts, 37
  for treating
    glaucoma, 106
    macular degeneration, 183, 184
Zinc
  for preventing cataracts, 39
  for treating
    diabetes, 70, 72
    erectile dysfunction, 89, 91
    hearing loss, 129
    hemorrhoids, 136
    influenza, 164
    macular degeneration, 184
    male menopause, 187, 189
    metabolic syndrome, 198
    prostate enlargement, 244
    prostatitis, 248
    shingles, 260
Zostavax vaccine, 260